Evidence-Based

Diagnostic Testing and Clinica

DATE DUE

Sep·30 2014	
SEP 2 1 2013	
FEB 0 9 2014	
APR 1 6 2014	

Website: Evidence-Based Medicine Series

The Evidence-Based Medicine Series has a website at:

www.evidencebasedseries.com

Where you can find:

- Links to companion websites with additional resources and updates for books in the series
- Details of all new and forthcoming titles
- Links to more Evidence-Based products: including the Cochrane Library, Essential Evidence Plus, and EBM Guidelines.

How to access the companion sites with additional resources and updates:

- Go to the Evidence-Based Series site:
  www.evidencebasedseries.com
- Select your book from the list of titles shown on the site
- If your book has a website with supplementary material, it will show an icon `Companion Website` next to the title
- Click on the icon to access the website

Evidence-Based Emergency Care

Diagnostic Testing and Clinical Decision Rules

Second Edition

Jesse M. Pines, MD, MBA, MSCE, FACEP, FAAEM

Director, Center for Healthcare Quality
Associate Professor of Emergency Medicine and Health Policy
George Washington University, Washington, DC, USA

Christopher R. Carpenter, MD, MSC, FACEP, FAAEM

Director, Evidence Based Medicine
Associate Professor of Emergency Medicine
Division of Emergency Medicine, Barnes Jewish Hospital
Washington University, St. Louis, MO, USA

Ali S. Raja, MD, MBA, MPH, FACEP, FAAEM

Director of Network Operations and Business Development
Assistant Professor of Medicine (Emergency Medicine)
Department of Emergency Medicine, Brigham and Women's Hospital
Harvard Medical School, Boston, MA, USA

Jeremiah D. Schuur, MD, MHS, FACEP

Director of Quality, Patient Safety and Performance Improvement
Assistant Professor of Medicine (Emergency Medicine)
Department of Emergency Medicine, Brigham and Women's Hospital
Harvard Medical School, Boston, MA, USA

WILEY-BLACKWELL

A John Wiley & Sons, Ltd., Publication

This edition first published 2013, © 2013 by John Wiley & Sons, Ltd.

Wiley-Blackwell is an imprint of John Wiley & Sons, formed by the merger of Wiley's global Scientific, Technical and Medical business with Blackwell Publishing.

Registered office: John Wiley & Sons, Ltd, The Atrium, Southern Gate, Chichester, West Sussex, PO19 8SQ, UK

Editorial offices: 9600 Garsington Road, Oxford, OX4 2DQ, UK
The Atrium, Southern Gate, Chichester, West Sussex, PO19 8SQ, UK
111 River Street, Hoboken, NJ 07030-5774, USA

For details of our global editorial offices, for customer services and for information about how to apply for permission to reuse the copyright material in this book please see our website at www.wiley.com/wiley-blackwell.

The right of the author to be identified as the author of this work has been asserted in accordance with the UK Copyright, Designs and Patents Act 1988.

Library of Congress Cataloging-in-Publication Data

Evidence-based emergency care : diagnostic testing and clinical decision rules
/ Jesse M. Pines ... [et al.]. – 2nd ed.
       p. ; cm.
   Includes bibliographical references and index.
   ISBN 978-0-470-65783-6 (pbk.)
   I. Pines, Jesse M.
   [DNLM: 1. Evidence-Based Emergency Medicine – methods. 2. Diagnostic
Techniques and Procedures. WB 105]
   616.02'5–dc23

**WB
105
P6515e
2013**

2012025774

A catalogue record for this book is available from the British Library.

Wiley also publishes its books in a variety of electronic formats. Some content that appears in print may not be available in electronic books.

Set in 9.5/12pt Minion by Laserwords Private Limited, Chennai, India.
Printed and bound in Malaysia by Vivar Printing Sdn Bhd

1 2013

To my wife, Lori Uscher-Pines, and to my children, Asher and Molly Pines, for all their support and encouragement.

J.M.P.

To Danielle, for putting up with everything and keeping me despite it all.

A.S.R.

To my wife, Lauraine, and our kids, Henry and Maggie, for their love and support.

J.D.S.

To my wonderful wife, Panechanh, and our fabulous children, Cameron and Kayla, thank you for your constant understanding and optimism. You are my daily inspiration. To the residents and faculty of Washington University in St. Louis, your passion to advance the science of emergency medicine continues to fuel my intellectual fires.

C.R.C.

Contents

Section 3: Cardiology

Section 4: Infectious Disease

Section 5: Surgical and Abdominal Complaints

Section 6: Urology

Section 7: Neurology

Section 8: Miscellaneous: Hematology, Ophthalmology, Pulmonology, Rheumatology, and Geriatrics

About the Authors

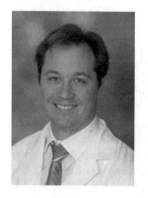

Jesse M. Pines, MD, MBA, MSCE, is the Director of the Center for Healthcare Quality and an Associate Professor of Emergency Medicine and Health Policy at George Washington University. He is also a board-certified emergency physician. Dr. Pines has served as a Senior Advisor to the Center for Medicare and Medicaid Innovation at the U.S. government's Center for Medicare and Medicaid Services. Dr. Pines holds a bachelor of arts degree and a master's of science degree in clinical epidemiology from the University of Pennsylvania as well as a medical degree and a master's of business administration degree from Georgetown University. He completed a residency in emergency medicine at the University of Virginia and a fellowship in research at the Center for Clinical Epidemiology and Biostatistics at the University of Pennsylvania. He has received grant funding from several government agencies and private foundations to conduct research, and is author of over 120 peer-reviewed academic publications. He lives in Fairfax, Virginia, with his wife, Lori, and two children, Asher and Molly.

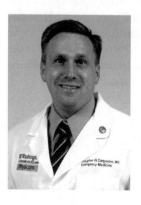

Christopher Carpenter, MD, MSc, FACEP, FAAEM, is the Director of Evidence Based Medicine for the Division of Emergency Medicine at Barnes Jewish Hospital at Washington University, St. Louis, Missouri. Dr. Carpenter completed an internal medicine–emergency medicine residency at Allegheny General Hospital in Pittsburgh, Pennsylvania, and a master's degree in clinical investigations at Washington University. Dr. Carpenter's research focuses on improving geriatric adult emergency care using evidence-based medicine and implementation science, and has been funded by federal agencies and foundations. Dr. Carpenter is Chair-Elect of the American College of Emergency Physicians' Geriatrics Section, as well as faculty at the McMaster University Evidence Based Clinical Practice course. Dr. Carpenter is an Associate Editor for *Academic Emergency Medicine* and formerly Chief Clinical Editor of *Emergency Physicians Monthly*. Dr. Carpenter has published over 40 peer-reviewed papers and has led the development of the "Evidence Based Diagnostics" series in *Academic Emergency Medicine*. Dr. Carpenter lives in St. Louis, Missouri, with his wife, Panechanh, and two children, Cameron and Kayla.

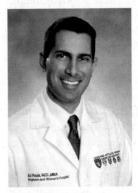

Ali S. Raja, MD, MBA, MPH is the Director of Network Operations and Business Development for the Department of Emergency Medicine and the Associate Director of Trauma for Brigham and Women's Hospital, an Assistant Professor of Medicine (Emergency Medicine) at Harvard Medical School, and on the faculty of the Center for Evidence-Based Imaging at BWH. He is a board-certified emergency physician who completed a residency in emergency medicine at the University of Cincinnati and holds a master's of public health degree from the Harvard School of Public Health as well as a medical degree and a master's of business administration degree from Duke University. The author of over 40 peer-reviewed journal articles, his federally funded research focuses on improving the appropriateness of radiology utilization and the management of patients with trauma. Dr. Raja has received both the BWH Outstanding Attending award from the Harvard-Affiliated Emergency Medicine Residency and the Exemplary Emergency Medicine Attending award from the BWH Emergency Department nurses. He serves as a national faculty member of the Difficult Airway Course, is a major in the US Air Force Reserve, and is the tactical physician for the Boston FBI SWAT team. Dr. Raja lives in Sudbury, Massachusetts, with his wife, Danielle, and son, Chase.

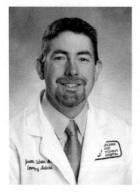

Jeremiah (Jay) Schuur, MD, MHS, FACEP, is the Director of Quality, Patient Safety and Performance Improvement for the Department of Emergency Medicine at Brigham and Women's Hospital and an Assistant Professor of Medicine (Emergency Medicine) at Harvard Medical School. Dr. Schuur completed an emergency medicine residency at Brown University in Providence, Rhode Island, and a fellowship as a Robert Wood Johnson Clinical Scholar at Yale University. Dr. Schuur's research has been funded by federal agencies and foundations and focuses on developing, evaluating, and improving measures of quality of care and patient safety in emergency medicine. Dr. Schuur chairs the Quality and Performance Committee of the American College of Emergency Physicians, is the emergency medicine representative to the American Medical Association Physician Consortium for Performance Improvement, and is an appointed member of the Medicare Evidence Development and Coverage Advisory Committee (MEDCAC). Dr. Schuur has published over 40 peer-reviewed papers and has led the development of seven quality measures that have been approved by the National Quality Forum. Dr. Schuur lives in Cambridge, Massachusetts, with his wife, Lauraine, and two children, Henry and Maggie.

About the Author

Foreword

Diagnosis correctly sorts truth and fiction into labeled bins. Diagnosis requires human intelligence, experience, and evidence. Intelligence may be inherited, and experience earned, but evidence must be acquired by reading. This second edition of *Evidence-Based Emergency Care: Diagnostic Testing and Clinical Decision Rules* provides a one-stop resource for the evidence of diagnosis in emergency care, continuing the tradition set by the first edition, except with greater depth and reach. To my knowledge, no other single resource offers a more comprehensive, contemporaneous, and parsimonious accumulation of the data to accelerate "clinical decisioning" at the bedside in emergency medicine. This book provides both an efficient pocket reference for daily practice and also expert interpretation to help us understand the context and rationale of key studies, as well as where the literature is lacking. The lean writing style respects its readers' time, but the scope of 58 chapters respects the breadth of emergency care. This textbook not only encompasses bread-and-butter topics, such as imaging patients with low-risk head injury, but also ventures into the unusual and provides useful data that I submit will surprise and inform veteran practitioners. What is the positive likelihood ratio for jaw claudication as a predictor of temporal arteritis? Should you care to know this datum, turn to chapter 53 and see the summary table that condenses each chapter for readers with limited time or attention spans.

I believe this book will improve and streamline my thought process at least once on every shift. It is often said that knowledge is power. And while this text conveys plenty of knowledge, more importantly, it may reduce practitioner stress by facilitating access to data, *thus helping transform knowledge into diagnostic knowhow.* So, for the next patient you see with chest pain, you need not spend your precious human computing power trying to remember where to find the decision rules for acute coronary syndrome, or the components of the various published decision instruments, or their authors, or levels of validation. Instead, you can relax (at least a little) and apply your mind power toward the good and valuable goal of listening to the patient and thinking about what he or she is telling you. And this attention provides the knowhow to correctly sort clinical truth and fiction. In the second edition of *Evidence-Based Emergency Care: Diagnostic Testing and Clinical Decision Rules*, Pines, Carpenter, Raja, and Schuur have provided a truly useful tool for the practice of emergency medicine. Keep a copy nearby for your next shift.

Jeffrey Kline
2012

Preface

One of the most vital skills in emergency medicine is the ability to differentiate patients who need emergency treatment from those who do not. The primary means of doing so include a detailed history, a skilled physical examination, and well-informed clinical judgment. While the skilled clinician acquires the basic tenets of taking a history, doing a physical examination, and developing reasonable clinical judgment through medical school and residency training, this knowledge is constantly updated through the experience of evaluating and treating patients in emergency care settings.

The technologies available to evaluate patients with emergency medical conditions have blossomed over the past 50 years and continue to evolve rapidly with a greater availability of advanced radiography and novel laboratory tests. The methods of conducting and reporting diagnostic research have also evolved significantly. In addition, clinicians now recognize the myriad forms of bias that impede confident interpretation of diagnostic studies, and methods to assess the quality of individual studies in diagnostic meta-analyses have been developed.

Modern emergency medicine is a delicate balance of practicing an evidence-based approach to diagnostic testing. The term that is often used is "appropriate use." Appropriate use means finding a balance between overuse (e.g., overtesting low-risk patients) and underuse (e.g., discharging people with undiagnosed, potentially life-threatening conditions). Appropriate testing should be patient centered, well reasoned, and evidence based. However, given the spiraling costs of healthcare, we need to also be cost conscious. This is one of the hardest parts of our jobs as emergency physicians.

Many disease processes can be safely and reliably excluded by clinical criteria alone. There has been a proliferation of research studies designed to guide test ordering; the best example of this is the use of radiography for ankle sprains, since only a small proportion of patients will have radiographs that demonstrate clinically significant fractures. These clinical decision rules for diagnostic testing can serve as guides for deciding which patients may or may not benefit from testing. Because this skill, the art and science of diagnostic testing, is so central to emergency medical practice, emergency physicians and other providers working in emergency care settings must be experts in this area.

The purpose of this book is to present relevant questions on diagnostic testing that arise in everyday emergency medicine practice and to comment on the best available evidence. The first part of the book serves as an overview of the science of diagnostic testing, reviewing the process behind the development of clinical decision rules and exploring the pressures that emergency practitioners will face in the coming years to increase the efficiency of diagnostic test utilization. Subsequent chapters focus on practical questions that have been addressed by original research studies. We provide a review of the current literature on a specific question, an interpretation of the clinical question in the context of the literature, and ?nally how we, as practicing clinicians, apply the evidence to the care of our patients. Importantly, we also try to provide the actual data, sample sizes, and statistics. As readers, you can come to your own conclusions about how to interpret the best available data by understanding not just the bottom-line study conclusions but also the limitations of various study designs. As a caveat, our comments section should not be interpreted as the standard of care. Not all emergency care settings have the same resources for testing or treatment, nor do all settings have the same availability of specialty consultation. Therefore, it is vital to evaluate our interpretation of the literature in the context of your local resources and practice patterns.

In this second edition of the book, we have expanded the book considerably, adding new evidence and many new chapters since the first edition was published in 2008. We hope that you enjoy and your patients benefit from this effort!

Jesse M. Pines
Christopher R. Carpenter
Ali S. Raja
Jeremiah D. Schuur
2013

Acknowledgments

We would like to thank the following individuals for their contributions to the second edition of *Evidence-Based Emergency Care: Diagnostic Testing and Clinical Decision Rules*: Worth W. Everett, MD, for his authorship and help writing the first edition of the book; Lisa Hayes at Washington University at St. Louis for helping with the image permissions; and Dorothea B. Hempel, MD, for help obtaining images from the Brigham and Women's Hospital Department of Emergency Medicine image library.

SECTION 1
The Science of Diagnostic Testing and Clinical Decision Rules

Chapter 1 **Diagnostic Testing in Emergency Care**

As emergency department (ED) physicians, we spend a good deal of our time ordering, interpreting, and waiting for the results of diagnostic tests. When it comes to determining who needs a test to rule out potentially life-threatening conditions, ED physicians are the experts. There are several reasons for this expertise. First and foremost, we see a lot of patients. Especially for those working in busy hospitals, the expectation is to see everyone in a timely way, provide quality care, and ensure patients have a good experience. If we order time-consuming tests on everyone, ED crowding and efficiency will worsen, costs of care will go up, and patients will experience even longer waits than they already do. In addition, the way ED physicians in the United States are paid may be changing over the coming years through mechanisms such as accountable care organizations and payment bundling. There may be more pressure to carefully choose who needs and who does not need tests in an evidence-based manner.

Differentiating which patients will benefit from further testing in the ED is a complex process. Over the past 30 to 40 years, science and research in diagnostic testing and clinical decision rules in emergency care have advanced considerably. Now, there is a greater understanding of test performance regarding the reliability, sensitivity, specificity, and overall accuracy of tests. Validated clinical decision rules exist to provide objective criteria to help distinguish who does and does not need a test. Serious, potentially life-threatening conditions such as intracranial bleeding and cervical spine (C-spine) fractures can be ruled out based on clinical grounds alone. There are also good risk stratification tools to determine a probability of disease for conditions like pulmonary embolism before any tests are even ordered.

How do we decide who to test and who not to test? There are some patients who obviously need tests, such as the head-injured patient who has altered mental status and who may have a head bleed where the outcome

Evidence-Based Emergency Care: Diagnostic Testing and Clinical Decision Rules, Second Edition.
Jesse M. Pines, Christopher R. Carpenter, Ali S. Raja and Jeremiah D. Schuur.
© 2013 John Wiley & Sons, Ltd. Published 2013 by John Wiley & Sons, Ltd.

may be dependent upon how quickly the bleeding can be detected with a computed tomography (CT) scan. There are also patients who obviously do not need tests, such as patients with a simple toothache or a mild upper respiratory tract infection. Finally, there is a large group of patients in the middle for whom testing decisions can sometimes be challenging. This group of patients may leave you feeling "on the fence" about testing. In this large middle category, it may not be clear whether to order a test or even how to interpret a test once you have the results. And when we receive unexpected test results, it may not be clear how best to use those results to guide the care of an individual patient.

Let's give some examples of how diagnostic testing can be a challenge in the ED. You are starting your shift and are signed out a patient for whom your colleague has ordered a D-dimer assay (a test for pulmonary embolism). She is 83 years old and developed acute shortness of breath, chest pain, and hypoxia (room air oxygen saturation = 89%). She has a history of a prior pulmonary embolism and her physical examination is unremarkable, except for mild left anterior chest wall tenderness and notably clear lung sounds. The D-dimer comes back negative. Has pulmonary embolism been satisfactorily ruled out? Should you perform a pulmonary angiogram or a CT scan of the chest, or maybe even consider a ventilation–perfusion (V/Q) scan? Was D-dimer the right test for her to begin with?

Let's consider a different scenario. Consider a positive D-dimer assay in a 22-year-old male with atypical chest pain, no risk factors, and normal physical examination including a heart rate of 70 beats per minute and an oxygen saturation of 100% on room air. What do you do then? Should he be anticoagulated and admitted? Does he have a pulmonary embolism? Should you move forward with further confirmatory testing before initiating treatment? Or is he so low risk that he's probably fine anyway? Of course, you might wonder why, if he was so low risk, was the D-dimer ordered in the first place?

As a third example, you are evaluating a 77-year-old female who has fallen down, has acute hip pain, and is unable to ambulate. The hip radiograph is negative. Should you pursue it? Possibly get a CT or magnetic resonance imaging (MRI)? But even though the hip radiograph is negative, will she be able to go home?

These are examples of when test results do not confirm your clinical suspicion. What do you do in those cases? Should you believe the test result or believe your clinical judgment before ordering the test? Were these the optimal tests in the first place? Remember back to conversations with your teachers in emergency medicine on diagnostic testing. Didn't they always ask, "How will a test result change your management?" and "What will you do if it's positive, negative, or indeterminate?"

The purpose of diagnostic testing is to reach a state where we are adequately convinced of the presence or absence of a condition. Test results are interpreted in the context of the prevalence of the suspected disease state: your clinical suspicion of the presence or absence of disease in the individual patient. For example, coronary artery disease is common. However, if we look for coronary disease in 25 year olds, we are not likely to find it because it is very uncommon in that population. There are also times when your clinical suspicion is so high that you do not need objective testing. In certain patients, you can proceed with treatment. For example, some emergency physicians may choose to treat a dislocated shoulder based on the clinical examination rather than first obtaining a radiograph. However, testing is often needed to confirm a diagnosis or to rule out more severe, life-threatening diseases.

The choice over whether to test or not test in the ED also depends upon the resources of the hospital and of the patient. Some hospitals allow easy access to radiographic testing and laboratory testing. In other hospitals, obtaining a diagnostic test may not be as easy. Some hospitals don't have CT scanners. Others do not have the staff available for certain types of tests at night or on weekends (like MRIs and ultrasounds). Sometimes patients may not need a test if you believe that they are reliable to return if symptoms worsen. For others, you may believe that a patient's emergency presentation may be the only time he or she will have access to diagnostic testing. For example, saying to a patient, "Follow up with your doctor this week for a stress test" may be impractical if the patient does not have a primary doctor or does not have good access to medical care. Many providers practice in environments where they cannot order a lot of tests (like developing countries). You also may practice in an office environment that simply does not have easy access to testing. However, regardless of the reason why we order tests in the ED or other acute settings, what is certain is that the use of diagnostic testing in many cases can change how you manage a patient's care.

Sometimes, you may question your choice of whether to test, to not test, or to involve a specialist early. Should you get a CT scan first or just call a surgeon in for a young male with right lower quadrant pain, fever, nausea, and possible appendicitis? How many cases have you seen where the CT scan has changed your management? What if the patient is a young, nonpregnant female? Does that change your plan?

How about using clinical decision rules in practice? By determining if patients meet specific clinical criteria, we can choose not to test some patients if they are low risk. Do all patients with ankle sprains need X-rays? Can you use the Ottawa ankle rules in children? What are the limits of clinical decision rules? Is it possible to apply the Canadian C-spine rules to a 70-year-old female? What is sufficiently "low risk"? These questions come up daily in the practice of emergency medicine. In fact, a major source of variability among physicians is whether or not they order tests. Remember back to your training when you were getting ready to present a patient to the attending physician. Weren't you trying to think to yourself, "What would she do in this case? What tests would she order?"

Access to test results helps us decide whether to treat a disease, initiate even more testing, or no longer worry about a condition. The cognitive psychology of clinical decision making has evolved rapidly over the last several decades. As ED physicians, we gain confidence in this process with experience. Much of the empirical science and mathematics behind testing that are described in this book become instinctive and intuitive the longer you practice emergency medicine. Sometimes we may think a patient does not need to be tested because the last hundred patients who had similar presentations all had negative tests. Maybe you or your colleagues were "burned" once when a subtle clinical presentation of a life-threatening condition was missed (like a subarachnoid hemorrhage). The next patient who presents with those symptoms is probably more likely to get a head CT followed by a lumbar puncture. Is this evidence based? Recognizing our individual diagnostic biases is one way to decrease the likelihood of erroneous decision making while increasing efficiency and effectiveness.

Step back for a moment and think about what we do when ordering a test. After evaluating a patient, we come away with a differential diagnosis of both the most common and the most life-threatening possibilities. The following approach to medical decision making was derived by Pauker and Kassirer in 1980.[1] Imagine diagnostic testing as two separate thresholds, each denoted as "I" (for *indeterminate*). The scale at the bottom of Figure 1.1 denotes pretest probability, which is the probability of the disease in question before any testing is employed. In practice, it is often a challenge to come up with a pretest probability, and frequently opinions on pretest probability differ considerably between experienced physicians. However, for the moment, assume that pretest probability is a known quantity.

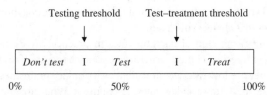

Figure 1.1 Pretest probability of disease. (Source: Data from Pauker and Kassirer (1980)).

In Figure 1.1, the threshold between "don't test" and "test" is known as the *testing threshold*. The threshold between "test" and "treat" is known as the *test–treatment threshold*. In this schema, treatment should be withheld if the pretest probability of disease is smaller than the testing threshold, and no testing should be performed. Treatment should be given without testing if the pretest probability of disease is above the test–treatment threshold. And, when our pretest probability lies between the testing and test–treatment thresholds, the test should be performed and the patients treated according to the test results. That is the theory. But now let's make this more clinically relevant.

Sometimes disease is clinically apparent and we do not need confirmatory testing before proceeding with treatment. If you are evaluating a patient with an obvious cellulitis, you may choose to give antibiotics before initiating any testing. How about a 50-year-old male with acute chest pain who on his electrocardiogram (ECG) has large inferior "tombstone" ST-segment elevations consistent with acute myocardial infarction (AMI)? Cardiac markers will not be very helpful in the acute management of this patient. This is an example of a situation in which it is important to treat the patient first: give the patient aspirin, anticoagulation, beta blockers, and oxygen, and send him off to the cardiac catheterization lab if your hospital has one or provide intravenous thrombolysis if cardiac catheterization is not readily available. Well, now imagine that the patient has a history of Marfan's syndrome and you think he is having an AMI, but you want to get a chest X-ray or even a CT scan to make sure he doesn't have an aortic dissection before you anticoagulate him. That might put you on the "test" side of the line.

Now imagine the scenario of the potential use for tissue plasminogen activator (tPA) in stroke, a situation frequently encountered in the ED. When a patient comes to the ED within the first few hours of the onset of her stroke symptoms, you rush to get her to the CT scanner. Why? The primary reason is to differentiate between ischemic and hemorrhagic stroke, which will make a major difference in whether or not the patient is even eligible to receive tPA.

Now imagine cases that fall below the testing threshold. You have a 32-year-old male with what sounds like musculoskeletal chest pain. Many would argue that the patient doesn't need any emergency tests at all if he is otherwise healthy and the physical examination is normal. Others might get a chest X-ray and an ECG to rule out occult things like pneumothorax and heart disease, while some others may even get a D-dimer to rule out pulmonary embolism. What is the right way to manage the patient? Is there any evidence behind that decision, or is it just the physician's preference? In some patients, at the end of the ED evaluation, you may not have a definitive answer. Imagine a 45-year-old female with atypical chest pain, a normal ECG, and normal cardiac markers, who you are evaluating at a hospital that does not perform stress testing from the ED. Does she need a hospital admission to rule out acute myocardial infarction and a stress test? The way that Pauker and Kassirer designed the test–treatment thresholds more than 30 years ago did not account for the proliferation of "confirmatory" diagnostic testing in hospitals. While the lower bound testing threshold is certainly lower than it has ever been, the upper bound threshold has also increased to the point where we are sometimes loath to treat before testing, even when the diagnosis seems apparent. The reason for this is that Occam's razor often does not hold true in emergency medicine. What is Occam's razor? Fourteenth-century philosopher William of Occam stated, "Plurality must not be posited without necessity," which has been interpreted to mean, "Among competing hypotheses, favor the simplest one."[2] When applied to test–treatment thresholds, what we find is that a patient with objective findings for what might seem like pneumonia (e.g., hypoxia, infiltrates, and a history of cough) likely does have pneumonia, and should be treated empirically, but may also have a pulmonary embolism. While finding that parsimony of diagnosis is important, often the principle of test–treatment thresholds means that if you're above the test–treatment threshold, then you should certainly treat the patient but also consider testing more, particularly in patients with objective signs of additional disease.

Think about how trauma surgeons practice. In the multi-injured trauma patient, isn't their approach to test, test, test? In a seriously injured patient trauma surgeons often default to scanning everything (aka the *pan-scan*). Some surgeons order CT scans of areas in which the patient has no complaints. They argue that this approach is not illogical. When a patient has been in a major car accident and has a broken left femur, a broken left radius, and mild abdominal tenderness, do they need more CT scans to rule out intra-abdominal injuries and intracranial injuries? Where Occam's razor dulls is that while the most parsimonious diagnosis (just radial and femoral fractures) is possible, patients with multiple traumatic injuries tend to have not only the obvious ones, but also occult injuries. This may necessitate a diagnostic search for the occult intra-abdominal, intrathoracic, and intracranial injuries in a patient with an obviously broken arm and leg.

Risk tolerance refers to the posttest probability at which we are comfortable with excluding or confirming a disease. That is, risk tolerance is where we are comfortable setting our own testing and test–treatment thresholds; it guides where we draw these thresholds and how much we do or do not search for the occult. When deciding on care plans, we develop our own risk tolerance based on our training, clinical expertise, and experiences, as well as local standard practice and the attitudes of the patient, family, or other physicians caring for the patient.

For example, consider possible acute coronary syndrome. After your ED evaluation with cardiac markers, an ECG, and a chest X-ray, you estimate that your patient has a 2% risk of having an unexpected cardiac event within 30 days if he is sent home without additional testing. Is it OK to send him home with this level of risk? Isn't 2% the published rate for missed AMI? What if the risk is 1%, or 0.5%, or 0.1%?

How do you make the decision about when to order a test or just treat? How do you assign a pretest probability? How do you apply test results to an individual patient? This is where research and the practice of evidence-based medicine (EBM) can influence practice by taking the best evidence in the literature about diagnostic testing or clinical decision rules and using that information to make an informed decision about how to care for patients. Chapters 2 and 3 provide an updated overview of the process of EBM as well as examples of the application of EBM to individual patients in the ED, levels of evidence, and how to evaluate a body of literature on diagnostic testing. Chapter 4 is a revised discussion of how we derive, validate, and study the impact of clinical decision rules in practice. Chapter 5, a new chapter in the second edition of this book, reviews recent trends in health policy that may force us to reduce test ordering and use clinical decision rules. Chapter 6 describes various forms of bias that can skew estimates of diagnostic accuracy in research settings.

Understanding the evidence behind diagnostic testing and using clinical decision rules to decide when not to test is at the core of emergency medicine practice. Think back to your last shift in the ED: how many tests did you order?

The purpose of this book is to demystify the evidence behind diagnostic testing and clinical decision rules in emergency care by carefully evaluating the evidence behind our everyday decision making in the ED. This book is written to provide objective information on the evidence behind these questions and our opinion on how we manage our patients with specific clinical problems given the best available evidence. It should be noted that we are writing this from the perspective of academic emergency physicians. We all work in academic EDs with abundant (although not always quick) access to consultants, state-of-the-art laboratories, and high-resolution imaging tests. As you read this, realize that not all emergency medicine practice is the same and you should interpret the literature yourself in the context of your own clinical practice environment.

We have designed each chapter around clinical questions that come up in everyday emergency medicine practice. In the second edition of the book, we have added more chapters and updated all of the old chapters to include new and relevant studies or insights that have emerged in the literature since the first edition was published in 2008. For each question, we present the objective data from published studies and then provide our "expert" comments on how we use these tests in our practice. While we try to provide insight into how we interpret the literature for each testing approach, again, our comments should not be interpreted as the standard of care in emergency medicine. Standard of care is based on practice guidelines and local practice patterns. Instead, these chapters should serve as a forum or basis for discussion. If you are a researcher, you can also think of this book as a roadmap to what is really "known" or "not known" with regard to diagnostic testing in emergency medicine and what needs further study. Finally, rigorous and sound research often takes months to years to accomplish, and sometimes longer to publish. Therefore the discussions we present are likely to change as newer, larger, more comprehensive studies are published, as new prediction or decision rules are validated and replicated, and as newer diagnostic technology is introduced.

References

1. Pauker SG, Kassirer JP. The threshold approach to clinical decision making. New England Journal of Medicine. 1980; 302: 1109–17.
2. Drachman DA. Occam's razor, geriatric syndromes, and the dizzy patient. Annals of Internal Medicine. 2000; 132: 403–4.

Additional Reading

1. Bossuyt PMM, Reitsma JB, Bruns DE, Gatsonis CA, Glasziou PP, Irwig L et al. The STARD statement for reporting studies of diagnostic accuracy: Explanation and elaboration. Annals of Internal Medicine. 2003; 138: W1–W12.
2. Brownlee S. Overtreated: Why too much medicine is making us sicker and poorer. New York: Bloomsbury; 2007.
3. Empey M, Carpenter C, Jain P, Atzema C. What constitutes the standard of care? Annals of Emergency Medicine. 2004; 44: 527–31.
4. Kovacs G, Croskerry P. Clinical decision making: An emergency perspective. Academic Emergency Medicine. 1999; 6: 947–52.
5. Schünemann AHJ, Oxman AD, Brozek J, Glasziou P, Jaeschke R, Vist GE et al. GRADE: Grading quality of evidence and strength of recommendations for diagnostic tests and strategies. British Medical Journal. 2008; 336(7653): 0.3. Available from: http://www.bmj.com/content/336/7654/0.3
6. Whiting P, Rutjes AWS, Westwood ME, Mallett S, Deeks JJ, Reitsma JB et al. QUADAS-2: A revised tool for the quality assessment of diagnostic accuracy studies. Annals ofInternal Medicine. 2011; 155: 529–36.

Chapter 2 **Evidence-Based Medicine: The Process**

The process we use in this book has been termed evidence-based medicine (EBM). The first question is "What is EBM?" EBM has been defined as "the conscientious, explicit and judicious use of current best evidence in making decisions about the care of patients."[1] However, evidence alone does not define EBM. Instead, EBM occurs within the context of our clinical expertise and incorporates each patient's unique circumstances and preferences. The best way to describe EBM in the emergency department (ED) is as a process by which we (i) ask relevant, focused clinical questions to answer a (ii) search for literature to answer this question, (iii) critically appraise the literature and make conclusions with an understanding of the strength of evidence behind a particular recommendation, and (iv) apply the evidence to the way that individual patients in the ED are managed. For this book, we use the process of EBM to answer important and relevant clinical questions regarding the use of diagnostic testing and clinical decision rules in the ED. Most of the questions we ask and attempt to answer in this book have to do with how to use, when to use, and how much to trust diagnostic testing and clinical decision rules, followed by how to apply published knowledge to individual patients. In this book, we will focus on diagnostic testing and clinical decision rules, however EBM can also be used for other applications in emergency medicine outside of diagnostic testing, such as the determination of which treatment is best for an individual patient.

The purpose of this chapter is to go through the steps of EBM in detail and to discuss how to use EBM in the practice of emergency medicine with regard to diagnostic testing. The practice of EBM is a process that follows four simple steps (see Table 2.1).

EBM queries can be broken down into two categories: (i) general medical questions (e.g., what is the sensitivity of urine dipstick testing in diagnosing urinary tract infections?) and (ii) specific patient-based questions (e.g., in

Evidence-Based Emergency Care: Diagnostic Testing and Clinical Decision Rules, Second Edition.
Jesse M. Pines, Christopher R. Carpenter, Ali S. Raja and Jeremiah D. Schuur.
© 2013 John Wiley & Sons, Ltd. Published 2013 by John Wiley & Sons, Ltd.

Table 2.1 The steps in practicing and applying evidence-based medicine (EBM) to diagnostic testing in the ED

Step 1: Formulate a clear question from a patient's problem. Does this patient need a test? Which test does she need? For example, does a patient with atypical chest pain who is otherwise low risk need a troponin? You may ask yourself, "How accurate is troponin I as a screening test for acute coronary syndrome in ED patients?" Ask yourself, "Is this an answerable question?"

Step 2: Search the literature for clinical articles that have addressed this question. Ideally, the sample will include ED patients with a similar complaint or disease process (i.e., patients with chest pain who are at low risk for acute coronary syndrome where troponin has been studied). You might start by doing searches on patients with chest pain in the ED and then narrow your search to articles that deal with the use of cardiac biomarkers.

Step 3: Read and critically appraise the articles for validity and applicability to the individual patient. That is, you can ask yourself, "Would the patient have met the inclusion criteria for this study?" or "Is this patient similar to patients who were included in the study?"

Step 4: Use the study findings and apply them to the care of an individual patient (e.g., does this patient need a troponin I? How should I approach use of cardiac troponins in the ED?).

---

a 45-year-old female without risk factors but with atypical chest pain and nonspecific electrocardiogram (ECG) changes, what is the value of a negative troponin?). In general, throughout this book, we ask the former: general medical questions. We recommend that you use our presentation of the literature as a model, from which you can use this same process to answer specific questions and apply your own interpretation of the literature to guide diagnostic plans within the context of your clinical environment.

The acronym PICO has been used to define the four elements of an answerable question regarding a diagnostic test.[2] PICO refers to (P) patient or population, (I) investigation, (C) comparison (i.e., what is the criterion standard?), and (O) outcome of interest. In our prior example, P = women in their 40s without cardiac risk factors, I = troponin I measurement, C = cardiac catheterization or possible coronary angiogram, and O = identification of an intervenable coronary artery lesion or the presence of coronary artery disease (for risk stratification).

Once you have come up with a clinical question that is answerable, the search begins. For those of you who have access to online databases (such as MEDLINE or others), it is probably best to start there because you can enter specific search criteria and narrow your search as appropriate. Websites such as PubMed (www.pubmed.com) allow free access to abstracts and some full-text articles; sometimes hospitals and universities will allow a greater level of access to full-text articles through institutional memberships. You may also choose to use other resources such as UpToDate, which examines the latest literature on a particular topic, and sometimes makes evidence-based treatment recommendations. Other resources include EMBASE, LILACS, CINAHL, the Cochrane Collaboration, and others. There are many other sources to use to search for medical information, and one way to get an idea of what your hospital or school offers is to sit down with a reference librarian in your local medical library and get a tour of all the resources. This is a rapidly evolving area, and it is important that 21st-century providers are aware of current diagnostic and treatment technologies, as well as the latest electronic search engines to best access information about evidence-based medicine.

OK, you're logged on to a MEDLINE database. What now? What you can do is either search by using a specific set of search criteria like *troponin* and *chest pain*, or use a more rigorous approach such as using the MeSH (Medical Subject Headings) system. MeSH is a vocabulary that is used to index articles in MEDLINE and PubMed. It is probably a more consistent way to search because sometimes different terminology is used for the same topic. Just as what the Brits call the *boot* is what Americans call a *trunk*, these differences are even more common in medical terminology. For example, you may want to know about shortness of breath, but these papers may describe shortness of breath in other ways, such as respiratory distress, dyspnea, or breathlessness. Another way to search PubMed more efficiently is by using a "Clinical Query," which allows the user to search for clinical research by study category: therapy, etiology, diagnosis, prognosis, or clinical prediction guide.[3] Another common trick to use is imposing "Limits" on your search, which allows you to search for articles by a specific type only, such as a review article, or to limit searches to specific age ranges, gender, publication dates, and language of publication. After finding the best evidence you can find on a clinical topic, you then need to do your own critical appraisal of the literature. Traditionally, assessment of the literature surrounding a clinical topic is good fodder for group discussion in either a conference or a residency journal club, but you can also go directly to the literature to answer important and relevant clinical questions.

Assessment of studies about diagnostic tests involves four critical steps.[4] These steps are detailed in Table 2.2. Assessing studies on clinical decision rules is similar and also involves four steps, which are detailed in Table 2.3.[5]

If you read a study or series of studies about a test or a clinical decision rule that do not meet the criteria detailed in either Table 2.2 or 2.3, you should be appropriately skeptical. However, in actual practice and as we found in writing this book, topics with research sufficient to fulfill all these specifications are the exception rather than the norm. In that case, what we need to do is interpret the literature cognizant of potential weaknesses and do our best to apply the results to how we practice medicine. Certainly, for some tests, there may be a huge literature from which we can make

Table 2.2 The steps in assessing studies on diagnostic testing

Step 1: Was there an independent, blind comparison with a criterion standard (i.e., gold standard) for diagnosis? Examples of relevant criterion standards in emergency medicine include surgical evaluation or biopsy results at laparotomy or laparoscopy for patients with appendicitis, cardiac catheterization results for patients with possible acute coronary syndrome, and pulmonary angiogram results for patients with potential pulmonary embolism. There may also be other ways to incompletely measure a criterion standard, like, in pulmonary embolism, the use of a negative chest CT scan followed by negative leg ultrasounds.

Step 2: Was the diagnostic test under question evaluated in the same population of patients as the patient in question? You can stratify this question by age, gender, location (e.g., were they ED patients?), or presenting symptoms (e.g., patients with chest pain). That is, when I read that the sensitivity for D-dimer is 95% in a meta-analysis, is my patient similar to the ones who were included in those studies?

Step 3: Did all patients have the reference standard test or follow-up whereby you can be convinced that the test was either positive or negative? An example of this is: if we perform the criterion standard test only on patients with positive tests, this may skew the results of our assessment of sensitivity. For example, if we do temporal artery biopsies only on patients with positive erythrocyte sedimentation rates (ESRs), we may miss some patients who had a negative ESR and would have had a positive biopsy. This is called *verification bias*.

Step 4: Has the test been validated in another independent group of patients? This is particularly concerning when the test is derived and validated in a specific population. For example, if a diagnostic test works well in Canada, does that mean it will have the same test characteristics in the U.S.?

Source: Data from [3].

Table 2.3 The steps in assessing studies on clinical decision rules

Step 1: Were the patients chosen in an unbiased fashion, and do the study patients represent a wide spectrum of severity of disease? For example, did the enrollment criteria for the Canadian head CT rule include patients ranging from those with minor bumps with a loss of consciousness to those with major head injuries?

Step 2: Was there a blinded assessment of the criterion standard for all patients? That is, did all patients who were enrolled in the study have CT scans?

Step 3: Was there an explicit and accurate interpretation of the predictor variables and the actual rule without knowledge of the outcome? Were the study forms filled out before the physicians had knowledge of the CT results? Was there an assessment of interrater reliability?

Step 4: Was follow-up obtained for 100% of patients who were enrolled? For patients who were discharged, did they follow them up to make sure that they did not have pain, any positive head CT, or poor outcome in a specific time period?

Source: Data from [4].

strong recommendations (e.g., for D-dimer or the Ottawa ankle rules). For others, like using erythrocyte sedimentation rates (ESRs) to rule out temporal arteritis, there may be no literature that meets all of these requirements.

The next step is to use these findings by applying them to individual patients. Chapter 3 describes in detail the terms *sensitivity, specificity, likelihood ratios,* and *Bayesian analysis* while illustrating the mathematics behind the practical application of what we learn from studies to individual patients. By determination of a specific pretest probability (or prevalence) of the disease in a particular patient, we are then able to not only calculate a posttest probability but also decide whether we need to perform the test at all.

The purpose of diagnostic testing in the ED is not necessarily to reach 100% certainty. Instead, we are trying to reduce the level of uncertainty to allow us to optimize medical decision making. In order to move between the test and test–treatment thresholds, we need to remember back to Chapter 1 and only order tests that ultimately change patient management by moving us over a specific threshold.

There are potential pitfalls in the application of EBM to diagnostic testing and clinical decision rules. The first potential pitfall is trying to describe the "P" component (patient or population) of the PICO question without being too exclusive. Let's say we are trying to determine what the sensitivity is for troponin I in a 45-year-old woman with atypical chest pain and a nondiagnostic ECG. There is likely not any specific study that describes sensitivity of troponin only in 45-year-old women with that exact description. On the other hand, if we are too vague in how we choose the "P" component, it can become similarly frustrating. For example, let's say we wanted to determine the test sensitivity for this patient by using a study that includes patients of different ages with all sorts of complaints. This would probably be too general to apply to a specific patient.

The "I" component (investigation) is generally fairly straightforward, but clinicians need to be aware that there is sometimes poor standardization in diagnostic testing. We need to be aware of which test our lab uses. Does your hospital use the D-dimer ELISA assay or the immunoassay? The reason why this is important is because the sensitivities for the two tests are actually different. Performance of a published assay is not necessary identical to what your hospital uses.

The "C" component is the comparison. A comparison is typically a criterion standard test for whatever you might be interested in studying. The criterion standard is the most definitive test there is. For example, for appendicitis, the criterion standard would be a histologic diagnosis of inflammation of the appendix in a surgical specimen. In some studies, criterion standard tests may not be ordered on all patients because the tests may have high risks of complications (like pulmonary angiogram for pulmonary embolism). In addition, for diseases like pelvic inflammatory disease, we may never get the criterion standard, which would be a positive culture for the right bacteria on an intraperitoneal lesion biopsied during laparoscopy. Because the criterion standard is not available, we need to use clinical findings to guide our treatment decisions in the ED. Researchers can also use a follow-up evaluation for patients who have not had the criterion standard, such as a 14-day follow-up phone call for patients with potential C-spine fractures. If they are not having pain at 14 days, they likely did not have a fracture.

The "O" component is the outcome. Outcomes should be objective and clear. For example, was the patient alive at 30 days? If the data were obtained in a valid way, survival is an outcome that is difficult to dispute. Some outcomes are not ideal in the emergency medicine literature, such as whether a patient was admitted or not. Because some admission decisions can be subjective, you should be skeptical of studies that use subjective outcomes where there is the possibility of interrater variability in the key outcome.

Once a question has been framed using PICO, literature searching is also straightforward. Care should be given to use "Limit" searches appropriately: for example, if you're studying children, use the age limits. When you are studying older adults, limiting the age to an upper bound can sometimes result in the exclusion of important studies.[6]

Once you've found studies, it is important to place them in the appropriate place in the "evidence pyramid" shown in Figure 2.1. Let's start at the top of the pyramid, with meta-analyses. *Meta-analyses* collect valid studies on a particular topic and use statistical methodology to test the studies together as if they were all from one large study. Systematic reviews focus on a clinical topic with a focused question, and are conducted using a methodologically sound, extensive literature review. Included studies are then reviewed and assessed, and the results are summarized. The Cochrane Collaboration has done considerable work with systematic reviews.

Next down on the evidence pyramid are randomized clinical trials, which are projects that study the effect of a therapy (or, in the case of this book, a diagnostic test or clinical decision rule) on real patients. The level of randomization may be at the level of the patient (e.g., every patient is randomized to receive test 1 versus test 2), or it may be at the level of the group (e.g., a hospital is randomized to a clinical decision rule intervention). Randomization reduces the potential for bias, and allows comparison between treatment (or test or clinical decision rule) and control groups where unmeasured confounders are balanced in the two study groups. Studies that examine the efficacy of a diagnostic test typically compare the test to a criterion standard study. For example, exercise stress testing may be compared to the results of cardiac catheterization (a criterion standard).

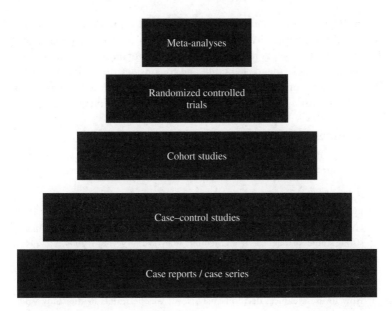

Figure 2.1 The evidence pyramid.

Cohort studies typically follow a large population of patients without a disease over a period of time and then examine the probability of developing a condition based on an exposure to a particular treatment or circumstances. Cohort studies are "observational" and generally are not as good as randomized controlled studies, because the two groups can differ in measured and unmeasured ways. Measured differences can be controlled for in multivariable analyses, while unmeasured differences cannot.

Case–control studies compare a group of patients who have a specific condition to another group of people who do not, and then assess the impact of a particular exposure in the two groups. They often rely on medical record review, or patient recall of a specific exposure (which can be subject to bias because often at the time of the study, patients may know whether they do or do not have the condition in question). For example, if you have brain cancer, you may be more likely to report having a specific exposure (like daily cell phone use) than if you don't have brain cancer. Case–control studies are usually seen as less reliable than randomized controlled trials and cohort studies.

Case reports and case series are either single reports or a series of reports on the treatment of an individual or group of patients. They both report cases and do not use control groups, so they have no statistical testing or comparisons.

In conclusion, understanding the process of EBM can allow you to apply our answers to the general medical questions in this book to the patients you see in the ED. Understanding the pitfalls of EBM is important, as is sitting down and practicing clinical scenarios to see if you can make this process work for you. It is important to recognize the limitations of the literature and where studies sit on the evidence pyramid, and to consider the limitations of the body of evidence on the literature surrounding a diagnostic test when coming up with conclusions both for clinical practice and in clinical guidelines.

References

1. Sackett DL, Rosenberg WM, Gray JA, Haynes RB, Richardson WS. Evidence based medicine: What it is and what it isn't. British Medical Journal. 1996; 312: 71–2.
2. Sackett et al. Chapter 1.2 in Evidence based medicine:How to practice & teach EBM. Edinburgh: Churchill Livingstone; 1998.
3. Haynes RB, Wilczynski NL: Optimal search strategies for retrieving scientifically strong studies of diagnosis from Medline: analytical survey. BMJ 2004, 328(7447): 1040.
4. How to use an article about a diagnostic test. A. Are the results of the study valid? Journal of the American Medical Association. 1994; 271: 389–91.
5. How to use a clinical decision analysis. A. Are the results of the study valid? Journal of the American Medical Association. 1995; 273: 1292–5.
6. Leeflang MM, Scholten RJ, Rutjes AW, Reitsma JB, Bossuyt PM: Use of methodological search filters to identify diagnostic accuracy studies can lead to the omission of relevant studies. J Clin Epidemiol 2006, 59(3): 234–240.

Additional Reading

1. Carpenter CR, Keim SM, Worster A, Rosen P. Brain natriuretic peptid in the evaluation of emergency department dyspnea:Is there a role? Journal of Emergency Medicine 2012; 42: 489–95.
2. Corrall CJ, Wyer PC, Zick LS, Bockrath CR. How to find evidence when you need it part I:Databases, search programs, and strategies. Annals of Emergency Medicine 2002; 39: 302–6.
3. Lijmer JG, Bossuyt PMM. Various randomized designs can be used to evaluate medical tests. Journal of Clinical Epidemiology. 2009; 62: 364–73.
4. Lijmer JG, Mol BW, Heisterkamp S, Bonsel GJ, Prins MH, van der Meulen JHP, et al. Empirical evidence of design-related bias in studies of diagnostic tests. Journal of the American Medical Association. 1999; 282: 1061–6.
5. Lord SJ, Irwig L, Simes RJ. When is measuring sensitivity and specificity sufficient to evaluate a diagnostic test, and when do we need randomized trials? Annals of Internal Medicine. 2006; 144: 850–5.
6. Mower WR. Evaluating bias and variability in diagnostic test reports. Annals of Emergency Medicine. 1999; 33: 85–91.
7. Newman TB, Kohn MA. Evidence-based diagnosis (practical guide to biostatistics and epidemiology). Cambridge: Cambridge University Press; 2009.

Chapter 3 **The Epidemiology and Statistics of Diagnostic Testing**

Throughout much of this book, we refer to diagnostic test characteristics including sensitivity, specificity, negative predictive value, positive predictive value, and likelihood ratios. There are also references to common epidemiological terms such as *incidence* and *prevalence*. Terms that denote risk are *odds* and *probability*. The odds ratio is commonly used in the literature to denote comparative risk among populations. Confidence intervals are also a frequently used but sometimes misunderstood concept. Two other more complex statistics that we will describe because they are frequently used in diagnostic testing are the receiver operator curve (ROC) and the interval likelihood ratio. This chapter will provide explanations of these terms that we use in this book and will offer examples of how they can be used in clinical practice in the emergency department (ED).

The 2 × 2 table

Throughout this chapter and in other areas of this book, we will be using the following 2 × 2 table that you may remember (and tried to forget) from your biostatistics class in medical school:

		Disease		
		+	−	Total
	+			
Test	−			
	Total			

On the top of the table the "disease" is listed, and on the left side of the table the "test" is listed. An easy way to remember the structure of the 2 × 2 table is to recall that "the truth is in the heavens," so the criterion standard

Evidence-Based Emergency Care: Diagnostic Testing and Clinical Decision Rules, Second Edition. Jesse M. Pines, Christopher R. Carpenter, Ali S. Raja and Jeremiah D. Schuur. © 2013 John Wiley & Sons, Ltd. Published 2013 by John Wiley & Sons, Ltd.

"truth" should always be on the top. Both "disease" and "test" are further broken down into "+" and "−" and "Total." For "disease," a "+" means that the disease is present (based upon the predefined criterion standard) and a "−" means the disease is absent; similarly for the "test," a "+" denotes a positive test and a "−" denotes a negative test.

Using information in these cells, all the common test characteristics, including sensitivity, specificity, positive predictive value, negative predictive value, and likelihood ratios, can be calculated. We can also take a pretest probability (probability that a patient has a specific condition before a test is applied) of disease, apply known sensitivity and specificity, and calculate a posttest probability. These 2 × 2 tables can be very helpful in the ED if you know how to use them properly. Their thorough understanding can allow you to apply "real-time" evidence-based medicine (EBM) as discussed in Chapter 2. First calculate a pretest probability, either based on a validated risk stratification tool or based on our own clinical judgment. Accurately assigning a pretest probability is both an art and a science. You have to think about the overall prevalence of disease. Is it common or rare? Then think about how prevalent the disease might be in the individual patient under question. However, aside from certain widely studied diseases like pulmonary embolism and acute coronary syndrome, it is often difficult to know if the pretest probability that you are assigning is correct. Often you must guess, which seems rather arbitrary given the calculations that ensue from this choice. A good way to determine how much variation there is in pretest probability is to do a simple experiment next time you are working a shift. After you and another team member (such as a nurse, resident, or medical student) evaluate a patient and decide upon a diagnostic testing plan, ask them what the probability is on a 0–100% scale that the patient will have the disease in question. Try this for 3–4 patients and what you'll see is that even experienced providers often will have dramatically different assessments of pretest probability after evaluating the same patient. You'll see that this will sometimes vary 10- to 20-fold. For example, some providers may think "low risk" is 20%, while others may think "low risk" is 1%. Different assessments in pretest probability become a real challenge when one is applying evidence-based test characteristics such as sensitivity and specificity because, depending on how "off" your initial assessment is, this can give you a posttest probability that is similarly flawed. What you may see is that for certain diseases, particularly where there is better evidence, assessment of pretest probability is more similar among providers.

After you've determined your pretest probability (although it's probably imperfect), the next step is to apply diagnostic test characteristics including sensitivity and specificity. From that, we can establish what the posttest probability is (i.e., the probability that a patient has a specific condition after test results are known). Using a posttest probability, we can then decide how to proceed with the care of an individual patient. Now, that is EBM in practice!

Sensitivity and specificity

Sensitivity refers to the ability of a test to detect a disease when it is actually present. A common acronym that has been used to remember sensitivity is PID (for *positive in disease*). Intuitively, sensitivity is an illogical marker of diagnostic accuracy since the test result can be interpreted only in a population of individuals known to have the disease. In other words, if we know the patient's disease status, why would we need the test? In the 2 × 2 table, sensitivity can be demonstrated as follows:

		Disease		
		+	−	Total
Test	+	85		
	−	15		
	Total	100		

In this example, of 100 people with a disease, 85 of them will have a positive test and 15 will have a negative test (also known as *false negatives*). The sensitivity of the test will therefore be 85/100, or 85%.

By contrast, **specificity** correctly identifies the absence of disease. That is, in people who do not have the disease, specificity denotes the percentage of those who will have a negative test. This can be easily remembered by the acronym NIH (for *negative in health*). Again, specificity can be interpreted only in a population known not to have the disease. In the 2 × 2 table, specificity can be demonstrated:

		Disease		
		+	−	Total
Test	+		20	
	−		80	
	Total		100	

In this case, of the 100 people without disease, 80% of those will test negative for the disease while 20% of patients will test positive (also known as *false positives*). The test specificity is therefore 80/100, or 80%.

Another problem with sensitivity and specificity is that they require data to be dichotomized, but many lab tests (e.g., D-dimer and brain natriuretic peptide (BNP)) are continuous data ranging from zero to infinity. Splitting continuous data into groups loses valuable diagnostic accuracy detail. This problem is eliminated by using interval likelihood ratios, which assign a specific value to each level of an abnormal test result, allowing calculation of a disease's posttest probability based on the specific test result.

Incidence and prevalence

The **prevalence** of disease is defined as the proportion of people who have a disease within a population at one time point. **Incidence** is related to prevalence but differs in that it refers to new cases of a disease over a certain period of time. For example, assuming that we have a healthy population of 1,000 people on January 1, and five had developed a specific disease by December 31, the disease incidence would be five per 1,000 per year.

But when it comes to diagnostic testing, prevalence is the more important property. Prevalence can be used interchangeably with the pretest probability of disease. In using our 2 × 2 table, we can demonstrate the concept of prevalence (or pretest probability) in the following way:

		Disease		
		+	−	Total
	+			
Test	−			
	Total	100	100	200

Of the total population of 200 people, 100 people have the disease (disease positive) and 100 people do not have the disease (disease negative). In this population, the overall prevalence is 100/200, or 50%. Sensitivity and specificity are independent of the prevalence of disease in the population, as you can see from the following table:

		Disease		
		+	−	Total
	+	85	20	105
Test	−	15	80	95
	Total	100	100	200

That is to say, sensitivity and specificity do not change when the prevalence changes. Predictive values, in contrast, always vary with prevalence.

Predictive values

Positive predictive value is the probability that the disease is present if the test is positive.

		Disease		
		+	−	Total
Test	+	85	20	105
	−			
	Total			

In this case, of the 105 people with positive tests, 85 actually have the disease; therefore, the positive predictive value is 85/105, or 81%.

The **negative predictive value** is the probability that the disease is present if the test is negative.

		Disease		
		+	−	Total
Test	+			
	−	15	80	95
	Total			

Of the 95 people with negative tests, 80 do not have the disease. Therefore, the negative predictive value is 80/95, or 84%.

Integrating concepts

Another way to integrate sensitivity and specificity with predictive values is the use of mnemonics. The mnemonics "Sn*out*" for sensitivity (to rule *out* disease) and "Sp*in*" for specificity (to "rule *in*" disease) have been proposed. When you want to rule out something (as in a clinical decision rule or a diagnostic test) for a low-risk patient, the ideal test should have near-perfect sensitivity. This will result in a correspondingly high negative predictive value (i.e., the disease is ruled out). Conversely, when you are trying to rule in something, ideal tests have near-perfect specificity that will correspond to a high positive predictive value (i.e., the disease will be ruled in).

Using 2 × 2 tables: an example

In contrast to sensitivity and specificity, positive and negative predictive values do change with changing disease prevalence. As an example, you go see a patient and based on your initial assessment, there is a high pretest probability of disease. Let's set the pretest probability estimate at 80%. If we take the same test characteristics that we had in the prior example, where sensitivity = 85% and specificity is 80%, what happens to the predictive values?

First, we start with the disease prevalence = 80%, where in a hypothetical population of 200 people, 160 have the disease and 40 do not.

		Disease		
		+	−	Total
Test	+			
	−			
	Total	160	40	200

We then add the known sensitivity = 85% and specificity = 80%. The number of true positives will be 136, false positives 8, true negatives 32, and false negatives 24:

		Disease		
		+	−	Total
Test	+	136	8	144
	−	24	32	56
	Total	160	40	200

Now, if we have a positive test in this population, the positive predictive value is 136/144 = 94% (which is higher than when the prevalence = 50%) and the negative predictive value is 32/56 = 57% (which is lower than it was if the prevalence = 50%). What tends to happen is that as your prevalence goes up, a positive test is *more* likely to be a true positive and a negative test is *less* likely to be a true negative.

How does this work if the disease prevalence is low? Let's assume a prevalence of 10%:

		Disease		
		+	−	Total
Test	+			
	−			
	Total	20	180	200

Now, if we apply the same test characteristics where sensitivity = 85% and specificity = 80:

		Disease		
		+	−	Total
Test	+	17	36	53
	−	3	144	147
	Total	20	180	200

In this case, the positive predictive value is 17/53 = 32% (which is less than it was when the population prevalence was 50%) and the negative predictive value is 144/147 = 98% (which is higher than when the population prevalence was 50%). In this case, because the prevalence is low, a positive test is less likely to be true positive and a negative test is more likely to be a true negative. As a general principle, as your disease prevalence goes up, positive predictive value increases. As disease prevalence goes down, your negative predictive value increases. In other words, if you are worried about a patient and you think she is at high risk for the disease, if the test is positive, it has a good chance of being a true positive. And, conversely, if a patient is probably OK and you're ordering an imperfect test (like an electrocardiogram to rule out acute coronary syndrome in a 25 year old), and the results are normal, the likelihood that it is a true negative is very high.

As described in this chapter, the other way to think about prevalence in a study setting is as the pretest probability for the disease in question. After you evaluate a patient, the prevalence is equal to the pretest probability for that individual patient. If you see 100 patients with the same presentation, what percentage will have the disease? In other words, clinicians can extrapolate the disease "+/−/Total" boxes to estimate pretest probability and to determine the predictive values for an individual patient.

Let's use an example of a specific patient to illustrate how we can use EBM at the bedside in emergency medicine. Imagine you are evaluating a 55-year-old female who presents with intermittent, sharp, right-sided chest pain and shortness of breath for one week. She has no traditional risk factors for pulmonary embolism or coronary artery disease. She has a normal physical examination except for tenderness to palpation over the right side of the chest. Vitals are within normal limits except for a heart rate of 110 beats per minute that is regular.

You are considering the diagnosis of pulmonary embolism in this patient, and you want to determine this patient's risk of pulmonary embolism. You pose your clinical question, you search the literature, and then you evaluate a study on the Wells criteria and decide to use it. The Wells criteria are a way to determine the pretest probability of disease in the case of pulmonary embolism (Table 3.1).[2]

According to the Wells criteria, you assign based upon your clinical judgment 1.5 points for a heart rate of >100 beats per minute. This assigns her to a "low-risk" category, and *a priori* before any testing, based on the Wells criteria, you assign her a pretest probability of 3.6%, which was the prevalence of pulmonary embolism in that category in the original study. While this is likely not exactly her specific pretest probability, you do agree that she is at relatively low risk for pulmonary embolism.

Table 3.1 The Wells criteria for pulmonary embolism

	Points	
Clinical symptoms or signs of deep vein thrombosis (DVT)	3	
PE more likely than other diagnosis	3	
Heart rate >100 beats per minute	1.5	
Immobilization or surgery within last 4 weeks	1.5	
History of DVT or pulmonary embolism (PE)	1.5	
Hemoptysis	1	
Malignancy	1	

Clinical probability of PE	Points	Probability of Disease
Low	<2	3.6%
Moderate	2–5	20.5%
High	>5	66.7%

Because she is low risk, you decide to order a D-dimer assay on her. You think back to one of two key questions, "What will you do if it's positive?" or "What if it's negative?" Let's go to the 2 × 2 tables to see. You first start by entering her pretest probability. Of every 200 patients you see who are identical to this one, roughly seven will have the disease.

		Disease		
		+	−	Total
Test	+			
	−			
	Total	7	193	200

Now, let's look up the sensitivity and specificity for D-dimer. We find a review article on MEDLINE that shows that in a meta-analysis, D-dimer sensitivity = 94% and the specificity = 45%.[3] Our hospital just so happens to use the same D-dimer assay that was studied in this meta-analysis. How convenient.

Let's enter the numbers and see what we get:

		Disease		
		+	−	Total
Test	+	6	106	112
	−	1	87	88
	Total	7	193	200

Well, it's not perfect, but let's say for simplicity that D-dimer will pick up 6/7 (85%) of the patients with disease to make the numbers fit.

OK, our test is positive, so what is the positive predictive value? We can calculate that $6/112 = 5.4\%$. This is not very good – with a positive D-dimer, we have moved from our pretest probability of 3.5% (7/200) to a posttest probability of 5.4%. This certainly does not push us over any treatment threshold. That is, we do not want to anticoagulate people with heparin or enoxaparin (the treatment for pulmonary embolism) with a 5.4% chance of having the disease because of the potential side effects of those medications. What if the test is negative? Well, then our negative predictive value $= 87/88 = 98.9\%$. That's a pretty good negative predictive value. So, given a negative test, we have moved from a pretest probability of 3.6% to a posttest probability of 1.2%. With a posttest probability of 1.2%, it may be reasonable to say that a diagnosis has been mostly excluded. As we can see from this example, D-dimer is a good rule-out test because the sensitivity is high. Remember: "Snout."

Odds, probability, and the odds ratio

We will be using two related terms that denote risk in this book: *odds* and *probability*. While people often use *odds* and *probability* interchangeably, they actually mean different things. To some, probability makes more intuitive sense than odds, but often in statistics, an odds ratio is typically used to represent the likelihood that one group will have the outcome in question over another group.

Let's start with probability because this is the easiest to understand. The probability is the expected number over the total number. An easy example is to use six-sided dice. The probability of rolling a "6" on any individual roll is $1/6 = 16.7\%$. Using a hypothetical clinical example, the probability that a 50-year-old male who has risk factors for coronary disease, acute chest pain, and new electrocardiographic changes is having an acute coronary syndrome (ACS) is high (let's say 80% as an estimate). That means that out of 100 identical patients, 80 will have ACS.

Odds are related but different. Odds are the ratio of the probability of occurrence to that of non-occurrence. Using the same example, the odds that you will roll a "6" are 1:6, while the odds that the 50-year old male will have ACS are 4:1.

You can convert odds to probabilities using the following formulas:

$$\text{Odds} = \text{Probability}/(1 - \text{Probability})$$

$$\text{Probability} = \text{Odds}/(1 + \text{Odds})$$

An odds ratio is a measure of the size of the difference between odds and is commonly used in the medical literature to denote risk. It is defined as a ratio of the odds of an event or outcome in one group to the odds of an event or outcome in another group. These groups are traditionally a dichotomous classification, like older people ($\geq$65 years old) versus younger people (<65 years old) or men versus women. It can also be the difference between a treatment group and a control group. When the odds ratio is equal to 1, this indicates that the event or outcome is equally likely in both groups. When it is greater than 1, the condition or outcome is more likely in the first group. Finally, when it is less than 1, it is less likely in the first group.

In an odds ratio, p = the probability of the outcome in group 1 and q is the probability of the outcome in group 2. As mentioned in this chapter, we can use the formula for odds to calculate an odds ratio in terms of probabilities:

$$\text{Odds ratio} = (p/(1 - p))/(q(1 - q))$$

As a clinical example, suppose that we have a sample of 100 male and 100 female ED patients with acute chest pain. This is only a theoretical example to demonstrate how to calculate an odds ratio and is not based on any studies. Of the 100 patients, 20 males and 10 females will have a serious cause for their pain. The odds of a male having a serious cause for this pain are 20 to 80 or 1:5, while the odds of a female having a serious cause for this pain are 10 to 90 or 1:9. Using the above formula, we can calculate the odds ratio:

$$\text{Odds ratio} = ((0.20)/(1 - 0.20))/(0.10/(1 - 0.10)) = 2.25$$

This calculation can be interpreted to mean that men have a 2.25 times higher odds of having a serious cause for their chest pain than women. This also illustrates how an odds ratio can be larger than the difference in probability. While men are two times more likely (in terms of probability), the odds ratio is higher (2.25).

Likelihood ratios and interval likelihood ratios

Likelihood ratios are a different way to incorporate sensitivity and specificity and provide a direct estimate of how much a test result (positive or negative) will change the odds of having a disease. The likelihood ratio for a positive result (LR+) tells you how much the odds of the disease increase when a dichotomous test is positive. The likelihood ratio for a negative result (LR−) tells you how much the odds of the disease decrease when a dichotomous test is negative.

In order to use likelihood ratios, you need to specify the pretest odds. The pretest odds are the likelihood that the patient would have a specific disease prior to any testing. Pretest odds are related to the prevalence of disease and may be adjusted upward or downward depending on the characteristics of your overall patient pool (is the disease likely in your community?) or of the individual patient (is the disease likely in the individual patient?).

In order to calculate likelihood ratios, you can use the following formulas:

$$\text{LR}+ = \text{Sensitivity}/(1 - \text{Specificity})$$

$$\text{LR}- = (1 - \text{Sensitivity})/\text{Specificity}$$

$$\text{Odds}_{\text{post}} = \text{Odds}_{\text{pre}} \times \text{LR} + \text{(a positive test)}$$

$$\text{Odds}_{\text{post}} = \text{Odds}_{\text{pre}} \times \text{LR} - \text{(a negative test)}$$

As a general rule of thumb, likelihood ratios >10 or <0.1 generate sizeable changes in posttest disease probability, while likelihood ratios of 0.5–2.0 have little effect. It is also possible to use likelihood ratios when considering a sequence of independent tests (e.g., electrocardiogram followed by troponin I testing for potential ACS). Likelihood ratios can be multiplied in series.

Presenting continuous data as dichotomous results neglects and oversimplifies valuable diagnostic detail. One advantage of likelihood ratios over sensitivity and specificity is that interval likelihood ratios can be computed for continuous data, whereas sensitivity and specificity are always reported as dichotomous "+" or "−" results. Stratifying continuous data into ranges of results captures additional diagnostic information for clinicians to more appropriately interpret test results. See "Receiver Operator Characteristic (ROC) Curves" section in this chapter for information on calculating interval likelihood ratios. Unfortunately, most research manuscripts do not report interval likelihood ratios.

Using odds, probabilities, and likelihood ratios: an example

The best way to describe odds, probabilities and likelihood ratios is by using a clinical example. Using D-dimer as an example, let's assume that the sensitivity = 94% and the specificity = 45%.

We can calculate the LR+ = 1.71 by the following calculation: (0.94)/(1−0.45); and the LR− = 0.13 through the following formula: (1−0.94)/(0.45).

Now let's go through the math.

Start with a pretest probability of 10%. The next step is to convert that to an odds of (0.10)/(1−0.10) = 0.1111. So our pretest odds are 0.1111. If we want to apply likelihood ratios, we need to know our test results. If the test is positive, given a LR+ of 1.71, we can calculate a posttest odds given a positive test = (1.71)(0.1111) = 0.1899. If the test is negative, we can apply a LR− of 0.13. So posttest odds given a negative test = (0.13)(0.1111) = 0.0144. Now, we need to convert these back to probabilities. An odds of 0.1899 is equal to a probability of (0.1899)/(1+0.1899) = 16.0%. An odds of 0.0144 is equal to a probability of (0.0144)/(1+0.0144) = 1.4%.

Translated into English: given a pretest probability of 10%, if you have a positive D-dimer, your posttest probability = 16%. Your posttest probability is also your positive predictive value. If you have a negative test, your posttest probability is 1.4%. Another way of expressing a posttest probability when there is a negative test is a negative predictive value. In this case, your negative predictive value is (1-posttest probability) = $(1-0.014) = 98.6\%$.

An even simpler way to work from a pretest probability, modified by a likelihood ratio, to a posttest probability is to use a likelihood ratio nomogram (Figure 3.1). Using a ruler, start from the pretest probability in the left column and intersect the likelihood ratio value in the middle column.

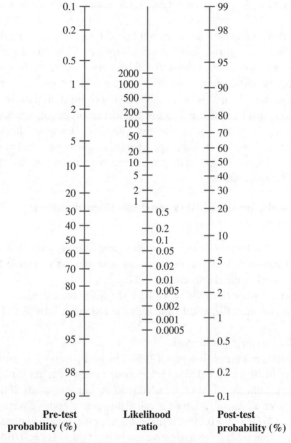

Figure 3.1 Likelihood ratio nomogram.
Note: Using a straight edge (such as a ruler), it is possible to move from pretest probability to posttest probability using the likelihood ratio of the test.

Extending the straight line from those two points out to the right-hand column results in the new posttest probability.

Bayes theorem

To make things even more complicated, in order to calculate a posttest probability given a pretest probability and known sensitivity and specificity, you can use the Bayes theorem and do it all in one step.

In the case of a positive test, you can calculate your posttest probability (or your positive predictive value) using the following formula:

Posttest probability = (Pretest probability × Sensitivity)/

[(Pretest probability × Sensitivity)

+ (1 − Pretest probability) × (1 − Specificity)]

In the case of a negative test, you can calculate your posttest probability (or one minus your negative predictive value) using the following formula:

Posttest probability = (1 − Pretest probability) × Specificity/

{[(1 − pretest probability) × specificity]

+ [pretest probability × (1 − sensitivity)]}

Let's go back to Chapter 1, when we mentioned the 83-year-old female with shortness of breath, chest pain, a history of pulmonary embolism, and a negative D-dimer. Given that her pretest probability for pulmonary embolism is 85%, we can calculate our posttest probability (and also our negative predictive value) using the Bayes theorem:

Posttest probability = (1 − 0.85) × 0.45/{[(1 − 0.85) × 0.45]

+ [0.85 × (1 − 0.94)]}

And after calculating it out, we get a posttest probability of 61.3% and our negative predictive value is (1−0.613) = 38.7%. Given that her chance of pulmonary embolism is 61.3% after a negative test result, we have not safely ruled out pulmonary embolism. Therefore, she needs further testing such as a chest CT or V/Q scan, or possibly even a pulmonary angiogram. Also, given that the pretest probability was so high, you could make an argument to just treat her. But given that anticoagulation is not without potential adverse effects, if you can order a confirmatory test, it is probably reasonable to do so.

So should we have ordered a D-dimer in the first place? The answer is probably not. In the case of a negative test, it did not help us because it did not move us over the test–treatment threshold.

Confidence intervals

Throughout this book, we make reference to confidence intervals. We will abbreviate 95% confidence intervals as CI. Confidence intervals are commonly used in statistics to give an estimated range of values that is likely to include a population parameter (like an odds ratio or a population mean) that is unknown. As an easy example, say we are trying to estimate the average age of everyone living in your county of 50,000 people. In order to do this, we randomly choose 100 houses and go door to door to ask people what their ages are, for a total sample of 322 people. From that, we find that the average age is 32 years old. But how certain are we that 32 is the real average for the population? Instead of saying that 32 is the average, what we can do is give a confidence interval. So we plug our numbers into our statistics program and what we find is that the average is indeed 32 but the 95% confidence interval is from 26 to 42 years old. What we can say is that we are 95% sure that whatever the real value is (if we sampled all 50,000) lies between 26 and 42. Intervals are usually reported with 95% confidence, but if we want to be really sure, we can report wider intervals such as 99% confidence intervals.

Let's use a clinical example. Like before, we want to know the odds of a male having a serious cause for chest pain compared to the odds for a female. What we would go out and do is collect sample data to answer the question by studying males and females with chest pain and estimating the odds ratio based on the sample data. Based on the data, we calculate an odds ratio of 2.25 with a 95% confidence interval of 1.5–3.5. Therefore, what we can say is that we are 95% confident that the real difference between men and women falls between 1.5 and 3.5. Since the lower bound of the confidence interval is greater than one, we can say that men are significantly at higher risk of having their chest pain be due to a serious cause than women.

Confidence interval width gives an idea about how uncertain we are about this unknown parameter. For example, if we reported an odds ratio of 2.3 (95% CI 2.0–2.5), we could be fairly confident in our estimate. However, if we reported 2.3 (95% CI 0.3–10.0), we would be less confident. A wide interval indicates that nothing very definite can be said about the parameter. As a rule of thumb, a parameter estimate with a small confidence interval is more reliable than a result with a large confidence interval.

Receiver operator characteristic (ROC) curves

Determination of sensitivity and specificity for a specific diagnostic test depends on the test values we define as "abnormal." The threshold value for an abnormal test that we set will determine the number of true positives, true negatives, false positives, and false negatives. For example, say that a patient with an abnormal D-dimer test is at a specific threshold, such as 500 ng/dL. If we were to set the cutoff at a higher level (e.g., 2000 ng/L), then the number of true positives would likely increase, but the number of false negatives would also increase. The purpose of ROC curves is to find the test cutoff that maximizes both sensitivity and specificity so that tests can be used and interpreted in clinically meaningful ways. Figure 3.2 shows an ROC curve.

ROC curves are a way to plot test sensitivity and specificity at different value thresholds for what defines a positive and negative test. Traditionally an ROC curve is a plot of the true positive rate (sensitivity) compared with the false positive rate (1−specificity). The accuracy of a test is dependent on how well the test distinguishes the group being tested into those with and without the disease. Test accuracy can be measured by the area under the ROC curve. If the area is 1, then the test is perfect. An area of 0.5 is a

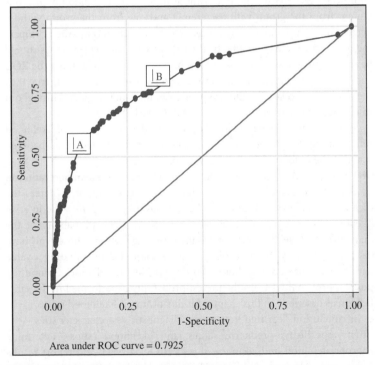

Figure 3.2 Receiver operator characteristic (ROC) curve.
Note: A and B are two specific points on the ROC curve. The slope of the line between the two is the interval likelihood ratio.

Table 3.2 Determining the accuracy of a diagnostic test using the area under the ROC curve

Value	Accuracy
0.90–1.00	Excellent
0.80–0.90	Good
0.70–0.80	Fair
0.60–0.70	Poor

worthless test. Table 3.2 provides a rough guide for classifying the accuracy of a diagnostic test using the area under the ROC curve.

Another way of describing the area under the ROC curve is test discrimination. It measures the ability of a test to correctly classify those with and without disease. Imagine a situation where we have two sets of patients, one with occult bacteremia and one without. If we were to randomly pick one patient from the group with bacteremia and one from the group without bacteremia and get a white blood cell (WBC) count on both, then compare the results for these two patients, the patient with the higher WBCs should be the one from the group with occult bacteremia. The area under the ROC curve is the percentage of randomly drawn pairs for which this is true (i.e., the test correctly classifies the two patients in the random pair). Throughout this book, we make reference to studies that use ROC curves.

Another way of using the ROC curve is to determine interval likelihood ratios. In Figure 3.2, the interval likelihood ratio for the test result between A and B is the slope of the line between those two points [$(Y_2 - Y_1)/(X_2 - X_1)$ or $(B_{sen} - A_{sen})/(B_{1-spec} - A_{1-spec})$]. The interval likelihood ratio can be determined between any two values of a diagnostic test. Whereas the dichotomous likelihood ratios are labeled *positive* or *negative*, the interval likelihood ratio is simply one value representing the probability of the diagnostic test yielding a value within this range among those who have disease, divided by the probability of the same test demonstrating a value within this range among those who do not have the disease. Computing posttest probabilities from the pretest probability is performed in the same fashion as described in this chapter for dichotomous likelihood ratios.

In conclusion, learning how to use diagnostic test characteristics (sensitivity, specificity, predictive values, and likelihood ratios), determine appropriate cutoff and accuracy of tests (ROC curves), and report results (odds ratios and confidence intervals), can be helpful in the practice of EBM in the ED. Thorough understanding of both the power and limitations of testing can aid in diagnosis and medical decision making.

References

1. Ramzi DW, Leeper KV. DVT and pulmonary embolism: Part I. Diagnosis. Am Fam Physician. 2004; 69: 2829–36.
2. Wolf SJ, McCubbin TR, Feldhaus KM, Faragher JP, Adcock DM. Prospective validation of Wells criteria in the evaluation of patients with suspected pulmonary embolism. Annals of Emergency Medicine. 2004; 44: 503–10.
3. Brown MD, Rowe BH, Reeves MJ et al. The accuracy of the enzyme-linked immunosorbent assay D-dimer test in the diagnosis of pulmonary embolism: A meta-analysis. Annals of Emergency Medicine. 2002; 40: 133–44.

Additional Reading

1. Hayden SR, Brown MD. Likelihood ratio: A powerful tool for incorporating the results of a diagnostic test into clinical decision making. Annals of Emergency Medicine. 1999; 33(5): 575–80.
2. Brown MD, Reeves MJ. Evidence-based emergency medicine skills for evidence-based emergency care. Interval likelihood ratios: Another advantage for the evidence-based diagnostician. Annals of Emergency Medicine. 2003; 42: 292–7.
3. Gallagher EJ. Evidence-based emergency medicine editorial: The problem with sensitivity and specificity. Annals of Emergency Medicine. 2003; 42: 298–303.
4. Pewsner D, Battaglia M, Minder C, Marx A, Bucher HC, Egger M. Ruling a diagnosis in or out with "SpPin" and "SnNout": A note of caution. British Medical Journal. 2004; 329: 209–13.
5. Phelps MA, Levitt MA. Pretest probability estimates: A pitfall to the clinical utility of evidence-based medicine? AcademicEmergency Medicine. 2004; 11: 692–4.
6. Smith C, Mensah A, Mal S, Worster A. Is pretest probability assessment on emergency department patients with suspected venous thromboembolism documented before SimpliRED D-dimer testing? Canadian Journal of Emergency Medicine. 2008; 10: 519–23.

Chapter 4 **Clinical Decision Rules**

Clinical decisions rules are practical tools intended to assist us in deciding whether a diagnostic test is needed, or what the likelihood is for the presence or absence of a particular disease or condition. They are designed to be simple and provide a practical decision-making guide to differentiate patients who require testing or treatment from those who do not. Clinical decision rules typically include at least three elements from the patient's history, a physical exam, and simple ancillary tests that can guide us at the bedside in the emergency department (ED) or in the office.[1] Decision rules are derived using a series of research studies on a specific clinical question. They then must be validated and tested in a different population. Each step in the derivation, validation, and external testing of a decision rule involves specific study designs and statistical analyses. At each stage in the development process, aspects of exactly how the study was conducted (i.e., the patient population tested and specific outcomes) impact how the rule should be interpreted and used in clinical practice. In this chapter, we describe the steps researchers take to derive (generate) and validate (show that it works) clinical decision rules.

The genesis of a decision rule is a specific research question. When related to diagnostic testing, it traditionally starts with a question like "XYZ is a disease that we often suspect but it has a low positive testing rate. Is there a way to clinically differentiate cases with negative tests where there is a risk for XYZ, so that XYZ can be ruled out clinically without ordering any tests?" *XYZ* may refer to common diseases that we want to exclude but that have a low prevalence of positives on test results, like intracranial bleeds, fractures, or infections. Decision aids have also been developed to risk-stratify patients for short-term adverse outcomes with presenting symptom complexes like chest pain, transient ischemic attack (TIA), and syncope. It is important to recognize that there are limitations for when a clinical decision rule can and should be used. For instance, consider the inclusion criteria for a rule. If the derivation and validation of a decision rule regarding whether a blunt trauma

Evidence-Based Emergency Care: Diagnostic Testing and Clinical Decision Rules, Second Edition. Jesse M. Pines, Christopher R. Carpenter, Ali S. Raja and Jeremiah D. Schuur. © 2013 John Wiley & Sons, Ltd. Published 2013 by John Wiley & Sons, Ltd.

patient should get a noncontrast head computed tomography (CT) scan to rule out intracranial pathology only included adult patients over the age of 18 years, then the results may not be applied to similarly injured pediatric patients unless the rule is validated in that specific population.

Decision rules are intended to include elements of the history, physical exam, or diagnostic tests that are reproducible and straightforward. Elements of clinical decision rules are also ideally binary (yes or no) or at least discrete with unambiguous options. We want to eliminate subjectivity as much as possible and maximize interrater reliability. This means that when two separate people assess an element of a rule, they have a high chance of agreeing on the results of that element. For example, consider a 72-year-old patient. Few would argue that the patient is 72 years old. If the criterion is "Is the patient 65 and older?", then there would likely be perfect agreement when two individuals assess this element. However, when we start using physical examination findings in a rule, such as "Does the patient have point tenderness over either malleolus of the ankle?", there is a greater chance for disagreement. This becomes further muddied when we try to use more subjective findings such as "Is there rebound or guarding on an abdominal examination?" This is where clinicians may have a high likelihood of obtaining different test results, depending on the way they conduct physical examinations or interpret clinical signs. Clinical decision rules also frequently do not take into context other intangible elements of the clinical setting. That is to say, clinical decision rules are not perfect. In the Canadian head CT rule, a rule that determines whether or not patients require head CT scans after blunt head trauma, one of the elements includes a failure to reach a Glasgow Coma Scale (GCS) of 15 within 2 hours. If you are assessing an individual with a GCS of 15 who is behaving strangely 30 minutes after a blunt head trauma, you probably should not wait the 2 hours to see whether she normalizes and should consider ordering a head CT scan early. Clinical decision rules often guide whether the likelihood of a disease is low enough to warrant the test. However, they are not necessarily binding. Even though clinical decision rules are designed to be theoretically 100% sensitive, when tested in real-life practice, they are almost always less than 100% sensitive. Clinical experience and gestalt are valuable assets in emergency medicine but are part of the intangible components that cannot be incorporated into clinical decision rules.

Over the past 15 years, many clinical decision rules have been introduced. The most notable and likely the most widely known are the sets of rules called the Ottawa rules (the knee rules and ankle rules). Dr. Ian Stiell and his research colleagues in Ottawa, Canada, have made a career of taking common clinical conditions where testing is frequently employed and positive tests are relatively rare, and then trying to figure out who needs tests and who doesn't. By asking very simple and straightforward questions, Dr. Stiell's research has aimed to reduce diagnostic variability via the elimination of unnecessary testing by deriving decision rules to identify low-risk patients who are unlikely to benefit from such tests. Other benefits of eliminating unnecessary testing using clinical decision rules include (i) reductions of time in the ED for the patients, (ii) reduced exposure to radiation (for imaging), and (iii) reduced costs to both patients and the health care system overall.

The clinical decision rule development process

A first step in creating a rule is to consider a clinical situation that is common enough to warrant a decision rule. Is there a discrete and finite clinical question? For instance, does every patient with ankle pain need an X-ray? How frequently are tests positive? Ankle injuries are common and widespread complaints presenting to EDs around the world, and ankle X-rays are frequently negative. Therefore, a rule that can identify low-risk criteria to reduce unnecessary ankle radiography would be clinically helpful. The clinical question is "Is there a fractured bone or not?" The practical question becomes "Is an X-ray needed?"

How do you go about creating a decision rule? The rest of this chapter will summarize the approach by describing the essential steps that researchers must undertake to develop a rule that is useful in practice. Several articles describing and discussing the methods for these components are available for those who want additional details.[1−3] As astute readers of the medical literature, developing a working understanding of each of these steps in order to determine if you should use the decision rule for your patients is essential.

The first step is *defining the outcome*. The outcome should be explicitly described and clinically relevant to the condition under study. Is there a fracture of either malleolus of the ankle? Does the patient have an acute appendicitis or a cervical spine (C-spine) fracture? All of these are discrete conditions with a binary yes or no answer. In describing the condition or test being examined, researchers also must define the patient population for the rule. Defining the outcome and the appropriate target patient population is essential because this determines the patient population to whom the rule can be applied. The outcome should be defined incorporating a global perspective that extends beyond the emergency physician to include pertinent specialists and patient-centric outcomes. For example, the Canadian head CT rule queried over 100 emergency and neurosurgery physicians to settle on the outcome of intracranial injury necessitating surgical management. Some clinicians discard the validated Canadian head CT rule based on this outcome because these physicians believe that even clinically inconsequential intracranial injuries should be identified with CT scans whenever possible.

Next, what are considered the most relevant and logical factors that might be used to predict an outcome or diagnosis? It is from the initial pool of *predictor variables* that the final decision rule is derived. The predictor variables usually include demographic factors, medical history, circumstances surrounding the patient's injury (mechanism of injury, or timing), physical exam findings, and sometimes blood test results, electrocardiogram findings, or results from imaging studies. Accurately and consistently determining the presence of the predictor variables is vital in determining which variables should be ultimately included in the decision rule. Both intra-observer agreement (between repeated measurements by the same clinician) and inter-observer agreement (in between measurements by different clinicians) should be high for inclusion in a decision rule. In terms of statistical measurement, researchers need to show that the predictor variables they are considering have sufficiently *high reproducibility*, in the form of a kappa statistic (κ). A κ statistic is a number from -1 to 1 where 0 indicates no agreement, -1 indicates perfect disagreement, and 1 indicates perfect agreement. Variables that are too subjective and have low κ values (<0.6) should not be included in the decision rule.

If the goal is to reliably exclude a fracture based on the history and physical exam findings of a patient with ankle pain, the predictor variables should be determined before knowledge of the X-ray results. Similarly, the X-ray results should not be interpreted with the knowledge of the history and physical exam findings of the patient. *Blinded assessment of the predictor variables and outcomes* from the imaging study ensures there is no observer or ascertainment bias on the validity of the findings. For instance, let's say we have examined a patient and know there is point tenderness over the medial malleolus. We may review an X-ray more carefully over the area of concern looking for a fracture in that specific area and may be more likely to call any irregularity a fracture. This is in contrast to a radiologist who is reading the similar X-ray but without knowledge or influence of the physical exam and who determines there is no fracture present.

The *derivation phase* of a decision rule is the process of collecting the data in a standardized way, including the predictor variables; assessing the reliability of those data; and determining the outcome(s) being studied (in the ankle examples, the outcome is fracture). Researchers then use statistical methods to distill the predictor variable down to those that are the most predictive of the outcome. The two most common methods are recursive partitioning and logistic regression analysis. Recursive partitioning takes patients and divides them sequentially into groups with a particular outcome. Subsets of patients are created with that particular outcome that have common predictor variables associated with the outcomes. Logistic regression analysis generates a model that predicts the outcome, which has to be binary (fracture or no fracture), by using the best statistical combination of predictor variables. Functionally, this type of analysis creates odds of the outcome event based on the presence or absence of the predictor variables. The end result of both methods is a set of best predictor variables that comprise the decision rule.

The next phase following the derivation stage is the *validation phase*. During the validation phase, the actual decision rule is applied to the patients for whom it is intended, and the outcomes are determined in a blinded fashion. The elements of the decision rule are assessed and recorded in a blinded format separate from the determination of the ultimate clinical outcome. The researchers then compare the performance of the decision rule with the outcome.

Validation usually takes the form of a 2 × 2 table (similar to the one we saw in Chapter 3) showing the results of the rule (rule positive or rule negative) compared to the outcome of the study (X-ray positive or X-ray negative).

	Outcome event (+)	Outcome event (−)
Clinical decision rule (+)	*a*	*b*
Clinical decision rule (−)	*c*	*d*

The results of the validation study should be clearly presented. When arranged in this format, we can then calculate the sensitivity and specificity for a rule.

Sensitivity, specificity, and likelihood ratios are performance characteristics of the rule or test being examined and are not influenced by the prevalence of the outcome event. Predictive values, both positive and negative, in contrast, change with the prevalence of the disease or outcome being studied, and therefore can and will change when the decision rule is applied to different populations or different settings. Statistical confidence in the results of the test performance should also be explicitly shown, usually in the format of 95% confidence intervals as described in Chapter 3.

Some studies combine data collection for the derivation and validation phases in order to streamline the process. In these studies, roughly half of the patient data are used to derive the best predictor variables to create a decision rule. The remaining patient data are then used to validate the decision rule. This split-sampling validation is acceptable, but it yields a clinical decision rule with a greater potential for bias which may limit its accuracy when used with other populations. Stiell et al have therefore suggested a hierarchy of clinical decision rule validation levels (Table 4.1).

Table 4.1 Clinical decision rule hierarchy

Level 1: Rules that are useful in a variety of settings with confidence that they change clinical behavior and improve outcomes. This includes prospectively validated rules in one or more different populations, and an impact analysis that demonstrates beneficial changes in clinical behavior.

Level 2: Rules that are useful in various settings and that have been validated by a demonstration of accuracy either in a large prospective study with a broad spectrum of patients and doctors or in several small different settings.

Level 3: Rules that clinicians may consider using with caution if study patients are similar to those in the clinician's setting. This may include studies that are validated in a single, narrowly defined prospective sample.

Level 4: Rules that need further application before clinical application. These include rules that are derived or validated in split samples, in retrospective databases, or by using statistical techniques.

Adapted from McGinn TG, Guyatt GH, Wyer PC, et al Users' Guides to the Medical Literature XXII: How to Use Articles About Clinical Decision Rules. JAMA 2000; 284 (1): 79–84. ©2000, American Medical Association, All Rights Reserved.

Issues of usability and practicality of the final rule also need to be taken into account. The ease of use of a decision rule will be linked to its acceptance and use in clinical practice. Therefore rules that have too many elements, are complicated to interpret or apply, or have vague or subjective variables are less likely to be widely accepted.

The final steps in the decision rule evolution are assessing the impact and cost effectiveness of the rule in actual clinical practice. Reports of the impact of a decision rule are described in implementation studies. They reveal if use of the rule results in changes in clinical practice and behavior patterns. Once effectiveness can be demonstrated, the economic effect can then be assessed. Demonstrating that resources are conserved, health savings are incurred, efficiencies are found, or, optimally, all of the above can determine the success or failure of a decision rule. These trials constitute Level 1 criteria for clinical decision rules. The trial design for an "impact analysis" is often a cluster randomized trial whereby entire hospitals are randomized to use or not use the clinical decision rule via various educational and real-time prompting methods. An example of a well-done impact analysis was conducted across 12 sites to test the impact of the implementation of the Canadian C-spine rule.[3] In the study, six sites were randomized to use active strategies to implement the Canadian C-spine rule (e.g., education, policy, and real-time reminders), while six sites were randomized to use no intervention. The study demonstrated a positive impact, in that the intervention group had a relative reduction of 13% (CI 9–16%) in imaging, while the control group had a 13% (CI 7–18%) increase in imaging rates. No adverse events occurred at any site. The process from concept to final decision rule often takes several years. The derivation and validation phases often are published separately. Implementation and cost-effectiveness studies on a clinical decision rule add additional years to a rule's long road to acceptance and use in clinical practice. Indeed, few decision rules have undergone these latter steps of testing. There is often a temptation to apply the results of a derivation study for a promising new decision rule based on the derivation study alone. We explicitly recommend this should not be done, no matter how great the results appear. The initial validation and derivation studies often employ highly trained research personnel to record and elicit the data used in these studies and are, in effect, efficacy studies. That is, under ideal clinical research terms and settings, can a rule be created and applied? This is different and distinct from effectiveness studies that examine how the rule works under regular routine clinical situations that are not study settings. The promising new decision rule should be examined critically and with caution. We should be sure to wait for external validation studies that replicate the findings in new or different settings from the initial sets of derivation and validation studies before incorporating a new decision rule into practice.

Few of the chapters in this book have a nice series of derivation, validation, external validation, implementation, and cost-effectiveness studies to describe and discuss. Instead, many of the common clinical questions have been only partially evaluated or are in the formative stages of evaluation. Since the first edition of this book was published in 2008, the science of clinical decision rules has advanced; however, future studies are still needed to fill in many gaps in the literature. Our goal is for these discussions to fuel new exploration of clinically relevant questions and the development of new, innovative decision rules.

References

1. Laupacis A, Sekar N, Stiell IG. Clinical prediction rules: A review and suggested modifications of methodological standards. Journal of the American Medical Association. 1997; 277(6): 488–94.
2. McGinn TG, Guyatt GH, Wyer PC, Naylor CD, Stiell IG, Richardson WS for the Evidence-Based Medicine Working Group. Users' guide to the medical literature XXII: How to use articles about clinical decision rules. Journal of the American Medical Association. 2000; 284(1): 79–84.
3. Stiell IG, Clement CM, Grimshaw J et al. Implementation of the Canadian C-spine rule: Prospective 12 centre cluster randomised trial. British Medical Journal. 2009 Oct 29; 339: b4146.

Additional Reading

1. Randolph AG, Guyatt GH, Calvin JE, Doig G, Scott RW. Understanding articles describing clinical prediction tools. Critical Care Medicine 1998; 26(9): 1603–12.

2. Reilly BM, Evans AT. Translating clinical research into clinical practice: Impact of using prediction to make decisions. Annals of Internal Medicine. 2006; 144(3): 201–9.

3. Stiell IG, Wells GA. Methodological standards for the development of clinical decision rules in emergency medicine. Annals of Emergency Medicine. 1999; 33(4): 437–47.

4. McGinn T, Wyer PC, Newman TB, Keitz S, Leipzig R, Guyatt G; Tips for learners of evidence based medicine: 3. Measures of observer variability (kappa statistic); CMAJ 2004; 171: 1369–1373.

Chapter 5 Appropriate Testing in an Era of Limited Resources: Practice and Policy Considerations

What role does physician decision-making around the use of diagnostic tests play in the debate around the rising cost of healthcare? Diagnostic testing makes up a significant and growing proportion of national healthcare expenditures. When ordered appropriately, diagnostic tests, such as computed tomography (CT) for abdominal pain, can help reduce resource use by identifying patients who do not need hospitalization or further interventions. Yet, in our search for certainty, we sometimes order tests that are unlikely to affect our medical decision making. Many tests add no information and do not affect decision making (e.g., "routine bloodwork" for the adult with gastroenteritis). Worse yet, out of tradition, habit, or the request of others we repeat tests that have been recently performed and are unlikely to have changed. Diagnostic tests that do not add useful information are a clear form of medical waste – directly visible to and controllable by clinicians. Less visible to emergency clinicians, but more important from a cost perspective, are the downstream costs of diagnostic testing. Unnecessary tests frequently yield false positive results requiring multiple follow-up tests or treatments to ensure the patent does not have conditions not initially suspected. Despite the overwhelming evidence that many diagnostic tests are of little or no value, changing practice is difficult. For example, routine preoperative testing of healthy adults is the norm across the United States despite strong evidence that it provides no value. We believe that improving the appropriateness of diagnostic testing is one way that medical professionals can reduce costs and improve value, as it can be done while improving the quality of patient care. Unfortunately, to date, many physicians have shown little interest or ability to do this. This is our challenge – apply the best evidence at the bedside and build systems to support us, before insurance and government regulators build them for us.

Evidence-Based Emergency Care: Diagnostic Testing and Clinical Decision Rules, Second Edition. Jesse M. Pines, Christopher R. Carpenter, Ali S. Raja and Jeremiah D. Schuur. © 2013 John Wiley & Sons, Ltd. Published 2013 by John Wiley & Sons, Ltd.

In this chapter, we discuss the role of diagnostic testing on healthcare costs, identify practice changes that physicians can implement to help improve the appropriateness of testing, and discuss policy approaches to reducing the use of testing.

Impact of diagnostic testing on healthcare expenditures

While discussions of healthcare costs and their effects abound in both the lay press and the medical literature, it is worth briefly reviewing some data to understand the importance of diagnostic testing. Healthcare spending is rising across the world at rates above the rate of economic growth or the willingness of societies to increase taxation. In the United States, national healthcare spending in 2010 was $2.6 trillion, or $8,402 per resident, accounting for 17.9% of GDP.[1] It is projected that by 2021, healthcare spending will be over $4.7 trillion or $14,000 per resident, and account for 19.6% of US GDP.[2] Why is this important? As a society, rising costs force us to choose between medical care and other worthy priorities. As healthcare is the single largest component of current and future deficit spending, rising costs are leading to political conflict and gridlock affecting many other areas. At the individual level, as healthcare costs rise, fewer people have access to care and more people suffer when they get sick, due to events such as medical bankruptcy. In this environment, healthcare providers should expect stable or shrinking resources and significant pressure to cut costs per patient for the foreseeable future. Put bluntly, if providers do not lead with solutions, politicians and businesses will be forced to implement controls. Political solutions to rising costs are unlikely to reflect the best available scientific evidence.

Diagnostic testing accounts for a significant and rising proportion of national health expenditures in Western industrialized countries, such as the United States. Exact calculations of spending on diagnostic testing are difficult, as testing can appear in several different categories of health expenditures (e.g. hospital care, physician services, and other professional services) and is sometimes bundled with other costs, such as during hospitalization. Estimates of the cost of diagnostic testing were around $100 billion per year from 2003 to 2007, or roughly 5% of total US healthcare spending. The cost of diagnostic imaging, one component of diagnostic testing, has risen dramatically in recent years. From 2003 to 2008, the use of diagnostic imaging among Medicare beneficiaries rose every year. Spending on the physician services associated with imaging, just one component of imaging costs, rose from $9.6 billion to $11.7 billion during this period, despite significant cuts in reimbursement per procedure during this time.[3] As a proportion of diagnostic tests are inappropriate and potentially avoidable, there is great potential to reduce the direct cost of diagnostic testing.

Downstream costs of diagnostic testing

Equally as important as the direct costs of diagnostic testing are the downstream costs of findings on unnecessary tests. While we should order diagnostic tests to answer a specific question, the results sometimes do not answer the question specifically. Instead, they provide a range of information that can influence the probability of disease. They may also provide additional information to other questions that we did not wish to ask. A false positive test result may not be in concordance with the rest of our thinking, yet still requires further downstream workup. For example, consider a patient admitted to hospital from the emergency department (ED) with community-acquired pneumonia and blood cultures that yield Gram-positive cocci in clusters, ultimately revealing *Staphylococcus aureus*. The blood culture may generate downstream testing such as repeat blood cultures and an echocardiogram. Studies have estimated that false positive blood cultures add tens of thousands of dollars to the overall hospital costs of patients compared to those without false positive blood cultures. Additionally, the diagnostic test may give answers to questions we did not wish to ask – the "incidentaloma." For example, when ordering a pulmonary angiogram computed tomography (CT) scan to evaluate a patient for pulmonary embolism, the scan will often reveal incidental findings in the thorax and upper abdomen such as pulmonary nodules or renal masses. Standard medical practice requires appropriate follow-up for these "incidentalomas," which usually involves repeat imaging and may require biopsies and eventual treatment. Thus indirect costs of the original test include workup and treatment of false positives and incidental findings. Although the indirect costs of many common diagnostic tests have not been formally assessed, they are likely greater than the direct costs of unnecessary tests.

Variation in testing and inappropriate testing

There is evidence that a significant proportion of diagnostic tests performed in the United States are potentially avoidable based on the patient's clinical condition and the best available evidence.[4] One way to look at this is to look at the indications for specific tests. Retrospective studies of diagnostic tests services show that a significant proportion of diagnostic tests do not have evidence to support their use in the patient. Studies of geographic variation also illustrate this vividly.[5] For example, patients in some areas of the United States are much more likely to undergo cardiac catheterization for stable angina or after an acute myocardial infarction than patients in other regions, regardless of the appropriateness of the procedure. Similar patterns have been shown with the use of laboratory tests and other diagnostic tests. Such variation also exists within hospitals, departments, and practices, even after adjustment for a patient's clinical condition and comorbidities. Such variation is reasonable for some diagnostic tests where there is little definitive evidence, such as abdominal CT for undifferentiated abdominal pain. It is hard to justify for conditions that have been well studied and for which validated clinical decision rules are available, such as ankle X-rays or CT for pulmonary embolism.

Causes of inappropriate testing

Inappropriate use of diagnostic tests can be classified into the categories of underuse, overuse, and misuse. Through his work describing unwanted variation in medical care, John Wennberg, MD, founder of the Dartmouth Atlas of Health Care defined these categories to classify the variation that they observed. *Underuse* refers to the failure to provide a healthcare service when there is evidence that it would have produced a favorable outcome for the patient. *Overuse* occurs when a test or treatment is used without medical justification – a diagnostic test without evidence to support its use in the condition, patient, or setting. *Misuse* of preference-sensitive care refers to situations in which there are significant trade-offs among the available options (such as the choice between CT and observation in a young woman with an atypical presentation for early appendicitis). Choices should be based on the patient's own values, but often they are not. Misuse results from the failure to accurately communicate the alternative's risks and benefits, and the failure to base the choice of diagnostic test on the patient's values and preferences. In this chapter we focus on overuse and misuse of diagnostic tests, as they are an important focus in the ongoing discussion of cost control in healthcare. Table 5.1 illustrates types of overuse and misuse of diagnostic testing.

Many forces contribute to the overuse of diagnostic tests in the United States, but chief among them is the clinician's quest for diagnostic certainty. Clinicians give many reasons why they order diagnostic tests that they acknowledge have little or no value, including fear of missing diagnoses ("defensive medicine"), patient's requests, and other physicians' requests. Additionally, there are financial incentives to encourage inappropriate testing, such as the fee-for-service medical system. Specifically, in emergency medicine in the United States, physician reimbursement is determined by the complexity of the visit. Ordering and interpretation of diagnostic tests are key determinants of complexity. For example, evaluating a patient with

Table 5.1 Categories of misuse and overuse of diagnostic testing in emergency medicine

Category	Rationale	Examples
Bad test	Evidence does not support the use of the diagnostic test for the clinical indication.	• Erythrocyte sedimentation rate (ESR) and C-reactive protein (CRP) to evaluate for septic arthritis • Abdominal series X-rays (KUB) for undifferentiated abdominal pain
Good test but wrong patient	Evidence does not support the use of the diagnostic test in the patient population.	• Blood culture for non–critically ill cases of community-acquired pneumonia • D-dimer for patients at very low clinical risk (PERC rule negative)
Good test but wrong time or setting	Evidence does not support the use of the diagnostic test at the time of the encounter.	• Lyme disease serology testing at the time of tick identification and removal
Lack of additive information in context to other tests being ordered	The test does not add information beyond other tests being performed.	• Amylase in addition to lipase to evaluate for pancreatitis • Creatinine kinase in addition to troponin to evaluate for acute myocardial infarction (MI) (excluding patients with recent MI)
Misuse of diagnostic test	The test is not appropriate based on available alternatives and the patient's preferences.	• Routine use of CT abdomen and pelvis in young women with early presentation of right lower quadrant pain that could be early appendicitis, when observation (at home or in an ED observation unit) is preferred

a mild traumatic head injury by routinely ordering a CT will generate a larger bill than using a clinical decision rule and not ordering a CT. While each of these plays a role in over-ordering diagnostic tests, none is as important as our cultural search for medical certainty. According to Sir William Osler, medicine at its heart is an art and science of uncertainty.

Advances in diagnostic testing have dramatically improved our ability to reduce uncertainty, but uncertainty will never be eliminated. In the United States, we have built a culture that expects diagnostic certainty, despite our knowledge of Bayesian theory and the limitations of specific diagnostic tests. This is reflected in our clinical language, such as "I am getting this test to rule out that diagnosis", our systems, such as having single cutoffs for normal and abnormal on continuous tests, our medical culture, such as morbidity and mortality conferences, and our legal system. A major casualty of this quest for diagnostic certainty is an appreciation and use of clinical evidence at the bedside. If diagnostic certainty is valued above all else, there is little incentive for physicians to learn and apply the available evidence when ordering tests. Unsurprisingly clinicians do not routinely apply the best evidence to the decision to order diagnostic tests – leading to inappropriate testing.

Medical liability and the fear of getting sued lead physicians to order more diagnostic tests, but these are not the main causes of *inappropriate* testing. Studies have not consistently found that a physician's fear of malpractice predicts inappropriate use of diagnostic testing.[6] It is worth noting that ordering tests that are not supported by medical evidence is unlikely to protect a practitioner from liability. Furthermore, inappropriate testing exposes clinicians to additional liability such as having incongruent and unexplained lab results (e.g., an elevated white blood cell (WBC) count in a patient without other signs of infection) and "incidentalomas" requiring outpatient follow-up.[7] While limiting medical liability could influence our quest for diagnostic certainty, it would not stop inappropriate testing by itself. We have trained patients and family members to expect diagnostic certainty. Reducing inappropriate testing will require us to acknowledge uncertainty with each other and our patients and build systems that allow clinicians to apply the best evidence to diagnostic decisions at the bedside. We hope this book is one step in that direction.

Improving appropriateness in diagnostic testing: practice considerations

Individual clinicians can take steps to improve the appropriateness of their diagnostic test ordering. Primarily, they can attempt to learn and apply the best evidence to their frequent decisions around diagnostic testing. This includes identifying good sources of information around diagnostic testing, regular reading, and applying the knowledge at the bedside. Use of handbooks such as this and websites will help in busy clinical situations.

Physician practices, including EDs, should implement systems to improve the appropriateness of test ordering. These systems include standardized

Table 5.2 Practice improvements to address inappropriate diagnostic testing

Intervention
Improved provider knowledge
• Better evidence: comparative effectiveness studies, systematic reviews, and guidelines
• Provider awareness: journal clubs and required reading
• Awareness of costs
Availability of evidence at time of ordering
• Tailoring guidelines to local practice, specific patients, and clinical situations
• Posters and pocket cards
• Computerized decision support systems
Performance monitoring and feedback
• Use of diagnostic testing and diagnostic yield
• Appropriateness of diagnostic testing
• Cost of diagnostic testing

pathways and guidelines, clinical decision support, and auditing practice with feedback to providers including data on the cost of testing. Table 5.2 lists approaches to improving appropriateness.

Standardized clinical pathways and guidelines are widely published but have had little effect on individual clinicians' practice behavior. The practice of medicine has been taught as an individual art with emphasis on provider autonomy and exceptionalism. Standardization of practice, such as through guidelines, is often seen as anathema to physician autonomy. Groups of physicians can overcome these barriers and successfully implement practice guidelines if they follow several steps. First, the guideline should be developed or modified locally, so it addresses local practice patterns and concerns. Second, clinical decision leaders (who can include either departmental leadership or well-respected peers) need to endorse and promote the guideline. Third, clinical systems need to be modified so that the practice guideline is available and integrated into the clinical workflow. Finally, practitioners need to receive data on their performance relative to the guideline the group. Intermountain Health, an integrated healthcare delivery system in Utah, has been a pioneer in the use of such pathways throughout multiple areas of care. Dr. Brent James, director for Intermountain Healthcare's Institute for Healthcare Delivery Research, has developed physician leaders to develop such guidelines and integrated them throughout Intermountain's clinical culture, information systems, and practices. They have been able to demonstrate reduced utilization of tests, shorter lengths of stay, decrease costs, and improved quality.[8] Yet, it is not easy work, and clinicians will need tools to support this practice change.

One critical tool is clinical decision support, which is a computer system that uses patient data to generate case-specific clinical advice. For example, a radiology ordering system's decision support would include validated clinical decision rules, and clinicians would be required to complete them prior to ordering tests (e.g., Wells criteria for pulmonary embolus). When clinicians want to order a test outside of the guideline, the system can impose varying degrees of interference, from a requirement that the clinician document the reason for deviation to a hard stop requiring a conversation with a supervisory physician. Decision support systems have been shown to improve appropriateness of test ordering and to decrease utilization of diagnostic testing.[9] One variation on decision support is to actively provide the cost of diagnostic tests to providers at the time of ordering. This makes the cost of testing visible, and has been shown to reduce use and improve appropriateness of testing.

Health policy considerations

In response to rising costs of US healthcare, payers and policy makers are implementing measures to reduce the use of diagnostic tests. Examples include funding comparative effectiveness research, publishing guidelines, implementing performance measures for public reporting and incentive-based compensation ("pay-for-performance"), and requiring preauthorization prior to ordering diagnostic tests. If physicians and hospitals cannot control the rising cost of diagnostic testing, we should be prepared for government to impose external controls on us.

Government and private payers are trying to improve the quality of evidence available to clinicians regarding diagnostic tests. It has long been noted that the majority of government research funding for healthcare goes into basic sciences and the development of new tests and treatments, the primary aims of the National Institutes of Health. Research on how to effectively apply available tests and treatments is funded at only a fraction of this level, primarily through the Agency for Healthcare Research and Quality. Recently, this debate has focused on increased funding for comparative effectiveness research, which compares more than one test or treatment and looks at patient-centered outcomes. While comparative effectiveness research has been strongly supported by the academic community, many policy makers are concerned that it is the first step in government healthcare rationing, and they oppose it on ideological grounds. While there is increased funding available for such research, the US Affordable Health Care Act of

2009 specifically stipulates that comparative effectiveness research should not be used to determine coverage of benefits by Medicare or other government-funded healthcare.

Public and private payers are developing and implementing performance measures of diagnostic testing for public reporting and pay-for-performance programs. These performance measures, also known as *quality measures*, aim to measure utilization or appropriateness of diagnostic testing. Utilization measures are easiest to develop and calculate, as they can be easily calculated from a large administrative database, such as Medicare claims. Alternatively, appropriateness measures attempt to use clinical information to determine if the diagnostic test was appropriate for the patient for whom it was ordered. Appropriateness measures require electronic medical records or chart review and are therefore more time-consuming and costly to implement. Payers and providers are at odds over the accuracy of utilization measures calculated from administrative claims – a debate that will intensify as the pressure over costs grows. An example is Medicare's new measure "OP-15: Use of Brain Computed Tomography (CT) in the Emergency Department for Atraumatic Headache." This measure uses Medicare claims to determine the appropriateness of brain CT scans performed in patients with headache, but providers are concerned that it does not accurately account for patients' clinical condition.[10]

The most direct way to control diagnostic test utilization is to require prior authorization. Private payers have increasingly implemented such authorizations for expensive tests and treatments. They are nearly universal for high-cost imaging tests such as CT and MRI. Although EDs were initially excluded, they are being increasingly required to obtain prior authorization or are subject to retroactive denials. MedPac proposed implementing prior authorization for Medicare in 2010, but to date this proposal has not progressed. Table 5.3 lists several policy and regulatory approaches to reducing diagnostic testing in the United States.

Table 5.3 Policy and regulatory approaches to reducing utilization of testing in the United States

Regulations on ordering of tests	Pre-authorization requirements for imaging
Cost sharing by patients	Co-pays for high-cost diagnostic tests (e.g., MRI)
Pay-for-performance programs around diagnostic testing	Medicare measures of imaging efficiency Head CT for atraumatic headache in the ED MRI for low back pain prior to conservative therapy

References

1. CMS National Health Expenditure Data: National Health Expenditures 2010 Highlights. Available from: http://www.cms.gov/Research-Statistics-Data-and-Systems/Statistics-Trends-and-Reports/NationalHealthExpendData/Downloads/highlights.pdf
2. CMS National Health Expenditure Data: National Health Expenditure Projections 2011–2021. Available from: http://www.cms.gov/Research-Statistics-Data-and-Systems/Statistics-Trends-and-Reports/NationalHealthExpendData/Downloads/Proj2011PDF.pdf
3. A Data Book: Health Care Spending and the Medicare Program (June 2010). MedPAC, Washington, DC. Available from: http://www.medpac.gov/chapters/Jun10DataBookSec8.pdf
4. Waste and Inefficiency in the U.S. Health Care System Clinical Care: A Comprehensive Analysis in Support of System-Wide Improvements. New England Healthcare Institute. February 2008. Available from: http://www.nehi.net/publications/27/waste_and_inefficiency_in_the_us_health_care_system_clinical_care
5. How Many More Studies Will It Take? NEHI Compendium on Overuse. New England Healthcare Institute. February 2008. Available from: http://www.nehi.net/publications/30/how_many_more_studies_will_it_take
6. Baicker K, Fisher ES, Chandra A. Malpractice Liability Costs And The Practice Of Medicine In The Medicare Program. Health Affairs. 2007; 26: 3841–852.
7. Gale BD, Bissett-Siegel DP, Davidson SJ, Juran DC. Failure to Notify Reportable Test Results: Significance in Medical Malpractice. Journal of the American College of Radiology. 2011; 8(11): 776–779.
8. Leonhardt D. Making Health Care Better. The New York Times. November 8, 2009.
9. Roshanov PS, You JJ, Dhaliwal J, Koff D, Mackay JA, Weise-Kelly L, Navarro T, Wilczynski NL, Haynes RB; CCDSS Systematic Review Team. Can computerized clinical decision support systems improve practitioners' diagnostic test ordering behavior? A decision-maker-researcher partnership systematic review. Implementation Science 2011; 6(88).
10. Mckenna M. CMS Head CT Rule Under Fire. Annals of Emergency Medicine. 2012: August; 60(1): 20–21.

Further Reading

1. Brody H. Medicine's ethical responsibility for health care reform – the top five list. *NEJM* 2010; 362: 283–5.
2. Kassirer JP. Our stubborn quest for diagnostic certainty: A cause of excessive testing. *NEJM*. 1989 Jun 1; 320(22): 1489–91.
3. National Guideline Clearinghouse website. Available from: http://www.guideline.gov
4. MDCalc website. Available from: http://www.mdcalc.com
5. National Quality Measures Clearinghouse website. Available from: http://quality measures.ahrq.gov

Chapter 6 **Understanding Bias in Diagnostic Research**

Chapter 2 describes the process of evidence-based medicine (EBM), including how to evaluate individual study quality and apply research to actual patient care. Learning this process requires mentoring and consistent practice just like any other skill set in medicine.[1] However, several tools developed over the past decade can help clinicians assess the quality of diagnostic research evidence for individual questions.

One such tool is the Standards for Reporting of Diagnostic Accuracy Studies (STARD) criteria. STARD is a systematic approach to conducting and reporting diagnostic research.[2,3] STARD provides a 25-item checklist of considerations that are important for diagnostic researchers and clinicians to consider while assessing the quality of a diagnostic manuscript (Table 6.1).

As described in Chapter 2, systematic reviews are at the top of the evidence pyramid (i.e., they are one of the least biased forms), but systematic review methods for diagnostic tests have only recently been developed and remain underused.[4] The Quality Assessment Tool for Diagnostic Accuracy Studies (QUADAS) methods provide an instrument for assessing four domains of bias that can skew an individual trial's estimates of diagnostic accuracy: patient selection, index test, criterion standard, and timing.[5-7] QUADAS is the preferred instrument for the evaluation of the quality of evidence in diagnostic meta-analyses. The Meta-Analysis of Observational Studies in Epidemiology (MOOSE) statement provides a structural framework for systematic reviews and meta-analyses of observational trials, which are the predominant design of diagnostic accuracy trials.[8] The Cochrane Collaboration provides the most explicit guidelines for diagnostic systematic reviews.[9] In this chapter, we will describe the forms of bias to consider in diagnostic research and provide suggestions for incorporating these data into guidelines.

Diagnostic research is vulnerable to several forms of bias that physicians should recognize while critically appraising the evidence (Table 6.2).[10-13]

Evidence-Based Emergency Care: Diagnostic Testing and Clinical Decision Rules, Second Edition.
Jesse M. Pines, Christopher R. Carpenter, Ali S. Raja and Jeremiah D. Schuur.
© 2013 John Wiley & Sons, Ltd. Published 2013 by John Wiley & Sons, Ltd.

Table 6.1 STARD criteria

Checklist item
Identify manuscript as a study of diagnostic accuracy.
Make explicit statement of research aim.
Describe study population including exclusions and location.
Describe participant recruitment.
Describe participant sampling.
Describe timing and method of data collection.
Describe the criterion standard and its rationale.
Describe technical specifications of material and methods employed for index and reference test.
Define and justify the units, cutoffs, and categories for the index test and criterion standard.
Describe the number and expertise of the study personnel interpreting the index test and criterion standard.
Describe whether interpreters of the index test and criterion standard were blinded to the results of the other test.
Describe methods for comparing measures of diagnostic accuracy and to quantify uncertainty.
Describe methods for calculating test reproducibility.
Make explicit statement of study timeframe.
Report clinical and demographic characteristics of the study population.
Flow diagram illustrating patients meeting inclusion criteria who did not obtain either the index test or the criterion standard.
Report time interval between the index test and criterion standard, and any treatment administered between them.
Report the distribution of disease severity in those with the target condition.
Cross-tabulate results of the index test (including indeterminate and missing results) by the results of the criterion standard, and for continuous data provide distributions of the index test result stratified by the criterion standard (to compute interval likelihood ratios).
Report adverse events from the index test or criterion standard.
Report estimates of diagnostic accuracy with confidence intervals.
Report how indeterminate results, missing responses, and outliers were handled.
Report estimates of variability for diagnostic accuracy between patient subgroups, outcome assessors, or medical centers.
Report estimates of test reproducibility.
Discuss the clinical applicability of the study findings.

Source: Data from [2,3].

For this discussion the new test being evaluated by researchers will be called the *index test*, whereas the standard upon which the presence or absence of the disease is determined will be called the *criterion standard*. The criterion standard is the most accurate test available for a particular indication. For example, in appendicitis, all diagnostic tests would be compared to the

Table 6.2 Description of bias in diagnostic research

Threats to diagnostic accuracy	Alternative names or subtypes	Description
Context bias	Prevalence bias	Outcome assessors influenced by overall disease prevalence or recent cases.
Double criterion standard bias	Verification bias, work-up bias, referral bias, sampling bias, or selection bias	Variable criterion standard applied based upon the index test.
Indeterminate criterion standard bias		Imperfect or poorly accepted criterion standard.
Interval bias		Extended time between index and criterion standard tests alters disease status or severity, outcome assessors' available diagnostic data, or both.
Review bias	Incorporation or interpretation bias	Outcome assessors' access to criterion standard while interpreting index test, vice versa, or both.
Spectrum bias*	Case-mix or subgroup bias	Test performance influenced by disease severity because diagnostic test characteristics are unique to subsets of patients.
Cutoff bias*		Thresholds to distinguish "normal" from "abnormal" for continuous data are defined arbitrarily or after data analysis.
Temporal bias*		Technological improvements, operator expertise, or both improve over time limiting the accuracy of earlier research.

Source: Drawn from [10–13].

*Spectrum bias, cutoff bias, and temporal bias skew estimates of diagnostic test performance in other populations based upon subsets tested, test thresholds defined, or time-period when the test was performed. However, the estimates of diagnostic performance within the populations tested are valid and accurate.

pathologic findings of appendiceal inflammation, which is the criterion standard for appendicitis.

Types of bias

Context bias is problematic when ambient conditions influence the outcome assessors while they are reviewing the data for the index test and the criterion standard. For example, if a clinician is assessing a constellation of symptoms for influenza-like illness (ILI) during a pandemic, he or she may be more likely to attribute malaise and fever to ILI than during periods of low ILI prevalence. The radiology literature often describes this form of bias, but it is difficult to detect and seldom reported.[14]

Double criterion standard bias is likely when investigators use one criterion standard for those with a positive index test and an alternative (usually less invasive and less accurate) criterion standard for those with a negative index test.[15,16] In this scenario, patients with a negative index test may have undetected disease because the most definitive criterion standard testing was not obtained.[17,18] Constellations of findings from history and physical exam leading to differential workup strategies also produce biased estimates of index test accuracy. For example, patients with chest pain, shortness of breath, and unilateral leg swelling are more likely to have definitive diagnostic testing for pulmonary embolism (PE) than are those with a productive cough, fever, and pulmonary infiltrate on chest X-ray. In clinical settings, this differential testing is logical, but in designing diagnostic accuracy studies, *workup bias* can skew the results. *Indeterminate criterion standard bias* occurs when the index test is superior to the historical criterion standard. When this bias is suspected, investigators should assess the discrepant cases to resolve disagreement using a third "umpire test" in addition to evaluating the prognostic and therapeutic consequences to these cases.[19]

Interval bias occurs when there is a clinically significant delay between the index test and the criterion standard, which is sufficiently long for the disease status to change. In general, this form of bias is applicable only in disease states that can change quickly over a short period of time such as infections. Chronic disease states such as dementia do not spontaneously reverse their pathological processes. Interval bias can also affect diagnostic accuracy estimates in acute disease states. For example, in subarachnoid hemorrhage, computed tomography (CT) is most sensitive immediately after the onset of a sentinel headache, with reduced sensitivities noted after 24 hours.

Subjective test interpretation can occur when study personnel are aware of other clinical information, a form of bias called *review bias*. There are three forms of review bias. If the criterion standard is available while interpreting the index test, then *test review bias* may distort estimates of diagnostic accuracy. In contrast, if the index test results are available to the outcome assessors who are interpreting the criterion standard, then *diagnostic review bias* may be problematic.[20] Finally, if the index test is one component of the criterion standard, then *incorporation bias* is possible.[21] To reduce the risk of any form of review bias, researchers blind clinicians who obtain and/or interpret the index test to the criterion standard while concurrently blinding outcome assessors (those who use the criterion standard to label the patient as "disease positive" or "disease absent") to the index test.

The last three forms of bias yield estimates of diagnostic test performance that are not necessarily inaccurate, but that apply only to subsets of patients or specific interpretations of the index test. Diseases often encompass a range of illness severity, and preliminary diagnostic research often targets a specific subset of patients based upon referral patterns or access to patients. This form of selection bias can yield *spectrum bias* with estimates of diagnostic test performance that are accurate only for patients with a similar profile of disease severity.[22,23] Strep pharyngitis is one example of spectrum bias, because rapid strep tests obtained on patients with a sore throat who have a higher Centor score (denoting a higher probability of a positive Group A streptococcal infection; see Chapter 29) will yield a higher sensitivity than situations in which the same assay is used to evaluate those less likely to have strep pharyngitis. Therefore, details about the methods of selecting patients and the case mix are essential in diagnostic research reports to gauge the potential for this form of bias. To minimize spectrum bias, diagnostic accuracy studies should enroll consecutive patients whenever possible. Alternatively, researchers can intentionally target well-defined and clinically relevant patient subsets for which the diagnostic test is likely to be particularly beneficial.

Cutoff bias occurs when different studies (or the same study) use variable and undefined thresholds to transform continuous data into dichotomous "disease-present" or "disease-absent" states. As described in Chapter 3, a receiver operator characteristic (ROC) curve can be used to identify an optimal cutoff value for continuous data that simultaneously maximizes sensitivity and specificity. However, researchers sometimes fail to explicitly state how or what cutoff values were used or assign these thresholds after data analysis.[24] *Temporal bias* is particularly problematic in diagnostic radiology since technological advances are continually improving, as is reader expertise.[25] For example, as discussed in Chapter 52, the diagnostic accuracy of CT for pulmonary embolism using first-generation scanners was

70%, while the more recent PIOPED II data demonstrated a sensitivity of 83% for newer generation scanners.[26]

Diagnostic systematic reviews and meta-analyses provide one method to assess the research evidence for new tests while contemplating the various forms of bias.[27] Another form of bias that systematic reviews reveal is publication bias.[28] The QUADAS and MOOSE guidelines provide a uniform framework for these manuscripts.[5-8] Diagnostic systematic reviews in other specialties are extremely useful to emergency medicine. For example, the *Journal of the American Medical Association*'s Rational Clinical Exam series provides two decades of diagnostic systematic reviews for a large variety of medical and surgical topics.[29] However, other specialties' diagnostic systematic reviews often fail to focus on ED populations, clinical situations, or diagnostic strategies. The Evidence Based Diagnostics series in *Academic Emergency Medicine* has introduced a venue for ED-based systematic reviews that also provide estimates of test–treatment thresholds and implications for future diagnostic research.[30,31]

Moving Beyond Bias to Effectiveness

Assessing bias in diagnostic accuracy research is essential, but it is only the first step since test accuracy is only a surrogate for patient-oriented outcomes. The implicit assumption is that if clinicians have a better idea of whether a disease is present or absent, outcomes will improve. The Grading of Recommendations Assessment, Development and Recommendations (GRADE) criteria comprise one approach to assess the overall patient-centric effectiveness of diagnostic testing based upon the available evidence.[32] The GRADE approach is to assess the diagnostic accuracy and clinical effectiveness data for a diagnostic test in order to make specific "actionable" recommendations for the use of these tests in guidelines. Although the least biased study design to assess a diagnostic strategy would be a randomized controlled trial (RCT), such trials are rare. Instead, most diagnostic studies are observational and calculate test characteristics based on a convenience sampling of patients who received both the index test and a criterion standard. According to the GRADE criteria, the most clinically relevant studies on diagnostic testing include representative and consecutive patients where diagnostic uncertainty exists. The focus has to be the patient for whom clinicians would reasonably apply a test in the course of practice: ED patients in whom the diagnostic impression is somewhere between the test and treatment thresholds described in Chapter 1.

Although diagnostic-testing RCTs are rare, criteria exist to establish when accuracy studies alone are insufficient.[33] The first step is to assess the sensitivity of the new test relative to the old test(s). If the sensitivities are similar, one can assume that either test will detect the same true cases of disease. In this scenario if the new test has superior specificity, then the potential adverse effects of additional testing or treatment of false positives will be reduced and an RCT is unnecessary. Additionally, when the new test is either cheaper or more readily available than the old test, RCTs are not needed.

If the new test is more sensitive than the old test with similar specificity, the benefit of the new test relates to the therapeutic responses of the additional true-positive cases as identified by RCTs of therapy. For example, CT colonography performed in the supine and prone positions is more sensitive (with equal specificity) than when performed in the prone position alone.[34] Therapeutic trials demonstrate improved survival associated with early detection and treatment of colorectal polyps on a similar spectrum of disease, so diagnosticians can reasonably assume that compared with supine positioning, dual-positioning CT colonography will improve survival without awaiting an RCT. However, when evaluating these therapeutic RCTs, clinicians need to contemplate whether the results apply to the new cases identified by the index test. Do the extra cases respond to therapy in the same manner as the cases identified by the older (less sensitive) test? For example, in the 1960s the diagnosis of pulmonary embolism occurred only in extreme life-threatening cases using older imaging strategies (or at autopsy), whereas modern CT technology identifies small and possibly clinically inconsequential emboli with high sensitivity. Do these peripheral emboli respond to anticoagulation therapy to the same degree as the massive PEs upon which we base the therapeutic management of PE?[35] If the newly identified cases do respond to the existing therapy and the new test has no negative attributes (e.g., safety, specificity, or cost), then use the new test without awaiting an RCT. If there are negative attributes, carefully contemplate the trade-offs before using the new test. In the situation where the more sensitive new test identifies additional cases that may not respond to therapy and one cannot deduce whether the extra cases represent the same spectrum of disease, awaiting RCTs is warranted.[33] Various RCT designs will evaluate the effect of emerging tests and testing strategies on patient-centric outcomes.[12] These diagnostic RCTs sometimes provide surprising results for accurate tests. For example, BNP is an accurate test to discriminate congestive heart failure from other etiologies of dyspnea (see Chapter 21), but multiple ED-based RCTs have not consistently identified significant patient-centric benefits to this new diagnostic technology.[36]

One proposal is to evaluate new tests using a hierarchical approach that groups research outcomes into six categories: technical efficacy, diagnostic accuracy efficacy, diagnostic thinking efficacy, therapeutic efficacy, clinical

Table 6.3 Hierarchical outcomes-based approach to diagnostic research

Level	Domain	Considerations
1	Technical efficacy	Acceptability
		Analytic sensitivity
		Intra- and interobserver reliability
		Feasibility
		Measurement inaccuracy and imprecision
		Operator dependence, training, and skill maintenance
2	Diagnostic accuracy efficacy	Area under the curve
		Likelihood ratios
		Predictive values
		Sensitivity and specificity
3	Diagnostic thinking efficacy	Confidence in diagnosis
		Cost of change in clinical diagnosis
		Differences in clinicians' posttest probability estimates before and after knowledge of test information
		Proportion of cases in which test was judged to be helpful
		Proportion of cases in which test changed the final diagnosis
4	Therapeutic efficacy	Proportion of cases in which further testing was avoided
		Proportion of cases in which management changed
		Total and per-patient cost with new diagnostic strategy
5	Patient outcome efficacy	Cost per unit of change in outcome variable
		Expected value of test in formation in quality-adjusted life years
		Functional status
		Morbidity avoided by testing
		Mortality
6	Societal efficacy	Cost-effectiveness analysis from societal perspective

Source: Drawn from [37,38].

outcome efficacy, and societal efficacy (Table 6.3).[37,38] These categories represent levels of diagnostic test assessment that progressively eliminate tests based upon their potential impact. Technical efficacy is the first level and serves to evaluate the operator and instrument characteristics, including reliability. The next level evaluates the diagnostic accuracy of the test using traditional measures. The third level is diagnostic thinking efficacy to assess the proportion of cases in which the final diagnosis changes because of the new test, as well as the costs entailed. The fourth level of research, therapeutic efficacy, evaluates the proportion of cases in which management changes based on the test information. The fifth level of research, patient outcome efficacy, evaluates the impact of the new test on symptom severity, functional status, and mortality including a cost-effectiveness analysis reporting the cost per unit change for each outcome variable using quality-adjusted life years. The sixth and final level of research evaluates the costs and benefits of the new test from a societal perspective.

The integration of most diagnostic tests into clinical practice occurs after the second level of assessment in this hierarchy. In fact, the evaluation of diagnostic tests in research settings is unlikely to follow this hierarchy in a linear fashion. Instead, this process is usually a cyclic and repetitive process.[38] This book will provide quantitative estimates of diagnostic accuracy while exploring the higher levels of diagnostic research whenever it exists. However, as the scientific methods for diagnostic research continue to evolve, readers must remain cognizant of ongoing studies that will continue to enhance clinicians' ability to accurately and reliably identify diseases in the ED.

References

1. Carpenter CR. Teaching lifelong learning skills: Journal club and beyond. In: Rogers RL, Mattu A, Winters M, Martinez J, editors. Practical teaching in emergency medicine. Oxford: Wiley-Blackwell; 2012.
2. Bossuyt PMM, Reitsma JB, Bruns DE, Gatsonis CA, Glasziou PP, Irwig L et al. The STARD statement for reporting studies of diagnostic accuracy: Explanation and elaboration. Annals of Internal Medicine. 2003; 138(1): W1–W12.
3. Smidt N, Rutjes AWS, van der Windt DAWM, Ostelo RWJg, Bossuyt PMM, Reitsma JB et al. Reproducibility of the STARD checklist: An instrument to assess the quality of reporting of diagnostic accuracy studies. BMC Medical Research Methodology. 2006; 6: 12.
4. Whiting P, Rutjes AWS, Dinnes J, Reitsma JB, Bossuyt PMM, Kleijnen J. A systematic review finds that diagnostic reviews fail to incorporate quality despite available tools. Journal of Clinical Epidemiology. 2005; 58(1): 1–12.
5. Whiting P, Rutjes AWS, Reitsma JB, Bossuyt PMM, Kleijnen J. The development of QUADAS: A tool for the quality assessment of studies of diagnostic accuracy included in systematic reviews. BMC Medical Research Methodology. 2003; 3: 25.
6. Whiting PF, Weswood ME, Rutjes AWS, Reitsma JB, Bossuyt PMM, Kleijnen J. Evaluation of QUADAS: A tool for the quality assessment of diagnostic accuracy studies. BMC Medical Research Methodology. 2006; 6: 9.
7. Whiting P, Rutjes AWS, Westwood ME, Mallett S, Deeks JJ, Reitsma JB et al. QUADAS-2: A revised tool for the quality assessment of diagnostic accuracy studies. Annals of Internal Medicine. 2011; 155(8): 529–36.

8. Stroup DF, Berlin JA, Morton SC, Olkin I, Williamson GD, Rennie D *et al*. Meta-analysis of observational studies in epidemiology: A proposal for reporting. Meta-Analysis of Observational Studies in Epidemiology (MOOSE) group. Journal of the American Medical Association. 2000; 283(15): 2008–12.

9. Macaskill P, Gatsonis C, Deeks JJ, Harbord RM, Takwoingi Y. Cochrane handbook for systematic reviews of diagnostic test accuracy. Version 0.9.0. London: The Cochrane Collaboration; 2010.

10. Ransohoff DF, Feinstein AR. Problems of spectrum and bias in evaluating the efficacy of diagnostic tests. New England Journal of Medicine. 1978; 299(17): 926–30.

11. Mower WR. Evaluating bias and variability in diagnostic test reports. Annals of Emergency Medicine. 1999; 33(1): 85–91.

12. Lijmer JG, Mol BW, Heisterkamp S, Bonsel GJ, Prins MH, van der Meulen JHP *et al*. Empirical evidence of design-related bias in studies of diagnostic tests. Journal of the American Medical Association. 1999; 282(11): 1061–6.

13. Newman TB, Kohn MA. Evidence-based diagnosis (practical guide to biostatistics and epidemiology). Cambridge: Cambridge University Press; 2009.

14. Egglin TK, Feinstein AR. Context bias: A problem in diagnostic radiology. Journal of the American Medical Association. 1996; 276(21): 1752–5.

15. Panzer RJ, Suchman AL, Griner PF. Workup bias in prediction research. Medical Decision Making. 1987; 7(2): 115–9.

16. Zhou XH. Correcting for verification bias in studies of a diagnostic test's accuracy. Statistical Methods in Medicine Research. 1998; 7(4): 337–53.

17. Diamond GA. Work-up bias. Journal of Clinical Epidemiology. 1993; 46(2): 207–9.

18. Kosinski AS, Barnhart HX. Accounting for nonignorable verification bias in assessment of diagnostic tests. Biometrics. 2003; 59(1): 163–71.

19. Glasziou P, Irwig L, Deeks JJ. When should a new test become the current reference standard? Annals of Internal Medicine. 2008; 149(11): 816–21.

20. Loy CT, Irwig L. Accuracy of diagnostic tests read with and without clinical information: A systematic review. Journal of the American Medical Association. 2004; 292(13): 1602–9.

21. Worster A, Carpenter C. Incorporation bias in studies of diagnostic tests: How to avoid being biased about bias. Canadian Journal of Emergency Medicine. 2008; 10(2): 174–5.

22. Mulherin SA, Miller WC. Spectrum bias or spectrum effect? Subgroup variation in diagnostic test evaluation. Annals of Internal Medicine. 2002; 137(7): 598–602.

23. Leeflang MMG, Bossuyt PMM, Irwig L. Diagnostic test accuracy may vary with prevalence: Implications for evidence-based diagnosis. Journal of Clinical Epidemiology. 2009; 62(1): 5–12.

24. Begg CB. Biases in the assessment of diagnostic tests. Statistics in Medicine. 1987; 6(4): 411–23.

25. Begg CB, McNeil BJ. Assessment of radiologic tests: Control of bias and other design considerations. Radiology. 1988; 167(2): 565–9.

26. Stein PD, Fowler SE, Goodman LR, Gottschalk A, Hales CA, Hull RD, *et al.* Multidetector computed tomography for acute pulmonary embolism. New England Journal of Medicine. 2006; 354(22): 2317–27.

27. Leeflang MMG, Deeks JJ, Gatsonis C, Bossuyt PMM. Systematic reviews of diagnostic test accuracy. Annals of Internal Medicine. 2008; 149(12): 889–97.

28. Deeks JJ, Macaskill P, Irwig L. The performance of tests of publication bias and other sample size effects in systematic reviews of diagnostic test accuracy was assessed. Journal of Clinical Epidemiology. 2005; 58(9): 882–93.

29. Simel DL, Rennie D. The rational clinical examination: Evidence-based clinical diagnosis. New York: McGraw-Hill; 2009.

30. Carpenter CR, Schuur JD, Everett WW, Pines JM. Evidence-based diagnostics: Adult septic arthritis. Academic Emergency Medicine. 2011; 18(8): 781–96.

31. Lang ES, Worster A. Getting the evidence straight in emergency diagnostics. Academic Emergency Medicine. 2011; 18(8): 797–9.

32. Schünemann AHJ, Oxman AD, Brozek J, Glasziou P, Jaeschke R, Vist GE *et al.* GRADE: Grading quality of evidence and strength of recommendations for diagnostic tests and strategies. British Medical Journal. 2008; 336(7653).

33. Lord SJ, Irwig L, Simes RJ. When is measuring sensitivity and specificity sufficient to evaluate a diagnostic test, and when do we need randomized trials? Annals of Internal Medicine. 2006; 144(11): 850–5.

34. Yee J, Kumar NN, Hung RK, Akerhar GA, Kumar PR, Wall SD. Comparison of supine and prone scanning separately and in combination at CT colonography. Radiology. 2003; 226(3): 653–61.

35. Newman DH, Schriger DL. Rethinking testing for pulmonary embolism: Less is more. Annals of Emergency Medicine. 2011; 57(6): 622–7.

36. Carpenter CR, Keim SM, Worster A, Rosen P. Brain natriuretic peptide in the evaluation of emergency department dyspnea: Is there a role? Journal of Emergency Medicine. 2012; 42(2): 197–205.

37. Pearl WS. A hierarchical outcomes approach to test assessment. Annals of Emergency Medicine. 1999; 33(1): 77–84.

38. Lijmer JG, Leeflang M, Bossuyt PMM. Proposals for a phased evaluation of medical tests. Medical Decision Making. 2009; 29(5): E13–E21.

SECTION 2
Trauma

Chapter 7 **Cervical Spine Fractures**

Highlights

- The prevalence of cervical spine injuries from blunt trauma is low (approximately 1–2%).
- Applying either of the clinical decision rules for bluntly injured patients (the Canadian C-spine rules or NEXUS low-risk rules) safely identifies low-risk patients in the ED who don't need neck radiography.
- CT imaging of the cervical spine is more sensitive than plain-film imaging, and should be the imaging modality of choice whenever available.
- Some seriously ill trauma patients who are neurologically intact with persistent midline tenderness and a negative CT have disco-ligamentous injuries and warrant MRI to definitively rule out injuries.

Background

More than 14 million patients undergo radiographic imaging of the cervical spine (C-spine) each year in the United States, with a clinically significant spine or cord injury found in less than 2% of all cases. As a result, many patients without injuries undergo negative radiographic evaluations. The development of sensitive clinical decision rules to help identify patients who are at extremely low risk of a cervical spine injury has been extremely useful for clinicians who hope to reduce unnecessary imaging.

Two rules have been developed using accepted clinical decision rule methodology: the National Emergency X-ray Utilization Study (NEXUS) criteria, referred to as the NEXUS low-risk rules (NLR), and the Canadian C-spine rules (CCR).[1,2] Each rule has been derived and validated in large and diverse populations of emergency department (ED) patients with very high sensitivity and negative predictive values (NPVs).

Evidence-Based Emergency Care: Diagnostic Testing and Clinical Decision Rules, Second Edition.
Jesse M. Pines, Christopher R. Carpenter, Ali S. Raja and Jeremiah D. Schuur.
© 2013 John Wiley & Sons, Ltd. Published 2013 by John Wiley & Sons, Ltd.

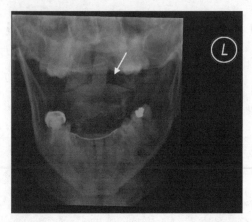

Figure 7.1 Open mouth odontoid cervical spine X-ray showing widening of the lateral pillar (arrow) of the first cervical vertebra, consistent with acute fracture.

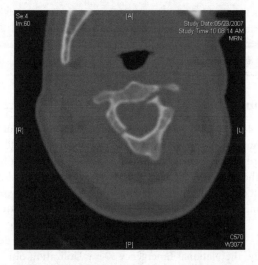

Figure 7.2 A second vertebral fracture is demonstrated on a cervical spine CT.

There are multiple radiographic modalities available to study the cervical spine, including plain films (Figure 7.1), computed tomography (CT) scan (Figure 7.2), and magnetic resonance imaging (MRI). While CT and MRI are more sensitive for fracture and are more accurate, plain films are more widely available and involve less radiation than CT. However, sometimes plain films are inadequate because of poor patient positioning, patient body habitus, or degenerative joint disease or age-related changes (such as osteophytes).

When the lateral view does not provide an adequate view of the C7–T1 space, repeat films with special (i.e., swimmer's) views are necessary in order to definitively rule out injuries. Instead of repeat films, physicians sometimes choose to perform CT scans on patients with inadequate X-rays. MRI provides additional information over the CT scan in that it can identify ligamentous and spinal cord injuries.

There is also an open question about what constitutes a significant C-spine injury. The two major decision rules for C-spine injuries were derived and validated using plain radiography, which is less sensitive than CT and MRI. Some clinicians may argue that the decision rules may not be sensitive enough and that any cervical spine fracture is important information, because patients with any fracture might be treated differently from those without a fracture through a better understanding of the prognosis, the treatment in terms of immobilization, or the provision of pain control. Examples of clinically insignificant fractures as defined by the derivation and validation studies of the NEXUS and Canadian C-spine rules include: spinous process fractures, simple wedge fractures without loss of 25% or more of vertebral body height, isolated avulsion fractures without accompanying ligamentous injury, Type 1 odontoid fractures, end plate fractures, fractures of osteophytes, trabecular bone injuries, and transverse process fractures. Finally, it is still an open question whether patients should receive an MRI to rule out ligamentous or spinal cord injury following another normal test (e.g., CT or plain radiography).

Clinical question

Which features of the history and physical exam identify patients at very low risk for clinically significant C-spine injuries who do not need radiography?

The NEXUS group used pilot study data and expert consensus to create a clinical decision rule that includes five elements (Table 7.1). The NEXUS criteria were assessed as present, absent, or unable to be assessed. Whenever a component of the NEXUS criteria was not able to be assessed, the patient was

Table 7.1 NEXUS low-risk criteria

- The absence of tenderness at the posterior midline of the cervical spine
- The absence of a focal neurologic deficit
- A normal level of alertness
- No evidence of intoxication
- The absence of clinically apparent pain that would distract a patient from the pain of a cervical injury

Source: Data from [1].

considered not to have met that criterion. Patients who met all five criteria were considered to be at low risk for clinically significant C-spine injury and to not require any radiography.

The initial study for the NEXUS criteria was a prospective observational study at 21 US medical centers that tested the hypothesis that blunt trauma patients who met all of the criteria would have an extremely low probability of C-spine injury. All patients who underwent imaging of the C-spine were included unless they had penetrating trauma or underwent imaging of the C-spine for a reason unrelated to trauma. Patients underwent either standard three-view imaging of the C-spine (lateral, anteroposterior, and open-mouth views) or advanced imaging (CT or MRI). The NEXUS criteria were applied in 34,069 patients who underwent imaging of the C-spine. The prevalence of radiographically documented C-spine injury was 2.4%. Table 7.2 shows the results of the study and the performance of the NEXUS criteria.

The criteria from this study missed a total of eight patients with documented C-spine injuries. Only two of those injuries were clinically significant as defined by the study; however, neither required surgical intervention or had any long-term clinical consequences. With 100% sensitivity and a 100% NPV, it was felt that patients meeting all of the criteria could safely be considered at extremely low risk for C-spine injury and did not need imaging.

Table 7.2 NEXUS low-risk criteria study results and test performance

Decision rule	Assessment result for any cervical spine injury		
	Positive	Negative	Totals
Positive	810	28,950	29,760
Negative	8	4,301	4,309
Totals	818	33,251	34,069
Sensitivity (CI)	99% (98–100%)		
Specificity (CI)	13% (13–13%)		
Positive likelihood ratio (LR+)	1.1		
Negative likelihood ratio (LR−)	0.08		
Decision rule	Clinically significant cervical spine injury		
	Positive	Negative	Totals
Positive	576	29,184	29,760
Negative	2	4,307	4,309
Totals	578	33,491	34,069
Sensitivity (CI)	100% (99–100%)		
Specificity (CI)	13% (13–13%)		
Positive likelihood ratio (LR+)	1.1		
Negative likelihood ratio (LR−)	0.03		

Source: Data from [1].

In a similar study performed at approximately the same time in Canada, Stiell and colleagues created the Canadian C-spine rules. This decision rule was first published as a derivation study in 2001.[2] Their goal was similar to that of the NEXUS investigators: to develop a prediction rule with extremely high sensitivity for detecting acute C-spine injuries in stable ED patients with blunt trauma. The authors conducted a prospective cohort study in 10 Canadian EDs and derived the clinical and historical factors that would optimize detection of a C-spine injury. In this, they differed from the NEXUS investigators, in that the NEXUS criteria did not consider the events surrounding the injury. Patients with blunt head or neck trauma were included in the study if they were alert (defined as a Glasgow Coma Scale (GCS) score of 15) and stable (defined as a systolic blood pressure >90 mm Hg and a respiratory rate greater than 10 but less than 24 breaths per minute). Patients were excluded if they met one of the following predefined criteria: age younger than 16 years, minor injuries not including blunt head or neck trauma (such as lacerations or abrasions), GCS <15, grossly abnormal vital signs, time since injury of greater than 48 hours, penetrating trauma, acute paralysis, known vertebral disease, return for reassessment of the same injury, or pregnancy.

Data were collected on 20 standardized clinical findings from the neurologic status, history, and physical exam. Patients underwent imaging of the C-spine at the discretion of the treating physician. Imaging of the C-spine was not mandatory; therefore, some patients did not undergo imaging. For those patients without C-spine imaging, a structured telephone follow-up was conducted to assess for missed injuries. The purpose of this hybridized criterion standard was to ensure that there were no missed injuries in patients who did not receive radiographs. Patients were considered not to have had a clinically significant C-spine injury if, during the telephone interview at 14 days, they met all of the following criteria: (i) neck pain rated as mild or none, (ii) restriction of neck movement rated as mild or none, (iii) use of a cervical collar not required, and (iv) neck injury did not prevent return of patient to usual occupational activities.

The Canadian C-spine rules include three sets of criteria that need to be evaluated in a stepwise manner. However, if a patient satisfies all of the criteria, the decision rule indicates a low risk of C-spine injury and radiography can be avoided. Table 7.3 lists the criteria that must be fulfilled in order to safely avoid imaging according to the Canadian C-spine rules.

For the derivation study, a total of 12,782 patients were eligible for the study; of those, 3,281 patients were not enrolled and another 577 patients were excluded because they did not undergo imaging and could not be reached for follow-up. A total of 8,924 patients were included in the final study group and had either radiographic imaging or the proxy 14-day telephone follow-up. The prevalence of documented cervical spine injury in

Table 7.3 The Canadian C-spine rules

- Criterion 1: Is there any high-risk factor that mandates radiography? Specifically, does the patient satisfy any of the following?
  - Age 65 years or older
  - Paresthesias in any extremity
  - Dangerous mechanism of injury (defined as a fall from 1 meter or greater, axial load to the head as in a diving injury, motor vehicle crash at high speed (>100 km/hr), rollover or ejection, or motorized recreational vehicle or bicycle collision)?

  If yes to any of these, radiographic imaging is recommended. If no, the second set of criteria is assessed.
- Criterion 2: Are there any low-risk factors that allow safe assessment of range of motion of the cervical spine? Specifically, are any of the following present: simple rear-end motor vehicle crash (excludes being pushed into oncoming traffic, hit by a bus or large truck, or hit by a high-speed vehicle, as well as rollovers), sitting position in the ED, ambulatory at any time, delayed onset of neck pain (defined as not immediate onset of neck pain), or absence of midline cervical spine tenderness? If none of these are present, radiographic imaging is recommended. If any one of these is present, the final criterion is assessed.
- Criterion 3: Is the patient able to actively rotate his or her neck 45 degrees to the left and right? If no, radiographic imaging is recommended. If yes, the patient meets all of the criteria to safely forgo imaging of the cervical spine.

Adapted from [2] Stiell IG, Wells GA, Vandemheen KL, et al The Canadian c-spine rule for radiography in alert and stable trauma patients. JAMA 2001; 286(15): 1841–1848 ©2001, American Medical Association, All Rights Reserved.
Source: Data from [2].

the study was 2%. Table 7.4 shows the study results and test performance. The stepwise nature of the CCR makes it more complicated than the NEXUS criteria and more difficult to remember; however, studies have shown that the rule can be used by paramedics in the field.[3]

Stiell and colleagues also compared both sets of rules in a large prospective study in the same EDs that participated in the derivation study for the Canadian C-spine rules.[4] The study aimed to compare the performances of the two rules (Canadian C-spine rules versus NEXUS) to determine which was more specific, and also to validate the Canadian C-spine rules. The methodologies for applying the clinical decision rules were the same as outlined in the original studies, but the inclusion and exclusion criteria of the Canadian C-spine rules derivation study were used and not all patients underwent imaging (consistent with the Canadian-C-spine rules study but in contrast to the NEXUS study). Criteria for both sets of rules were prospectively determined and recorded prior to C-spine imaging. The authors achieved their objective of validating the CCR. Among the 8,283 patients enrolled, 7,438 had complete data from both sets of rules and

Table 7.4 Canadian C-spine rules study results and test performance

Decision rule	Radiographically documented injury		
	Positive	Negative	Totals
Positive	151	5,041	5,192
Negative	0	3,732	3,732
Totals	151	8,773	8,924
Sensitivity (CI)	100% (98–100%)		
Specificity (CI)	43% (40–44%)		
Positive likelihood ratio (LR+)	1.8		
Negative likelihood ratio (LR−)	0		

Source: Data from [2].

underwent either C-spine imaging or the 14-day telephone proxy instrument. The incidence of C-spine injury in this study was 2%. Table 7.5 shows the test results and test characteristics. In comparing the performances of the NEXUS and the Canadian C-spine rules, the authors found the Canadian C-spine rules to have a higher sensitivity, NPV, and specificity. Table 7.6 shows the results and performances of the NLR.

Finally, in a study that assessed the effectiveness of a strategy to implement the CCR in multiple EDs using a matched-pair clustered-randomized design in 11,824 patients in 12 Canadian hospitals, patients seen at intervention sites had a relative reduction in C-spine imaging of 12.8% (CI 9–16%; 61.7% versus 53.3%; P = 0.01), and the control group had a relative increase of 12.5% (CI 7–18%; 52.8% versus 58.9%; p = 0.03).[5] In addition, the changes were significant when both groups were compared directly: there were no missed fractures and no adverse outcomes in either group. The authors

Table 7.5 Validation results of the Canadian C-spine rule and test performance

Decision rule	Radiographically documented injury		
	Positive	Negative	Totals
Positive	161	3,995	4,156
Negative	1	3,281	3,282
Totals	162	7,276	7,438
Sensitivity (CI)	100% (96–100%)		
Specificity (CI)	45% (44–46%)		
Positive likelihood ratio (LR+)	1.8		
Negative likelihood ratio (LR−)	0.01		

Source: Data from [4].

Table 7.6 NEXUS low-risk criteria test performance

Decision rule	Radiographically documented injury		
	Positive	Negative	Totals
Positive	147	4,599	4,746
Negative	15	2,677	2,692
Totals	162	7,276	7,438
Sensitivity (CI)		91% (85–94%)	
Specificity (CI)		37% (36–38%)	
Positive likelihood ratio (LR+)		1.4	
Negative likelihood ratio (LR−)		0.24	

Source: Data from [4].

concluded that implementation of the CCR could lead to a significant decrease in imaging without missing injuries.

Clinical question

How do the test performances of plain radiography and CT of the cervical spine compare for identifying cervical spine injuries after blunt trauma?
The increased availability of CT technology has resulted in more widespread use for C-spine imaging. An important question is how the test performance of CT compares to that of plain films, especially given that it is sometimes difficult to obtain adequate plain film images to rule out spinal fractures. A meta-analysis in 2005 examined the English language literature from 1995 to 2004 and found seven studies in which both types of imaging were performed.[6] Studies had to have C-spine plain imaging with at least three standard views (anteroposterior, lateral, and open-mouth odontoid) and CT scanning that extended from the occiput to the first thoracic vertebra with the distance between images of <5 mm. The analysis examined 3,834 patients and the criterion standards used were the final radiologist interpretation of all imaging studies for five of the studies and the CT results themselves in two of the studies. The prevalence of C-spine injury in the studies was 12%, which is notably higher than in a general population of ED patients. Given the heterogeneity of the studies, there was no consistent definition of what constituted an injury among all the pooled studies. The pooled sensitivity of plain radiography for detecting C-spine injury was 52% (CI 47–56%) while the pooled sensitivity of CT scanning of the C-spine was 98% (CI 96–99%) but, due to the lack of independent criterion standards in many of the studies, specificities could not be calculated for XR and CT.

A more recent study tried to further define this question by stratifying injuries into clinically significant injuries (defined as those requiring an operative procedure, halo application, or rigid cervical collar), and further defined them into high risk, moderate risk, and low risk in a single Level I trauma center, based on the type of injury.[7] Patients were included who met one or more of the NEXUS criteria. In 1,505 patients, 78 (5%) had an injury on either plain C-spine radiography or C-spine CT. Of those, 50 (3% of the total) had clinically significant injuries. CT was 100% sensitive for clinically significant injuries, while C-spine radiography only detected 18, yielding a 36% sensitivity. For high-risk, moderate-risk, and low-risk C-spine injuries, plain radiography was 46%, 37%, and 25% sensitive, respectively.

Clinical question

Which alert, neurologically intact patients with negative radiography should receive an MRI to assess for ligamentous and spinal cord injury?

A recent study examined this precise question, specifically to find factors associated with cervical disc or ligamentous injury found on MRI in alert trauma patients with a negative CT and persistent midline tenderness on physical examination.[8] The study was performed in one Australian hospital (a Level I trauma center) and studied patients who underwent a CT and an MRI for persistent tenderness. The outcomes in the study were the presence and extent of MRI-detected injury of the cervical ligaments, intervertebral discs, spinal cord, or associated soft tissues. In 178 patients with negative CT imaging, 78 (44%) had acute cervical injuries found on MRI. Thirty-eight patients (21% of the overall sample) required intervention: thirty-three patients with cervical collars ranging from 2 to 12 weeks and five patients with operative management, one of whom had delayed instability. Factors associated with a higher number of spinal columns injured included CT-detected advanced cervical spondylosis (OR 11.6, CI 3.9–34.3%), minor isolated thoracolumbar fractures (OR 5.4, CI 1.5–19.7%), and multidirectional C-spine forces (OR 2.5, CI 1.2–5.2%).

Comment

The NEXUS and the Canadian C-spine rules have both been validated in large cohorts of ED patients with blunt trauma to the neck. In the validation cohorts, both have high sensitivities (>99.3%) and negative predictive values (>99.9%) making both decision rules safe. In addition, a recent multicenter study has found that implementation of the CCR is associated with lower use of spine radiography.

When comparing the two rules, Stiell and colleagues concluded that the Canadian C-spine rules performed better than the NEXUS criteria. We feel that there are sufficient differences between the two rules and the studies supporting them to make the issue not as clear cut. Table 7.7 compares and contrasts the differences in the derivation, validation, and implementation of these rules.

Given the differences, we believe both rules are useful for assessing the stable patient with blunt trauma. Overall, the NEXUS criteria are somewhat easier to use clinically because they are less difficult to remember. The Canadian C-spine rules are more complex and must be employed in a stepwise fashion. In our experience, the most common reason for failure of the NEXUS criteria and for requirement of cervical radiography is midline tenderness. The Canadian C-spine rules are more specific than the NEXUS criteria, and patients with midline tenderness can be identified who do not otherwise meet criteria for cervical radiography.

Because of the higher specificity of the Canadian C-spine rules, we propose that the CCR criteria be applied as a first step in the ED. While both the NEXUS and the Canadian rules have roughly equal high sensitivity and high negative predictive values, Canadian rules will have many fewer false positives. This is not to say that the NEXUS criteria should not be used, but you should be aware that while the NPV is very high with both sets of rules, the very low specificity of the NEXUS criteria will lead to more unnecessary imaging (i.e., false positives in which the prediction rule indicates the patient is not low risk and therefore recommends imaging). We would point out that either rule was not designed to be used in isolation of other clinical information. If there are historical or exam findings that lead you to have a high suspicion for C-spine injury, then you should proceed to imaging and not apply any clinical decision rule. Regarding whether or not plain films or CT C-spine should be the initial test of choice in blunt cervical trauma, it appears in the limited studies of highly selected trauma patients that CT C-spine has a higher sensitivity for detecting C-spine injury compared to plain-film imaging. However, in these studies, the overall prevalence of C-spine injury was much higher than is seen in everyday ED practice. In fact, it was nearly six times higher than in the NEXUS and Canadian studies. This selection bias makes it difficult to generalize the patients in these studies (patients were enrolled at primary trauma centers) to the typical patient after a minor motor vehicle crash who is seen in the ED outside of the trauma bay. Regardless, at this time, in patients suspected of C-spine injury, our opinion is that you should consider CT imaging over plain radiographs, especially in high-risk cases. However, radiation exposure and cost are the two factors that have not been sufficiently explored. While there may be subgroups of patients who would benefit from CT scanning over plain radiography (such

Table 7.7 Comparison of NEXUS criteria and the Canadian C-spine rule

	NEXUS low-risk criteria (NLR)	Canadian C-spine rule (CCR)	Comment
Explicit description for each criterion in the rule	Intoxication and painful distracting injury left undefined	High-risk mechanism defined by the authors	NLR • Authors felt that intoxication and painful distracting injury were best determined clinically and that strict definitions would limit use in clinical practice. CCR • Intoxication not included as it was found in the preliminary studies to not be predictive of injury. • Provided list of high-risk mechanisms, but many others exist that are not explicitly listed.
Patient enrollment	Patients with blunt trauma undergoing cervical imaging	Patients with complete data (undergoing either imaging or 14-day proxy telephone survey)	NLR • Risk of selection bias based on whether or not at-risk patients got initial imaging, possibly limiting generalizability. CCR • Not all patients had criterion standard (imaging), but proxy tool accounted for those patients without imaging.
Exclusion criteria	Patients with penetrating trauma or who had cervical imaging for reasons other than blunt trauma	Excluded conditions explicitly listed	NLR • These are reasonable given the emphasis on blunt trauma. CCR • Exclusion criteria limit generalizability.

(continued)

Table 7.7 (*continued*)

	NEXUS low-risk criteria (NLR)	Canadian C-spine rule (CCR)	Comment
Age criteria	None	Age 16 years or older	NLR • No age limitation. CCR • Excluded patients younger than 16 years, limiting generalizability.
Prevalence of clinically significant injury	2%	2%	–
Study size (validation study)	>34,000 patients in 21 US medical centers	>7,400 patients in nine Canadian medical centers	Diverse ED patient populations make results generalizable.
Sensitivity, % (validation study)	99% (CI 98–100%)	100% (CI 96–100%)	Comparable sensitivities, with correspondingly high negative predictive values (NPVs).
Specificity, % (validation study)	13% (CI 12.8–13.0%)	45.1% (CI 44–46%)	The CCR has a significantly higher specificity and therefore fewer false positives.
Decision rule usability	Five elements to determine as present or absent	A total of three sets of criteria, totaling 14 elements to determine; some dictate imaging, others dictate no imaging.	NLR • With fewer elements and a straightforward interpretation, it is simpler to use. CCR • Many elements make it cumbersome to use. • Age criteria simplify approach for older patients.

as patients with obesity, a history of degenerative joint disease, advanced age, or prior surgery), there are not good data on this topic.

Finally, performing MRI in stable, awake trauma patients with persistent C-spine tenderness and a negative CT may detect important injuries, particularly because of the relatively high prevalence of injuries for which a different management plan may be indicated. However, it is important to understand that the referenced study was conducted in a select group of patients seen by the trauma team (i.e., already very high-risk patients). Therefore, we do not recommend performing an MRI in relatively low-risk ED patients who have midline tenderness without other injuries. In addition, it is important to note that the study was performed in just one hospital, and the editor's note attached to the article opined that the results should be replicated before any clinical practice is changed based on the results of the study.

References

1. Hoffman JR, Mower WR, Wolfson AB *et al.* Validity of a set of clinical criteria to rule out injury to the cervical spine in patients with blunt trauma. New England Journal of Medicine. 2000; 343(2): 94–9.

2. Stiell IG, Wells GA, Vandemheen KL *et al.* The Canadian c-spine rule for radiography in alert and stable trauma patients. Journal of the American Medical Association. 2001; 286(15): 1841–8.

3. Vaillancourt C, Stiell IG, Beaudoin T *et al.* The out-of-hospital validation of the Canadian C-spine rule by paramedics. Annals of Emergency Medicine. 2009 Nov; 54(5): 663–71.

4. Stiell IG, Clement CM, McKnight RD *et al.* The Canadian C-spine rule versus the NEXUS low-risk criteria in patients with trauma. New England Journal of Medicine. 2003; 349(26): 2510–18.

5. Stiell IG, Clement CM, Grimshaw J *et al.* Implementation of the Canadian C-spine rule: prospective 12 centre cluster randomised trial. British Medical Journal. 2009 Oct 29; 339: b4146.

6. Holmes JF, Akkinepalli R. Computed tomography versus plain radiography to screen for cervical spine injury: A meta-analysis. Journal of Trauma. 2005; 58: 902–5.

7. Bailitz J, Starr F, Beecroft M *et al.* CT should replace three-view radiographs as the initial screening test in patients at high, moderate, and low risk for blunt cervical spine injury: A prospective comparison. Journal of Trauma. 2009 Jun; 66(6): 1605–9.

8. Ackland HM, Cameron PA, Varma DK *et al.* Cervical spine magnetic resonance imaging in alert, neurologically intact trauma patients with persistent midline tenderness and negative computed tomography results. Annals of Emergency Medicine. 2011 Dec; 58(6): 521–30.

Chapter 8 Cervical Spine Fractures in Children

Highlights

- The prevalence of traumatic cervical spine injuries in children who sustain blunt trauma is approximately 1%.
- The NEXUS criteria can be used in all children but were developed from a dataset with very few injuries in children ≤8 years old.
- In children needing cervical spine imaging after blunt trauma, X-ray should be the modality of choice.
- If imaging is needed in children ≤8 years old, those having a head CT performed or in whom an adequate odontoid X-ray cannot be obtained should have a CT of the occiput to C3, given their higher risk for high-cervical-spine injury.
- New decision rules for younger children are being developed but have not yet been prospectively validated.

Background

Cervical spine (C-spine) injuries occur rarely in the pediatric blunt trauma population; their overall prevalence is approximately 1.3%, increasing in a stepwise fashion from 0.4% in infants to 2.6% in adolescents.[1] Despite this, C-spine computed tomography (CT) imaging of injured children continues to increase, especially outside of Level I pediatric trauma centers.[2] In order to minimize unnecessary ionizing radiation exposure in children and to ensure the appropriateness of C-spine imaging while also maximizing patient safety, emergency physicians need to be able to identify a subset of patients at very low risk of clinically significant injury who can have their C-spines safely cleared without imaging.

Evidence-Based Emergency Care: Diagnostic Testing and Clinical Decision Rules, Second Edition.
Jesse M. Pines, Christopher R. Carpenter, Ali S. Raja and Jeremiah D. Schuur.
© 2013 John Wiley & Sons, Ltd. Published 2013 by John Wiley & Sons, Ltd.

Table 8.1 The NEXUS low-risk criteria

- The absence of tenderness at the posterior midline of the cervical spine
- The absence of a focal neurologic deficit
- A normal level of alertness
- No evidence of intoxication
- The absence of clinically apparent pain that would distract a patient from the pain of a cervical injury

Source: Data from [3].

Clinical question

Which features of the history and physical exam identify children who are at very low risk of clinically significant cervical spine injury and do not need radiography?

There is one large multicenter prospective study that examines a clinical decision rule for obtaining C-spine radiographs in pediatric patients with blunt trauma.[3] The study was a prespecified analysis of patients enrolled in NEXUS in which the NEXUS criteria were applied to patients <18 years of age (Table 8.1).

The NEXUS cohort comprised 34,069 patients and included 3,065 pediatric patients (9% of the total study cohort).[4] The incidence of C-spine injury in the pediatric subgroup was 1.0% (n = 30) and Table 8.2 shows the performance of the NEXUS criteria in children. A perfect sensitivity was achieved, but due to the low number of actual injuries, the confidence intervals are wide (88–100%). The authors pointed out that of the 603 (approximately 20%) patients who the NEXUS criteria classified as low risk (the decision rule was negative), no C-spine injury occurred. They do note, however, that while 817 of the 3,065 (27%) patients were 3–8 years old, only four of them (0.5%) had C-spine injuries. Similarly, 88 (2.8%) of the 3,065

Table 8.2 Test characteristics for the NEXUS low-risk rules in children

Decision rule	Radiographically documented injury		
	Positive	Negative	Totals
Positive	30	2,432	2,462
Negative	0	603	603
Totals	30	3,035	3,065
Sensitivity (CI)		100% (88–100%)	
Specificity (CI)		20% (19–21%)	
Positive likelihood ratio (LR+)		1.3	
Negative likelihood ratio (LR−)		0.08	

Source: Data from [3].

Table 8.3 PECARN factors associated with cervical spine injury in children after blunt trauma

- Altered mental status
- Focal neurologic findings
- Neck pain
- Torticollis
- Substantial torso injury
- Conditions predisposing to cervical spine injury
- Diving
- High-risk motor vehicle crash

Source: Data from [5].

patients were 0–2 years old and none of them sustained C-spine injuries. The authors concluded that, while the NEXUS criteria can safely be used in children older than 8 years, they should be used with caution in children aged 8 years or younger, due to the low number of injuries recorded in their study population.

While NEXUS is the largest prospectively collected dataset of children at risk for C-spine injury, two recent studies have also focused on the development of decision instruments designed to identify a subset of patients at low risk for injury. Leonard et al conducted a case–control study of children younger than 16 years who received C-spine X-rays after blunt trauma in hospitals in the Pediatric Emergency Care Applied Research Network (PECARN).[5] They reviewed 540 patients with C-spine injuries (defined as injuries to the cervical vertebrae, ligaments, or spinal cord as well as any spinal cord injury without radiographic association) and matched them to controls without injury, identifying eight factors associated with C-spine injury (Table 8.3). Having one or more of the factors was 98% (CI 96–99%) sensitive and 26% (CI 23–29%) specific for C-spine injury, with a LR+ of 1.3 and a LR− of 0.08. While the use of these factors as a decision rule needs validation, they show promise as a decision rule with discriminative ability similar to that of NEXUS.

Pieretti-Vanmarcke et al reviewed trauma registries from 22 Level I or Level II trauma centers, focusing on children <3 years old who had sustained blunt trauma.[6] They found 12,537 patients meeting these criteria, developed a decision rule with two-thirds of this population, and then validated it on the remaining one-third. Their population contained 83 (0.66%) confirmed C-spine injury patients (defined as any osseous or ligamentous injury to the cervical spine seen on CT, radiograph, or MRI), and their decision rule (Table 8.4) had a range from 0 to 8; a score of 0 or 1 had a sensitivity of

Table 8.4 Decision rule to identify children <3 years old who are at low risk for cervical spine imaging

Patients with total scores of 0 or 1 point may not need cervical spine imaging performed:	
• GCS < 14	(3 points)
• Motor vehicle accident	(2 points)
• GCS (eye) = 1	(2 points)
• Age > 2 years	(1 point)

Source: Data from [6].

93%, a specificity of 70%, a LR+ of 3.1, and a LR− of 0.10 for excluding C-spine injury. While the rule was developed retrospectively from a trauma registry and clearly needs refinement and multicenter prospective validation before it is applied, it shows promise in a younger age group that has not yet been the focus of an imaging decision rule, and which was specifically underrepresented in NEXUS.

Clinical question

Which cervical spine–imaging modality should be used when evaluating pediatric patients with blunt trauma who cannot be clinically cleared?

Given the increased risks of radiation exposure in children, the choice of which imaging modality to use in pediatric blunt trauma patients who cannot be clinically cleared by NEXUS is an important one.[7] Pediatric anatomy, especially increased head size in young children, places greater torque and accelerational stress higher in the C-spine than in adults, increasing the likelihood of upper C-spine injury in these patients. In order to balance radiation exposure with this increased risk of high-C-spine injury, CT imaging of the occiput to C3 is often recommended in these younger children who cannot be clinically cleared.[8]

Garton and Hammer retrospectively reviewed records over a 20-year period from their institution and found 239 pediatric blunt trauma patients with final diagnoses of C-spine injury based on billing codes, 187 (78%) of whom had adequate radiologic records.[9] In the 157 patients aged 8 years or older, X-rays were 93% sensitive for the detection of C-spine injuries, while the addition of occiput to C3 CT scans increased this sensitivity to 97%. In the smaller group of 33 (22%) patients younger than 8 years old, X-rays were only 75% sensitive, and sensitivity increased to 94% with the limited CT described in this chapter. While this study is limited by its retrospective nature and reliance on billing codes (since they included only patients with known diagnoses, specificities could not be calculated, and the true number of missed injuries is unknown), it is the largest set of children with blunt traumatic C-spine injuries in the literature.

Although their study contained fewer injuries in children 8 years old or younger, Viccellio et al noted that all of the children were diagnosed by X-rays, and one 16-year-old girl had a C7 fracture missed by CT examination.[3] Similarly, Hernandez et al performed a retrospective review of 606 children undergoing emergency department C-spine imaging at their institution, 459 (76%) of whom were cleared using clinical examination and X-ray findings.[10] Of the remaining 147 patients evaluated with CT, only four (2.7%) had positive findings of fracture, dislocation, or instability, and all of them also had positive findings on their X-rays.

Comment

In the only prospective study examining a decision rule regarding risk determination for C-spine injury in children with blunt trauma, Viccellio et al validated the NEXUS criteria as being highly sensitive. Exploration of their data also found no cases of spinal cord injury without radiographic abnormality (SCIWORA) in any child, which is a lingering concern in the minds of clinicians. The authors were careful to note that there were 3,065 patients with only 30 C-spine injuries, resulting in wide CIs around the test parameters, despite their having not missed any cases of C-spine injury. They further reported that it would require a study of nearly 80,000 children to narrow the CIs to within 0.5%, making it unlikely that another study will improve on the current performance of the NEXUS criteria.

A major concern that clinicians may have is applying the NEXUS criteria to infants (0–2 years) and toddlers (2–8 years) as they may be nonverbal or it may be difficult to accurately determine whether any individual item is present or absent. While only four of the 30 C-spine injuries occurred in patients ≤8 years old, at least one criterion was positive in each of those four patients. Until a new decision rule focusing on this younger population is developed and validated, we recommend using the NEXUS in all pediatric patients, with the caveat that the inability to obtain certain NEXUS criteria on very young patients should not imply their absence.

In children needing radiographic evaluation for C-spine injury after blunt trauma, we recommend X-ray as the modality of choice. In patients ≤8 years old who are also obtaining head CT or in whom an odontoid view is unobtainable, we recommend a CT of the occiput to C3, given the increased incidence of high-C-spine injuries in this population.

References

1. Mohseni S, Talving P, Branco BC *et al*. Effect of age on cervical spine injury in pediatric population: A National Trauma Data Bank review. Journal of Pediatric Surgery. 2011; 46(9): 1771–6.

2. Mannix R, Nigrovic LE, Schutzman SA *et al*. Factors associated with the use of cervical spine computed tomography imaging in pediatric trauma patients. Academic Emergency Medicine. 2011; 18(9): 905–11.

3. Viccellio P, Simon H, Pressman BD *et al*. A prospective multicenter study of cervical spine injury in children. Pediatrics. 2001; 108(2): e20.

4. Hoffman JR, Mower WR, Wolfson AB, Todd KH, Zucker MI. Validity of a set of clinical criteria to rule out injury to the cervical spine in patients with blunt trauma: National Emergency X-Radiography Utilization Study Group. New England Journal of Medicine. 2000; 343(2): 94–9.

5. Leonard JC, Kuppermann N, Olsen C *et al*. Factors associated with cervical spine injury in children after blunt trauma. Annals of Emergency Medicine. 2011; 58(2): 145–55.

6. Pieretti-Vanmarcke R, Velmahos GC, Nance ML *et al*. Clinical clearance of the cervical spine in blunt trauma patients younger than 3 years: A multi-center study of the American Association for the Surgery of Trauma. Journal of Trauma. 2009; 67(3): 543–9; discussion 549–50.

7. Brenner DJ, Elliston CD, Hall EJ, Berdon WE. Estimated risks of radiation-induced fatal cancer from pediatric CT. American Journal of Roentgenology. 2001; 176(2): 289–96.

8. Chung S, Mikrogianakis A, Wales PW *et al*. Trauma Association of Canada Pediatric Subcommittee National Pediatric Cervical Spine Evaluation Pathway: Consensus guidelines. The Journal of Trauma: Injury, Infection, and Critical Care. 2011; 70: 873–84.

9. Garton HJL, Hammer MR. Detection of pediatric cervical spine injury. Neurosurgery. 2008; 62(3): 700–8.

10. Hernandez JA, Chupik C, Swischuk LE. Cervical spine trauma in children under 5 years: Productivity of CT. Emergency Radiology. 2004; 10(4): 176–8.

Chapter 9 **Cervical Spine Fractures in Older Adults**

Highlights

- The prevalence of traumatic cervical spine injury in older adults (≥65 years of age) is approximately double that of younger patients.
- Clinicians should have a low threshold for imaging the cervical spine in older adults due to anatomic and physiologic changes that are less tolerant of even minor trauma.
- The NEXUS low-risk criteria's sensitivity in the subgroup of older adults rivals its sensitivity for all patients.

Background

Older adults (≥65 years of age) who present to the emergency department (ED) for evaluation after blunt trauma should be evaluated for potential cervical spine (C-spine) injuries. Anatomic and physiologic factors associated with these older patients, including osteopenia, osteophytes, and relative immobility, predispose them to C-spine injuries even by low-impact or minimal-energy mechanisms. In addition, one of the most commonly used decision rules to identify patients who are at low risk for clinically significant C-spine injury (the Canadian C-spine rules) identifies patients who are 65 years and older as a high-risk group who should all receive imaging. The overall one-year mortality for older adults who sustain C-spine fractures is between 24% and 28%, necessitating that emergency physicians evaluating these patients remain acutely aware of the significance of these injuries in this population.[1,2]

Evidence-Based Emergency Care: Diagnostic Testing and Clinical Decision Rules, Second Edition.
Jesse M. Pines, Christopher R. Carpenter, Ali S. Raja and Jeremiah D. Schuur.
© 2013 John Wiley & Sons, Ltd. Published 2013 by John Wiley & Sons, Ltd.

Clinical question

Are there decision rules for determining which older adult patients are at low risk for cervical spine injury?

There are three studies that address the issue of a clinical decision rule to identify older adults with a low risk of C-spine injury. Two of these examine subsets of patients from the NEXUS low-risk criteria study: one evaluates the very elderly (age ≥80 years),[3] and the other evaluates the population of older adults typically classified as elderly (age ≥65 years).[4] A third study examined patients 65 years and older in order to stratify C-spine injury risk and guide appropriate imaging.[5]

The first of the studies is a subgroup analysis of 1,070 patients from the NEXUS study who were 80 years of age or older.[3] The NEXUS low-risk criteria state that C-spine radiography can be avoided if five clinical criteria are met (Table 9.1). The predefined study objective was to test the performance of the NEXUS criteria in this very elderly patient population. In addition, the injury patterns were examined to determine how injuries sustained in this subgroup differed from those of the entire study population. Their results demonstrated that the prevalence of C-spine injury in this patient group was 4.7%, almost twice that of the total NEXUS cohort (2.4%). Table 9.2 shows the test performance in this subgroup.

No injuries were missed in this cohort. A total of 13% of patients were correctly identified as being low risk, representing those who could have forgone cervical imaging. Injuries of the first and second cervical vertebrae accounted for nearly half of all injuries (47%), in contrast to younger patients in whom the lower C-spine was injured more frequently.

The second study is a subgroup analysis of the 2,943 patients from the NEXUS study who were 65 years or older.[4] The prevalence of C-spine injury in this subgroup was 4.6%, which is similar to that of the very elderly population in the first study. The authors examined the performance of the NEXUS criteria among this group and found that they had an overall

Table 9.1 The NEXUS low-risk criteria

- The absence of tenderness at the posterior midline of cervical spine
- The absence of a focal neurologic deficit
- A normal level of alertness
- No evidence of intoxication
- The absence of clinically apparent pain that would distract a patient from the pain of a cervical injury

Source: Data from [4].

Table 9.2 Performance of the NEXUS criteria among patients 80 years and older

| Decision rule | Radiographically documented injury | | |
	Positive	Negative	Totals
Positive	50	888	938
Negative	0	132	132
Totals	50	1,020	1,070
Sensitivity (CI)	100% (93–100%)		
Specificity (CI)	13% (11–15%)		
Positive likelihood ratio (LR+)	1.1		
Negative likelihood ratio (LR−)	0		

Source: Data from [4].

Table 9.3 Performance of NEXUS among patients 65 years and older

	Sensitivity, % (CI)	Specificity, % (CI)	Positive likelihood ratio (LR+)	Negative likelihood ratio (LR−)
Assessment result for any cervical injury	99% (95–100%)	15% (15–15%)	1.2	0.07
Clinically significant cervical injury	100% (97–100%)	15% (15–15%)	1.2	0

Source: Data from [4].

sensitivity of 99% for any cervical injury and 100% for clinically significant cervical injury (Table 9.3).

Cervical spine injuries occurred in a total of 135 elderly patients, with the NEXUS criteria identifying all but two injuries. Neither of the two injuries misclassified by the NEXUS criteria required surgical intervention. Analysis of the specific types of injuries occurring in this population aged 65 years or older revealed that fractures of C1 and C2 represented more than half of all cervical fractures, similar to the very elderly population noted in the first study. Among the individual NEXUS criteria not met and thus responsible for patients not being classified as low risk, midline tenderness (present in 53% of patients) and distracting injury (present in 44%) were the most frequent.

In the most recent study, performed specifically to examine C-spine fractures in elderly patients, Bub et al performed a case–control study

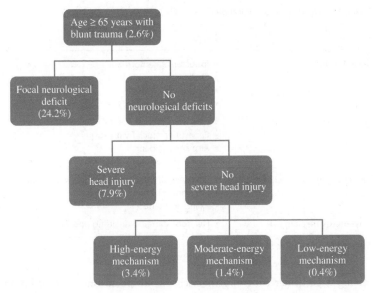

Figure 9.1 Schematic of clinical prediction rule for cervical spine fractures in elderly patients in a trauma registry. The risk of cervical spine fractures in each subgroup is shown in parentheses. (Source: Reproduced from [5]. Percentages correspond to absolute cervical fracture risk).

among trauma registry patients in Seattle, Washington, from 1995 to 2002.[5] Their objective was to derive and validate a clinical decision rule that identified C-spine fracture, using clinical and historical elements to guide imaging in patients aged 65 years or older.

Cases were identified for inclusion from their inpatient trauma registry. Only patients 65 years or older with nonpenetrating trauma who had confirmatory cervical imaging prior to death were eligible. Patients transferred to the trauma center were excluded in an effort to minimize referral bias. Controls were chosen from among ED patients seen between 1995 and 2002 (admitted or discharged) who were age 65 years or older, had blunt trauma with the absence of cervical fracture, and were also not transferred to the ED. Statistical methods adjusted for confounding. The prevalence of C-spine fracture was 2.6% among all the trauma registry patients meeting the inclusion criteria during the study period (n = 3958). One hundred and three cases and 107 control patients were identified and included in the analysis. The final clinical prediction rule (Figure 9.1) is able to stratify patients according to cervical fracture risk and uses the author definitions listed in Table 9.4. The authors do not give recommendations for or against

Table 9.4 Definitions for clinical prediction rule

Criterion	Definition
Severe head injury	• Intracranial hemorrhage • Skull fracture • Unconsciousness • All intubated patients
High-energy mechanism	• Falls from 10-foot height • Pedestrian struck by an auto • Airplane accident • High-speed motor vehicle injury ($\geq$ 30 mph)
Moderate-energy mechanism	• Low-speed motor vehicle injury ($<$ 30 mph) • Fall from $<$10 feet • Skiing accident
Low-energy mechanism	• Fall from standing or sitting position

Source: Reproduced from [5].

imaing a particular subgroup themselves, but aimed only to develop an understanding of the risk for cervical fracture in each subgroup, allowing individual clinicians to use that risk when deciding who to image.

Comments

It is clinically intuitive that older patients can sustain C-spine injuries from traumatic mechanisms that might not cause injury in younger patients, such as falling out of a chair or from standing height. Furthermore, older patients may not report symptoms or circumstances in as clear a manner as younger patients because of underlying medical illnesses or cognitive impairment. However, we would exercise caution in using the clinical prediction rule developed by Bub et al[5] It was derived and validated in the same setting, done so retrospectively from chart review of a preselected trauma registry population, and identified only cervical spine fractures rather than all types of clinically significant injury. The simple conclusion that all older patients are at risk of cervical fractures does nothing to support a more selective approach to imaging, which was the goal of both the NEXUS and Canadian C-spine studies (discussed in Chapter 7).

In contrast to the NEXUS criteria, the Canadian C-spine rules have an age criterion and do not allow for avoidance of imaging in patients $\geq$65 years old. To date, no subset analysis of elderly patients from the Canadian dataset has been published. Nevertheless, the two secondary analyses from the NEXUS study reveal that using the NEXUS criteria allows identification of patients at low risk of cervical spine injury with a very high sensitivity in both the elderly (≥65 years) and the very elderly (≥80 years). While there has been one published case report in which the application of the NEXUS criteria to a 101-year-old patient resulted in misclassification of the patient as low risk for cervical spine injury, the case (and the few others like it that remain unpublished) should not deter emergency physicians from applying the well-validated NEXUS criteria to elderly patients given the two subset analyses noted in this chapter.[3,4,6]

References

1. Harris MB, Reichmann WM, Bono CM *et al.* Mortality in elderly patients after cervical spine fractures. Journal of Bone and Joint Surgery, American Volume. 2010; 92(3): 567–74.

2. Damadi AA, Saxe AW, Fath JJ, Apelgren KN. Cervical spine fractures in patients 65 years or older: A 3-year experience at a level I trauma center. Journal of Trauma. 2008; 64(3): 745–8.

3. Ngo B, Hoffman JR, Mower WR. Cervical spine injury in the very elderly. Emergency Radiology. 2000; 7(5): 287–91.

4. Touger M, Gennis P, Nathanson N *et al.* Validity of a decision rule to reduce cervical spine radiography in elderly patients with blunt trauma. Annals of Emergency Medicine. 2002; 40(3): 287–93.

5. Bub LD, Blackmore CC, Mann FA, Lomoschitz FM. Cervical spine fractures in patients 65 years and older: A clinical prediction rule for blunt trauma. Radiology. 2005; 234(1): 143–9.

6. Barry TB, McNamara RM. Clinical decision rules and cervical spine injury in an elderly patient: A word of caution. Journal of Emergency Medicine. 2005; 29(4): 433–6.

Chapter 10 **Blunt Abdominal Trauma**

Highlights

- There are many diagnostic tests available to evaluate for the presence of intra-abdominal injury in patients with blunt abdominal trauma including CT scan, focused assessment with sonography for trauma (FAST), and diagnostic peritoneal lavage (DPL).
- FAST is highly sensitive and accurate in adult patients and is a useful, rapid, non-invasive adjunct used routinely in the evaluation of blunt abdominal trauma.
- FAST is particularly useful in patients who are too unstable for CT imaging.
- High clinical suspicion in the setting of a negative FAST should prompt further evaluation by CT scanning or surgical exploration.
- FAST should be used with caution in pediatric trauma patients due to its poor sensitivity in this population.

Background

In the acutely injured patient with abdominal trauma, there are a number of diagnostic modalities available in the emergency department (ED) to detect the presence of solid organ injury and intra-abdominal hemorrhage. There have been many studies comparing abdominal ultrasound with computed tomography (CT) scan, most of which have shown that CT is superior to ultrasound in detecting intra-abdominal injuries. However, CT does have drawbacks, primarily that it cannot be safely performed in unstable patients. In these hemodynamically unstable patients, a diagnostic peritoneal lavage (DPL) was historically used the detect the presence of intra-abdominal blood. Over the past 10 years, however, diagnostic ultrasound in the form of a focused assessment with sonography for trauma (FAST) exam has emerged

Evidence-Based Emergency Care: Diagnostic Testing and Clinical Decision Rules, Second Edition.
Jesse M. Pines, Christopher R. Carpenter, Ali S. Raja and Jeremiah D. Schuur.
© 2013 John Wiley & Sons, Ltd. Published 2013 by John Wiley & Sons, Ltd.

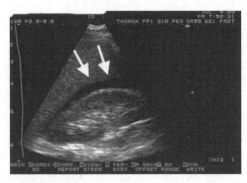

Figure 10.1 A focused assessment by sonography in trauma (FAST) reveals fluid in Morison's pouch (arrows). (Courtesy of Anthony J. Dean, MD).

as a safe, rapid, and non-invasive alternative to DPL in unstable patients treated in hospitals at which ED ultrasound is available (Figure 10.1). While the FAST exam is not 100% sensitive and thus cannot completely rule out the presence of intra-abdominal injuries, it is often used during the initial evaluation of trauma patients to provide early information and rule in intra-abdominal bleeding.

Clinical questions

How accurate is FAST compared to CT scan in adult patients with blunt abdominal trauma?
An early study that compared diagnostic peritoneal lavage to ultrasound and CT scan was performed in China.[1] Liu et al prospectively compared the accuracy of the three modalities for the detection of significant intra-abdominal injuries. Patients with stable vital signs after their initial resuscitation and who had equivocal physical examination findings underwent CT and ultrasound, followed by DPL. If any of the three exams were positive, the investigators performed a laparotomy. They compared surgical findings (the criterion standard) to the results of the diagnostic tests. For the 55 patients studied, the sensitivity, specificity, and accuracy are shown in Table 10.1.

Since then, many studies have been performed evaluating the use of ultrasound in adults with blunt abdominal trauma (Table 10.2).

A systematic review performed in 2001 aimed to determine the precision and reliability of ultrasound in blunt abdominal trauma.[7] The authors performed a statistical analysis and reported summary receiver operating characteristic (SROC) curves using weighted and robust regression models, with Q* denoting the overall accuracy of the curve, the highest point at

Table 10.1 Comparison of test sensitivity, specificity and accuracy of computed tomography (CT) scan, diagnostic peritoneal lavage (DPL), and ultrasound in 55 patients using surgical findings as the criterion standard

	Sensitivity, %	Specificity, %	Accuracy, %
CT	97.2	94.7	96.4
DPL	100	84.2	94.5
Ultrasound	91.7	94.7	92.7

Source: Data from [1].

Table 10.2 Test performance summaries of ultrasound to detect intra-abdominal injury in blunt abdominal trauma

Authors	N	Patients	Sensitivity, %	Specificity, %	Accuracy, %
Hoffman et al[2]	291	Severely injured (ISS > 20)	89	97	94
McKenney et al[3]	1,000	Patients with blunt trauma	88	99	97
Rothlin et al[4]	312	Blunt thoracic and abdominal injuries	90*	100	NR
Rozyski et al[5]	476	Blunt abdominal trauma	79	96	NR
Dolich et al[6]	2,576	Blunt abdominal trauma	86	98	97

*98% for intra-abdominal fluid and 41% for solid organ injuries. NR = Not reported.

which sensitivity and specificity are both equal. They calculated posttest probabilities as a function of pooled likelihood ratios (LRs). They found that 30 of 123 trials were eligible for their enrollment; these included data on 9,047 patients. Their results demonstrated that ultrasound had a summary Q* value of 0.91 (where 1.0 is perfect sensitivity and specificity) and that its negative predictive values ranged from 72% to 99%. For screening for free fluid, the SROC was calculated at Q* = 0.89. However, while ultrasound did detect the presence of organ injury, it could not adequately exclude injuries (LR− = 0.2). They calculated that given a pretest probability of 50% (0.5) for blunt abdominal injury, a posttest probability of nearly 25% remains in the case of a negative ultrasound due to the fact that, despite high specificity, ultrasound has a low sensitivity for the detection of both free fluid and solid organ lesions. In cases where there is a suspicion for true intra-abdominal injury (i.e., cases with a high pretest probability), they concluded that another assessment (e.g., CT) must be performed regardless of the initial ultrasound findings. The authors reported that a considerable issue in the use of ultrasound was the potential to miss small intestinal perforations.

Clinical question

Can FAST exclude intra-abdominal injuries in pediatric patients with blunt trauma?

Three studies have examined the sensitivity of FAST for the detection of intra-abdominal injuries in pediatric patients requiring laparotomy.[8-11] In these studies, sensitivities ranged from 33% to 55%. Another study by Luks et al reported a higher ultrasound sensitivity of 89% in a pediatric population; however, a criterion standard examination was not performed in all patients.[12]

Comment

The FAST examination performs with relatively high sensitivity for the detection of hemoperitoneum and is therefore useful in blunt abdominal trauma patients who are unstable. In many Level I trauma centers, FAST has become a useful adjunct in nearly all patients with blunt abdominal trauma, not just unstable patients, and is part of the evaluation process during the primary and secondary surveys. In centers where ultrasound is readily available, it has all but replaced DPL in unstable trauma patients with potential hemoperitoneum. However, FAST's inadequate LR− means that it cannot be used to rule-out significant intra-abdominal injury and it should not be used as a criterion standard. In patients in whom a high pre-test probability exists, further testing or laparotomy should be considered in consultation with a trauma surgeon.

References

1. Liu M, Lee CH, P'eng FK. Prospective comparison of diagnostic peritoneal lavage, computed tomographic scanning, and ultrasonography for the diagnosis of blunt abdominal trauma. Journal of Trauma. 1993; 35: 267–70.
2. Hoffmann R, Nerlich M, Muggia-Sullam M *et al*. Blunt abdominal trauma in cases of multiple trauma evaluated by ultrasonography: A prospective analysis of 291 patients. Journal of Trauma. 1992; 32: 452–8.
3. McKenney MG, Martin L, Lentz K *et al*. 1,000 consecutive ultrasounds for blunt abdominal trauma. Journal of Trauma. 1996; 40: 607–10; discussion 611–12.

4. Rothlin MA, Naf R, Amgwerd M *et al.* Ultrasound in blunt abdominal and thoracic trauma. Journal of Trauma. 1993; 34(4): 488–95.
5. Rozycki GS, Ochsner MG, Jaffin JH *et al.* Prospective evaluation of surgeons' use of ultrasound in the evaluation of trauma patients. Journal of Trauma. 1993; 34: 516–26; discussion 526–7.
6. Dolich MO, McKenney MG, Varela JE *et al.* 2,576 ultrasounds for blunt abdominal trauma. Journal of Trauma. 2001; 50(1): 108–12.
7. Stengel D, Bauwens K, Sehouli J *et al.* Systematic review and meta-analysis of emergency ultrasonography for blunt abdominal trauma. British Journal of Surgery. 2001; 88(7): 901–12.
8. Patel JC, Tepas JJ. The efficacy of focused abdominal sonography for trauma (FAST) as a screening tool in the assessment of injured children. Journal of Pediatric Surgery. 1999; 34: 44–7; discussion 52–4.
9. Mutabagani KH, Coley BD, Zumberge N *et al.* Preliminary experience with focused abdominal sonographyfor trauma (FAST) in children: Is it useful? Journal of Pediatric Surgery. 1999; 34: 48–52; discussion 52–4.
10. Coley BD, Mutabagani KH, Martin LC *et al.* Focused abdominal sonography for trauma (FAST) in children with blunt abdominal trauma. Journal of Trauma. 2000; 48: 902–6.
11. Fox JC, Boysen M, Gharahbaghian L, Cusick S, Ahmed SS, Anderson CL, Lekawa M, Langdorf MI. Test characteristics of focused assessment of sonography for trauma for clinically significant abdominal free fluid in pediatric blunt abdominal trauma. Academic Emergency Medicine. 2011; 18: 477–82.
12. Luks FI, Lemire A, St-Vil D *et al.* Blunt abdominal trauma in children: The practical value of ultrasonography. Journal of Trauma. 1993; 34: 607–11.

Chapter 11 Acute Knee Injuries

Highlights

- Acute knee fractures are identified in only a small proportion of ED patients with acute knee injuries,
- The Ottawa knee rule and Pittsburgh knee rule are highly sensitive in guiding the need for imaging in adults and children with acute knee injury.

Background

Acute knee pain is a common complaint in the emergency department (ED). Prior to the advent of clinical decision rules, plain radiographs of the knee were typically obtained to rule out a fracture after blunt knee trauma in which there was any clinical suspicion of fracture. However, similar to ankle injuries, knee fractures are identified in only a small proportion (approximately 7%) of knee injuries. Two clinical decision rules have been created to identify patients in whom knee radiography may be deferred in the setting of an acute knee injury: the Ottawa knee rule and the Pittsburgh knee rule. The Ottawa knee rule and the Pittsburgh knee rule are described in Table 11.1.

Clinical question

How well does the Ottawa knee rule identify patients requiring knee radiography?
A systematic review of studies on the Ottawa knee rule directly addressed this question.[1] The authors included articles that reported patient-level information to determine sensitivity and specificity. Two independent reviewers independently tallied data on study samples, the details about how the Ottawa knee rule was used, and methodological characteristics. Of the 11 studies identified, data were collected from six, resulting in a set of 4,249 adult patients who were considered appropriate for pooled analysis. The aggregate negative likelihood ratio was 0.05 (CI 0.02–0.23), sensitivity was 99% (CI 93–100%), and specificity was 49% (CI 43–51%). Given a knee fracture

Evidence-Based Emergency Care: Diagnostic Testing and Clinical Decision Rules, Second Edition. Jesse M. Pines, Christopher R. Carpenter, Ali S. Raja and Jeremiah D. Schuur.
© 2013 John Wiley & Sons, Ltd. Published 2013 by John Wiley & Sons, Ltd.

Table 11.1 Clinical decision rules to defer radiography in patients with blunt knee trauma

---

The Ottawa knee rule

The Ottawa knee rule recommends radiography if any of the following is present in the context of an acute knee injury:

1. Age > 55 years
2. Tenderness at the head of fibula
3. Isolated tenderness at the patella
4. Inability to flex knee to 90 degrees
5. Inability to transfer weight for four steps, both immediately after the injury and in the ED.

Exclusion criteria for the Ottawa knee rule include: age < 18 years, superficial skin injuries, injuries more than 7 days old, reevaluation of recent injuries, altered levels of consciousness, paraplegia, or multiple injuries.

The Pittsburgh knee rule

The Pittsburgh knee rule recommends radiography if:
The mechanism of injury is either blunt trauma or a fall AND either

1. Age is < 12 years or > 50 OR
2. There is an inability to walk four weight-bearing steps in the ED.

Exclusion criteria for the Pittsburgh knee rule are knee injuries > 6 days prior to presentation, only superficial lacerations and abrasions, a history of previous surgeries or fractures on the injured knee, and patients being reassessed for the same injury.

---

prevalence of 7%, a negative Ottawa knee rule resulted in a probability of knee fracture of 1.5%. Table 11.2 shows data from the six studies reviewed with reported sensitivities and specificities.

Clinical question

How does the Ottawa knee rule compare with the Pittsburgh knee rule?
A prospective study conducted at three academic centers investigated this question.[8] The decision whether to order radiographs was made using

Table 11.2 Six studies reporting sensitivity and specificity of the Ottawa knee rule

Reference	Year	Sensitivity, %	Specificity, %
Steill et al [2]	1996	100% (CI 94–100%)	50% (CI 46–53%)
Steill et al [3]	1997	100% (CI 94–100%)	48% (CI 45–51%)
Richman et al [4]	1997	85% (CI 65–96%)	45% (CI 39–52%)
Emparanza and Aginaga [5]	2001	100% (CI 96–100%)	52% (CI 50–55%)
Szucs et al [6]	2001	100% (CI 63–100%)	47% (CI 36–58%)
Ketelslegers et al [7]	2002	100% (CI 87–100%)	32% (CI 26–38%)

physician judgment. All patients who underwent radiography had a three-view knee series (anterior-posterior, lateral, and obliques), with a sunrise view added in patients with suspected patellar fractures. The performance of the Ottawa knee rule and Pittsburgh knee rule was determined by using appropriate variables from the data sheets and film reports from board-certified radiologists. There were a total of 934 patients evaluated, and the Ottawa knee rule and the Pittsburgh knee rule were applicable to 745 and 750 patients, respectively. The main results of the study are detailed in Table 11.3.

The difference in sensitivity was not significant; however, the Pittsburgh knee rule was considerably more specific (33% difference; CI 28–38%). However, two elements of this study bring into question its validity. First, the authors did not follow patients who did not undergo radiography, introducing a potential selection bias. However, in a previous study, 357 patients with knee pain who did not have radiography were reevaluated by a formal telephone interview 2 weeks later, and none required clinical reassessment. Second, two of the three clinical sites were University of Pittsburgh–affiliated hospitals and the physicians making the initial determination of imaging need may have already been using the Pittsburgh knee rule or the Ottawa knee rule, leading to selection bias in the population of patients enrolled in the study.

Clinical question

How well does the Ottawa knee rule work in pediatric patients?
A recent study aimed to determine the sensitivity and specificity of the Ottawa knee rule in children.[9] The authors performed a prospective, multicenter validation study and included children aged 2 to 16 years presenting to the ED with a knee injury sustained within 7 days. Physicians ordered radiographs according to their usual practice. The outcome measure was any fracture and patients with negative films were followed for 14 days. A total of 750 were

Table 11.3 Study comparing the Ottawa knee rule with the Pittsburgh knee rule

	Sensitivity	Specificity	Positive predictive value (PPV)	Negative predictive value (NPV)	LR+	LR−
Pittsburgh knee rule	99% (CI 94–100%)	60% (CI 56–64%)	24%	100%	2.5	0.02
Ottawa knee rule	97% (CI 90–99)	27% (CI 23–30%)	15%	99%	1.3	0.11

Source: Data from [4].

enrolled; 670 had radiography, and fewer than 10% (n = 70) had fractures. The Ottawa knee rule was 100% sensitive (CI 95–100%), with a specificity of 43% (CI 39–47%). The authors concluded that the Ottawa knee rule is valid for use in children.

Comment

Both the Pittsburgh knee rule and the Ottawa knee rule can be used (in the ED) to identify adults and children who do not need X-rays following acute knee injury. The Pittsburgh knee rule is considerably more specific and includes the mechanism of injury, which is important since blunt knee trauma, including direct blows to the knee and falls, accounts for 80% of knee fractures. With this mechanism, patients are four times more likely to have fractures.[10] While the specificity of the Pittsburgh knee rule is higher and may therefore result in less unnecessary radiography, the sensitivity for both rules is near 100%, making them safe for use in the ED. In addition, one study validated the use of the Ottawa knee rule in children between 2 and 16 years of age.

References

1. Bachmann LM, Haberzeth S, Steurer J et al. The accuracy of the Ottawa knee rule to rule out knee fractures: A systematic review. Annals of Internal Medicine. 2004; 140: 121–4.
2. Stiell IG, Greenberg GH, Wells GA, McDowell I, Cwinn AA, Smith NA et al. Prospective validation of a decision rule for the use of radiography in acute knee injuries. Journal of the American Medical Association. 1996; 275: 611–15.
3. Stiell IG, Wells GA, Hoag RH, Sivilotti ML, Cacciotti TF, Verbeek PR et al. Implementation of the Ottawa knee rule for the use of radiography in acute knee injuries. Journal of the American Medical Association. 1997; 278: 2075–9.
4. Richman PB, McCuskey CF, Nashed A, Fuchs S, Petrik R, Imperato M et al. Performance of two clinical decision rules for knee radiography. Journal of Emergency Medicine. 1997; 15: 459–63.
5. Emparanza JI, Aginaga JR. Validation of the Ottawa knee rules. Annals of Emergency Medicine. 2001; 38: 364–8.
6. Szucs PA, Richman PB, Mandell M. Triage nurse application of the Ottawa knee rule. Academic Emergency Medicine. 2001; 8: 112–16.
7. Ketelslegers E, Collard X, Vande Berg B, Danse E, El-Gariani A, Poilvache P et al. Validation of the Ottawa knee rules in an emergency teaching centre. European Radiology. 2002; 12: 1218–20.
8. Seaberg DC, Yealy DM, Lukens T et al. Multicenter comparison of two clinical decision rules for the use of radiography in acute, high-risk knee injuries. Annals of Emergency Medicine. 1998; 32: 8–13.

9. Bulloch B, Neto G, Plint A *et al*. Validation of the Ottawa knee rule in children: A multicenter study. Annals of Emergency Medicine. 2003; 42: 48–55.
10. Dalinka MK, Alazraki NP, Daffner RH *et al*. Expert panel on musculoskeletal imaging: Imaging evaluation of suspected ankle fractures. Reston (VA): American College of Radiology (ACR); 2005.

Chapter 12 **Acute Ankle and Foot Injuries**

Highlights

- The prevalence of ankle fractures among ED patients with ankle sprain is approximately 15%.
- The Ottawa ankle rules are widely used, well-validated clinical decision rules that accurately identify patients at low risk for fractures.
- The Ottawa ankle rules have been shown to be highly sensitive in children; however, they should be used only in patients who can communicate verbally and were able to ambulate prior to their injuries.

Background

Patients with acute foot and ankle injuries often present to the emergency department (ED), most commonly with injuries occurring after over-inversion of the ankle. Regardless of mechanism, these injuries can result in either ankle fractures (typically seen on a three-view ankle series) or foot fractures (seen on a three-view foot series). Historically, depending on the sites of swelling and tenderness, patients might have obtained an ankle series, a foot series, or both. However, the low overall prevalence of fractures (about 15%) led to the development of the Ottawa ankle and foot rules. The Ottawa ankle and foot rules were derived to have a sensitivity of 100%; if the criteria for the rules (listed in Figures 12.1 and 12.2) are met, fractures can be effectively ruled out based on clinical evaluation, and radiography can be deferred.

In the studies that formed the basis for the Ottawa ankle and foot rules, patients were excluded if they had a delayed presentation of injury (greater than one week), had altered mental status, or were pregnant.

The Ottawa ankle and foot rules are probably the best studied decision rules in emergency medicine. The rules have been validated in multiple settings across multiple cultures. The purpose of this chapter will be to

Evidence-Based Emergency Care: Diagnostic Testing and Clinical Decision Rules, Second Edition.
Jesse M. Pines, Christopher R. Carpenter, Ali S. Raja and Jeremiah D. Schuur.
© 2013 John Wiley & Sons, Ltd. Published 2013 by John Wiley & Sons, Ltd.

An ankle X-ray series is only necessary if there is
pain near the malleoli and any of these findings:

1. Inability to bear weight both
   immediately and in emergency
   department (four steps)
       or
2. Bone tenderness at the posterior
   edge or tip of either malleolus

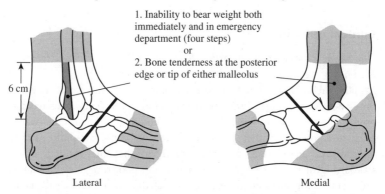

Lateral   Medial

Figure 12.1 The Ottawa ankle rules. (Reproduced with permission from Shell IG , Greenberg GH , McKnight RD, et al Decision Rules for the Use of Radiography in Acute Ankle Injuries: Refinement and Prospective Validation. JAMA 1993; 269 (9): 1127–1132. ©1993, American Medical Association).

A foot X-ray series is only necessary if there is pain
in the mid-foot and any of these findings:

1. Inability to bear weight both
   immediately and in emergency
   department (four steps)
       or
2. Bone tenderness at the navicular
   or the base of the fifth metatarsal

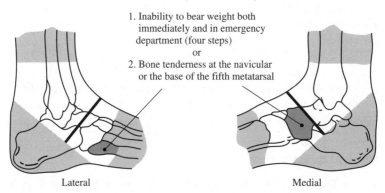

Lateral   Medial

Figure 12.2 The Ottawa foot rules. (Reproduced with permission from Shell IG , Greenberg GH , McKnight RD, et al Decision Rules for the Use of Radiography in Acute Ankle Injuries: Refinement and Prospective Validation. JAMA 1993; 269 (9): 1127–1132. ©1993, American Medical Association).

briefly review the evidence behind the Ottawa ankle and foot rules and to examine their use in children.

Clinical question

How strong is the evidence supporting the use of the Ottawa ankle and foot rules to clinically exclude fractures of the ankle and midfoot?

In 2003, Bachmann et al performed a systematic review and meta-analysis of the evidence regarding the Ottawa ankle and foot rules.[1] They extracted data on the study populations and the study methodologies. Their intent was to calculate a pooled sensitivity for the decision rules. A bootstrapping method for statistical analysis was performed to ensure that their estimate of the standard error was correct, they calculated and pooled negative likelihood ratios (LR−) for many subgroups, they adjusted for methodological quality, and they excluded retrospective studies and those that did not specifically blind the radiologists involved. Of the 32 studies that met the inclusion criteria, the data from 27 were pooled, resulting in an evaluation of 15,581 patients. The authors calculated a LR− of 0.08 (95% CI 0.03–0.18) for the ankle rule and 0.08 (95% CI 0.03–0.20) for the midfoot rule. In children, the pooled LR− was 0.07 (95% CI 0.03–0.18). Data were tabulated as boot-strapped sensitivities and specificities with a focus on specific populations, prevalence of fracture, and time to referral in Table 12.1 – the *n* denotes the number of studies used to calculate the point estimate for the sensitivity or the median specificity.

They calculated that applying these ratios to a population with a 15% fracture prevalence would yield a less than 1.4% probability of actual fracture and that the evidence supports the use of the Ottawa ankle and foot rules as accurate tools to exclude fractures of the midfoot and ankle, with an almost 100% sensitivity and low specificity.

Clinical question

Can the Ottawa ankle and foot rules be safely used in children to exclude ankle and foot fractures?

Safe application of the Ottawa ankle and foot rules in children has been the subject of recent debate. Three major considerations differentiate the use of the Ottawa ankle and foot rules in children from their safe use in adults. The first issue is that children may not be as reliable regarding the verbal histories of their injuries. Second, the most common missed fracture type, a Salter–Harris type I fracture (defined as a separation of the bone 0.3 mm through the physis) is often associated with trauma in infants and children,

Table 12.1 Sensitivities and specificities of the Ottawa ankle rules in pooled studies

Category	Sensitivity (95% CI)	Median specificity (interquartile range)
All studies (n = 39)	97.6% (96.4–98.9)	31.5% (23.8–44.4%)
Type of assessment		
Ankle (n = 15)	98.0% (96.3–99.3%)	39.8% (27.9–47.7%)
Foot (n = 10)	99.0% (97.3–100%)	37.8% (24.7–70.1%)
Combined (n = 14)	96.4% (93.8–98.6%)	26.3% (19.4–34.3%)
Population		
Children (n = 7)	99.3% (98.3–100%)	26.7% (23.8–35.6%)
Adults (n = 32)	97.3% (95.7–98.6%)	36.6% (22.3–46.1%)
Prevalence of fracture		
<25th centile (n = 7)	99.0% (98.3–100%)	47.9% (42.3–77.1%)
25th–75th centile (n = 22)	97.7% (95.9–99.0%)	30.1% (23.8–40.1%)
>75th centile (n = 10)	96.7% (94.2–99.2%)	27.3% (15.5–40.0%)
Time to referral (hours)		
<48 (n = 5)	99.6% (98.2–100%)	27.9% (24.7–31.5%)
>48 (n = 34)	97.3% (95.9–98.5%)	36.6% (19.9–46.8%)

Source: Data from [1].

and point tenderness will be present only if patients are able to communicate effectively. Third, application of the Ottawa ankle and foot rules requires that children be able to walk prior to their injuries, excluding infants and children who are not yet able to ambulate.

In addition to the high estimate for the sensitivity of the Ottawa ankle and foot rules in the seven pediatric studies in the systematic review by Bachmann et al a more recent review has included more data confirming the excellent sensitivity of the Ottawa ankle and foot rules in children.[2] With the addition of more recent data, its authors calculated an overall sensitivity of 97% (CI 93–100%) and a specificity of 29% (CI 18–40%). In all the studies examined, a prevalence of 12% was calculated. While one article in their review showed that a total of five patients who were rule negative actually had fractures yielding a sensitivity of 83% (CI 65–94%),[3] most articles had zero or one missed fracture in their pediatric populations.

Comment

Use of the Ottawa ankle and foot rules allows for the clinical exclusion of fractures in both adult and pediatric populations and has been validated in multiple settings. In applying the Ottawa ankle and foot rules to children, it is important to use the rule only in children who are able to communicate verbally and had the ability to walk prior to the injury. In the pooled studies reviewed in this chapter, a small percentage of patients who did not receive x-rays based on the Ottawa ankle and foot rules actually had fractures. However, given a prevalence of 12% in pediatric studies and 15% in adult studies, a very low percentage of patients (less than 1.4%) will fall into this category. The clinical relevance of these subtle missed ankle fractures is also unknown. Therefore, in the case of either negative or deferred (due to the Ottawa ankle and foot rules) ankle radiography in patients with significant soft tissue injury, we recommend that patients be splinted; use ice, elevation, and crutches; and obtain close follow-up and reevaluation.

In the pediatric population, missed fractures will most likely be Salter–Harris type I fractures, which typically have almost no long-term consequences. As a note of caution, because the sensitivity for the rule is not 100%, in patients in whom the rule is negative and whose pretest probability is high, clinicians should use their best judgment in the decision to order foot and ankle X-rays.

References

1. Bachmann LM, Kolb E, Koller MT et al. Accuracy of Ottawa ankle rules to exclude fractures of the ankle and mid-foot: Systematic review. British Medical Journal. 2003; 326(7386): 417.

2. Myers A, Kanty K, Nelson T. Are the Ottawa ankle rules helpful in ruling out the need for x ray examination in children? Archives of Disease in Childhood. 2005; 90: 1309–11.

3. Clarke KD, Tanner S. Evaluation of Ottawa ankle rules in children. Pediatric Emergency Care. 2003; 19: 73–8.

Chapter 13 **Blunt Head Injury in Children**

Highlights

- Blunt head trauma in children is associated with significant morbidity and mortality, but the need to diagnose clinically significant intracranial injuries must be balanced with the risks of radiation exposure in children.
- The PECARN decision rules are the only clinical decision rules to have been validated. The two rules (for children <2 years old and ≥ 2 years old) are highly sensitive for the detection of clinically important intracranial injury in children.
- Four additional decision rules have been derived but not yet validated: CATCH, CHALICE, NEXUS II, and the Italian pediatric head CT rule.

Background

Traumatic brain injury is a leading cause of morbidity and mortality in children and accounts for a significant proportion of the > 1 million annual emergency department (ED) visits and hospitalizations due to trauma-related head injuries.[1] The concern on the part of emergency physicians evaluating a child who has been involved in trauma is establishing the presence or absence of an intracranial injury. Because the radiation risks of computed tomography (CT) are greater in children, North American and European researchers have developed clinical decision rules for imaging children with blunt head trauma. The objectives of these pediatric head injury clinical decision rules are to identify patients who are either at low risk for injury and can thus be evaluated without imaging or at great risk for injury to require imaging.

Evidence-Based Emergency Care: Diagnostic Testing and Clinical Decision Rules, Second Edition.
Jesse M. Pines, Christopher R. Carpenter, Ali S. Raja and Jeremiah D. Schuur.
© 2013 John Wiley & Sons, Ltd. Published 2013 by John Wiley & Sons, Ltd.

Clinical question

Can elements of the history and physical exam identify children with minor head injury who are at low risk for intracranial injury and who do not need CT imaging?

There are five large prospective studies of children that have derived clinical decision rules to identify those who are at low risk of intracranial injury.[2-6] The only one of these to have been validated is by the Pediatric Emergency Care Applied Research Network (PECARN).[2] They enrolled 42,412 children younger than 18 years old who presented within 24 hours of blunt trauma and had Glasgow Coma Scale scores of 14 or 15, 14,969 (35%) of whom had head CTs performed. Patients were enrolled at 25 EDs, and their outcome of clinically important traumatic brain injury was defined *a priori* as death from traumatic brain injury, neurosurgery, intubation for more than 24 hours for traumatic brain injury (designed to exclude children intubated for imaging), or hospital admission of two nights or more associated with traumatic brain injury on CT. Medical records were reviewed for the outcomes, and telephone follow-up was performed between seven and 90 days after ED visits to identify any missed injuries. The PECARN rule was derived in a population of 33,785 patients and then validated in 8,627 patients by continued data collection at the same sites.

The PECARN investigators analyzed preverbal (<2 years old) and verbal (≥2 years old) children separately in order to account for differences in communicative ability, mechanisms, and risks for intracranial injury. Of the 8,502 preverbal children in the derivation cohort, there were 73 cases (0.86%) of intracranial injury and, of the 25,283 verbal children, there were 215 (0.85%) cases of intracranial injury. The PECARN decision rule for children <2 years old (Table 13.1) had a sensitivity of 99%, a specificity of 54%, a LR+ of 2.2, and a LR− of 0.02. Similarly, the rule for children≥2 years old (Table 13.2) had a sensitivity of 97%, a specificity of 59%, a LR+ of 2.4,

Table 13.1 The PECARN head CT rule for children <2 years old

Children without any of the following are at very low risk of clinically important traumatic brain injury, and CT can routinely be obviated:
• Altered mental status
• Scalp hematoma
• Loss of consciousness (either no or <5 seconds)
• Mild or moderate mechanism of injury
• Palpable or unclear skull fracture
• Acting abnormally per parent.

Source: Data from [2].

Table 13.2 The PECARN head CT rule for children ≥ 2 years old

Children without any of the following are at very low risk of clinically important traumatic brain injury, and CT can routinely be obviated:
- Altered mental status
- Loss of consciousness
- History of vomiting
- Mild or moderate mechanism of injury
- Clinical signs of basilar skull fracture
- Severe headache.

Source: Data from [2].

Table 13.3 Performance of the PECARN head CT rule in children <2 years old

Derivation cohort	PECARN-defined clinically important traumatic brain injury		
Decision rule	Injury	No injury	Totals
Positive	72	3,901	3,973
Negative	1	4,528	4,529
Totals	73	8,429	8,502
Sensitivity (CI)	99% (93–100%)		
Specificity (CI)	54% (53–55%)		
Positive likelihood ratio (LR+)	2.2		
Negative likelihood ratio (LR−)	0.02		
Validation cohort	PECARN-defined clinically important traumatic brain injury		
Decision rule	Injury	No injury	Totals
Positive	25	1,015	1,040
Negative	0	1,176	1,176
Totals	25	2,191	2,216
Sensitivity (CI)	100% (86–100%)		
Specificity (CI)	54% (52–56%)		
Positive likelihood ratio (LR+)	2.2		
Negative likelihood ratio (LR−)	0		

Source: Data from [2].

and a LR− of 0.05. Test characteristics were similar in the validation cohorts (Tables 13.3 and 13.4).

The 2009 PECARN rules were the first validated CT clinical decision rules for pediatric blunt trauma, but they were not the first rules to be derived. In 2006, three independent groups published decision rules designed to answer this same question.[3–5] The first of these, a preplanned analysis of

Table 13.4 Performance of the PECARN head CT rule in children ≥ 2 years old

Derivation cohort	PECARN-defined clinically important traumatic brain injury		
Decision rule	Injury	No Inijury	Totals
Positive	208	10,412	10,620
Negative	7	14,656	14,663
Totals	215	25,068	25,283
Sensitivity (CI)	97% (93–99%)		
Specificity (CI)	59% (58–59%)		
Positive likelihood ratio (LR+)	2.4		
Negative likelihood ratio (LR−)	0.05		
Validation cohort	PECARN-defined clinically important traumatic brain injury		
Decision rule	Injury	No injury	Totals
Positive	61	2,550	2,611
Negative	2	3,798	3,800
Totals	63	6,348	6,411
Sensitivity (CI)	97% (89–100%)		
Specificity (CI)	60% (59–61%)		
Positive likelihood ratio (LR+)	2.4		
Negative likelihood ratio (LR−)	0.05		

Source: Data from [2].

Table 13.5 The NEXUS II low-risk head CT rule for children

Children without any of the following are at very low risk of clinically important traumatic brain injury, and CT can routinely be obviated:
- Evidence of significant skull fracture
- Altered level of alertness
- Neurologic deficit
- Persistent vomiting
- Presence of scalp hematoma
- Abnormal behavior
- Coagulopathy.

Source: Data from [3].

the NEXUS II investigation by Oman et al studied patients ≤18 years old to examine the performance of the NEXUS II low-risk head CT rule on this population.[3] The NEXUS II HCT (head CT) rules are shown in Table 13.5. In an adaptation suited for the study of children, only seven of the eight variables were evaluated (the age > 65 criterion was dropped). NEXUS II enrolled 1,666

Table 13.6 Performance of the NEXUS II HCT rule in children

Decision rule	NEXUS II head CT rule-defined clinically important intracranial injury		
	Injury	No injury	Totals
Positive	136	1,298	1,434
Negative	2	230	232
Totals	138	1,528	1,666
Sensitivity (CI)	98% (95–100)%		
Specificity (CI)	15% (13–17%)		
Positive likelihood ratio (LR+)	1.2		
Negative likelihood ratio (LR−)	0.13		

Decision rule	NEXUS II head CT rule-defined clinically important intracranial injury (age <3y)		
	Injury	No injury	Totals
Positive	25	269	294
Negative	0	15	15
Totals	25	284	309
Sensitivity (CI)	100% (86–100%)		
Specificity (CI)	5% (3–9%)		
Positive likelihood ratio (LR+)	1.0		
Negative likelihood ratio (LR−)	0		

Source: Data from [3].

children, all of whom underwent head CT. The outcomes evaluated were the same as for the larger NEXUS II study: clinically important intracranial injury requiring neurosurgical intervention or likely to lead to significant long-term neurological impairment. The prevalence of clinically significant intracranial injury was 8.3% (138/1,666). The performance of the adapted NEXUS II HCT rules is shown in Table 13.6 and, given the fact that this population was a subset of the original population from which the NEXUS II rule was derived, the test characteristics (high sensitivity and low specificity) are similar to those of the rule when it was applied to the population as a whole.

Another group (from Italy) examined a cohort of children <16 years old with blunt head trauma presenting to pediatric EDs to determine predictors of the diagnosis of intracranial injury and death.[4] They enrolled 3,806 patients from 1996 to 1997, 22 (0.58%) of whom had intracranial injuries. All patients discharged from the ED were followed up by phone after 10 days. All patients underwent routine care, but head CTs were only obtained at the discretion of the treating physician. The seven variables included in their prediction model are listed in Table 13.7. Patients were classified as high risk

Table 13.7 Criteria associated with traumatic brain injuries in children with closed head trauma

Children with any of the following are at risk of intracranial injury and should have a head CT performed:
- Abnormal Glasgow Coma Scale
- Abnormal neurological examination
- Clinical signs of skull base fracture or of skull fracture in nonfrontal area
- Prolonged loss of consciousness
- Persistent headache
- Persistent drowsiness
- Amnesia.

Source: Data from [4].

Table 13.8 Test performance of the Italian pediatric head CT rule

Decision rule	Clinically significant intracranial injury or death		
	Positive	Negative	Totals
Positive	22	478	500
Negative	0	3,298	3,298
Totals	22	3,776	3,798*
Sensitivity (CI)	100% (84–100%)		
Specificity (CI)	87% (86–88%)		
Positive likelihood ratio (LR+)	7.7		
Negative likelihood ratio (LR−)	0		

*Eight children with negative outcomes had no initial evaluation and therefore are not included.
Source: Data from [4].

for death or intracranial injury by the presence of any one of these variables, necessitating imaging. The absence of these variables classified a patient as low risk for these outcomes. The performance of the derived model is shown in Table 13.8.

British researchers created the Children's Head Injury Algorithm for the Prediction of Important Clinical Events (CHALICE) rule.[5] From 2000 to 2002, the CHALICE study examined all children <16 years old who presented to EDs in 10 hospitals in northwest England with any history or sign of head injury (not just blunt trauma). Data were collected on 40 clinical variables. The primary outcome was a composite of death from head injury, requirement for neurosurgical intervention, or marked abnormality on head CT. CT abnormalities were defined as acute, new traumatic intracranial injuries that included intracranial hematomas, cerebral contusions, cerebral edema,

Table 13.9 The Children's Head Injury Algorithm for the Prediction of Important Clinical Events (CHALICE) rule

A head computed tomography (CT) is indicated if any of the following are present:

History
- Witnessed loss of consciousness (LOC) > 5 min
- History of amnesia > 5 min duration
- Drowsiness
- ≥ 3 episodes of vomiting after injury
- Suspicion of nonaccidental injury
- Seizure after injury (in patients without epilepsy).

Exam
- Glasgow Coma Scale (GCS) <14 (or GCS <15 if <1 year old)
- Suspicion of penetrating or depressed skull fracture, or bulging fontanelle
- Signs of skull base fracture
- Focal neurological finding
- Bruise, swelling, or laceration > 5 cm if <1 year old.

Mechanism
- High-speed road traffic injury (> 40 mph)
- Fall from > 3 meters (10 feet) height
- High-speed injury from projectile or object.

Source: Data from [5].

and depressed skull fractures. Nondepressed skull fractures were specifically excluded as they were deemed not significant injuries that do not normally require intervention or hospitalization. Similar to the Canadian CT head rule, the study did not mandate that all patients undergo CT. Patients who were admitted for inpatient stays, had a head CT or skull radiographs, or underwent neurosurgery were followed up. At the end of the study, all participating hospital radiology records were reviewed for skull radiographs and head CTs and cross-referenced with enrolled patients. The National Office of Statistics was also contacted regarding the deaths of children with head injury.

The CHALICE study, which was the largest of its kind dedicated to examining children when it was published, enrolled 22,772 patients. Only 744 patients (3.2%) underwent head CT. The prevalence of clinically significant head injuries was 1.2% (281/22,772).

The CHALICE rule is shown in Table 13.9. It consists of 14 criteria, with a head CT being indicated when any item is present. In this derivation study, the clinical prediction rule for detecting any clinically significant head injury performed with a sensitivity of 98.6% and specificity of 86.9% (Table 13.10).

The most recently developed clinical decision rule for children with minor head injury was published by the Pediatric Emergency Research Canada (PERC) Head Injury Study Group.[6] Their rule, the Canadian assessment of tomography for childhood head injury (CATCH) rule, was derived in a

Table 13.10 Test performance of the CHALICE rule

| Decision rule | Clinically significant head injury | | |
	Injury	No injury	Totals
Positive	277	2,933	3,210
Negative	4	19,558	19,562
Totals	281	22,491	22,772
Sensitivity (CI)	99% (96–100%)		
Specificity (CI)	87% (87–87%)		
Positive likelihood ratio (LR+)	7.6		
Negative likelihood ratio (LR−)	0.02		

Source: Data from [5].

population of children 0–16 years old enrolled consecutively at 10 Canadian pediatric teaching EDs. All patients had been injured within 24 hours of presentation, had a GCS of 14 or 15 at presentation, and had blunt trauma to the head resulting in witnessed loss of consciousness, definite amnesia, witnessed disorientation, persistent vomiting (two or more distinct episodes of vomiting 15 minutes apart), or persistent irritability in the ED (for children under 2 years of age). The primary outcome was the need for neurologic intervention, and their secondary outcome was intracranial injury on CT. Patients who did not undergo CT were followed up at 14 days with a phone call, and those who could not be reached were excluded from the final analysis.

The CATCH investigators enrolled 3,866 patients, 159 (4.1%) of whom had intracranial injury. Their rule consists of four high-risk factors and three medium-risk factors (Table 13.11). The high-risk factors predict the need

Table 13.11 The Canadian Assessment of Tomography for Childhood Head injury (CATCH) rule

A head CT is required only for children with minor head injury and any one of the following:

High-risk factors (predict need for neurological intervention):
1. Glasgow Coma Scale (GCS) <15 at 2 hours after injury
2. Suspected open or depressed skull fracture
3. History of worsening headache
4. Irritability on examination

Medium-risk factors (predict brain injury on computed tomography (CT) scan):
1. Any sign of basal skull fracture (e.g., hemotympanum, "raccoon" eyes, otorrhea or rhinorrhea of the cerebrospinal fluid, or Battle's sign)
2. Large, boggy hematoma of the scalp
3. Dangerous mechanism of injury (e.g., motor vehicle crash, fall from elevation ≥ 3 ft (≥ 91 cm) or five stairs, or fall from bicycle with no helmet)

Source: Data from [6].

Table 13.12 Test performance of the CATCH rule

Decision rule	Injury requiring neurological intervention		
	Injury	No injury	Totals
Positive	24	1,144	1,168
Negative	0	2,698	2,698
Totals	24	3,842	3,866
Sensitivity (CI)	100% (86–100%)		
Specificity (CI)	70% (69–72%)		
Positive likelihood ratio (LR+)	3.3		
Negative likelihood ratio (LR−)	0		
Decision rule	Presence of brain injury on computed tomography (CT) scan		
	Injury	No injury	Totals
Positive	156	1,851	2,007
Negative	3	1,856	1,859
Totals	159	3,707	3,866
Sensitivity (CI)	98% (95–99%)		
Specificity (CI)	50% (49–52%)		
Positive likelihood ratio (LR+)	2.0		
Negative likelihood ratio (LR−)	0.04		

Source: Data from [6].

for neurological intervention, while the addition of the medium-risk factors to the high-risk factors predicts any brain injury on CT scan. The test's performance is described in Table 13.12.

Comments

Children with head injuries present commonly to EDs, and clinicians have to decide whether or not to perform head CTs, with their associated risk of ionizing radiation. The prevalence of intracranial injury in the studies ranged from 0.58% to 8.3%, and differs partially due to the varying definitions of intracranial injury used by the studies. In addition, the studies can be divided into two groups based on their stated goals; while PECARN and NEXUS II were derived to identify children who do not require imaging, the other studies explicitly identify those children who do. While this may seem like an academic distinction, it is not. For example, the presence of a PECARN predictor variable does not mandate CT imaging. Rather, the PECARN investigators recommend observation if certain predictor variables are present and imaging if others are present, leaving much to individual clinician direction.[2] A later study by the PECARN group demonstrated that children with blunt trauma who undergo observation are less likely to end up receiving head CTs, suggesting that a period of ED observation might decrease head CT use.[7]

While all of these clinical decision rules have favorable test characteristics, to date only the PECARN rules have been validated. We recommend their use for the identification of children with blunt head trauma who are at very low risk for intracranial injury in order to avoid the overuse of imaging.

References

1. Langlois JA, Rutland-Brown W, Thomas KE. Traumatic brain injury in the United States. Atlanta (GA): US Department of Health and Human Services; 2006.
2. Kuppermann N, Holmes JF, Dayan PS *et al.* Identification of children at very low risk of clinically-important brain injuries after head trauma: A prospective cohort study. Lancet. 2009; 374(9696): 1160–70.
3. Oman JA, Cooper RJ, Holmes JF *et al.* Performance of a decision rule to predict need for computed tomography among children with blunt head trauma. Pediatrics. 2006; 117(2): e238–46.
4. Da Dalt L, Marchi AG, Laudizi L *et al.* Predictors of intracranial injuries in children after blunt head trauma. European Journal of Pediatrics. 2006; 165(3): 142–8.
5. Dunning J, Daly JP, Lomas J-P *et al.* Derivation of the children's head injury algorithm for the prediction of important clinical events decision rule for head injury in children. Archives of Disease in Childhood. 2006; 91(11): 885–91.
6. Osmond MH, Klassen TP, Wells GA *et al.* CATCH: A clinical decision rule for the use of computed tomography in children with minor head injury. Canadian Medical Association Journal. 2010; 182(4): 341–8.
7. Nigrovic LE, Schunk JE, Foerster A *et al.* The effect of observation on cranial computed tomography utilization for children after blunt head trauma. Pediatrics. 2011; 127(6): 1067–73.

Chapter 14 **Blunt Head Injury**

Highlights

- The Canadian CT head rule and the New Orleans criteria are both highly sensitive and well validated clinical decision rules that identify patients at low risk for clinically significant head injuries and in whom noncontrast head CT can be deferred.
- The Canadian CT head rule has proven to be more specific than the New Orleans criteria, and its use will reduce inappropriate imaging to a greater extent.
- No decision rules have yet identified a population of older adults who are at low risk for intracranial injuries following head trauma.

Background

There are approximately 1.74 million cases of traumatic brain injury annually in the U.S. with a mortality rate of 3–4%.[1] Patients with minor head injury, typically described as those having a Glasgow Coma Scale (GCS) score of 14–15 and a nonfocal neurological examination, comprise the majority of these traumatic head injury cases who are seen and evaluated in emergency departments (EDs).[2] While these patients can be evaluated for intracranial injuries using computed tomography (CT), the risk of radiation exposure and the cost of CT imaging necessitate that emergency physicians attempt to image appropriate, rather than all, patients with minor head injury. Blunt head injury in children was reviewed in Chapter 13, however a number of clinical decision rules have been developed to help guide clinicians in making this decision in adults as well.

Evidence-Based Emergency Care: Diagnostic Testing and Clinical Decision Rules, Second Edition.
Jesse M. Pines, Christopher R. Carpenter, Ali S. Raja and Jeremiah D. Schuur.
© 2013 John Wiley & Sons, Ltd. Published 2013 by John Wiley & Sons, Ltd.

Clinical question

Can elements of the history and physical exam identify adult patients with minor head injury who are at low risk for intracranial injury and who do not need CT imaging?

The first clinical decision rule that addressed this question was published by Haydel et al in 2000.[3] Dubbed the New Orleans criteria, the rule was derived in a single inner-city ED and enrolled patients ≥3 years old who had loss of consciousness or amnesia, a normal neurological examination, and a GCS of 15, and who presented within 24 hours of the injury. A total of 1,429 patients were enrolled in the study and all underwent head CT. The initial portion of the study was a derivation phase that included 520 patients. Eight clinical findings were determined *a priori* by the study authors as being associated with significant head injury; these included headache, age > 60 years old, vomiting, drug or alcohol intoxication, deficits in short term memory, posttraumatic seizure, coagulopathy, or evidence of trauma above the clavicles. The authors explicitly defined each criterion. The presence or absence of each factor was determined before the head CT was performed, and blinded radiologists interpreted the head CTs. Their study outcome was positive findings on CT, defined as the presence of an acute traumatic intracranial lesion (a subdural, epidural, or parenchymal hematoma; subarachnoid hemorrhage; cerebral contusion; or depressed skull fracture) (Figure 14.1). An analysis of the eight clinical factors determined

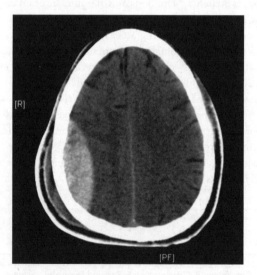

Figure 14.1 Acute epidural hematoma.

Table 14.1 The New Orleans criteria for patients with minor head injury

If none of the following are present, patients are unlikely to have a positive CT
and do not need CT imaging:
- Age > 60 year old
- Vomiting
- Drug or alcohol intoxication
- Short-term memory loss
- Seizure after the injury
- Evidence of trauma above the clavicles.

Source: Data from [3].

Table 14.2 Performance of the New Orleans criteria in the derivation and validation cohorts

Derivation cohort	New Orleans criteria defined positive findings on head computed tomography (CT)		
Decision rule	Injury	No injury	Totals
Positive (≥ 1 criterion present)	36	368	404
Negative (all criteria absent)	0	116	116
Totals	36	484	520
Sensitivity (CI)		100% (90–100%)	
Specificity (CI)		24% (20–28%)	
Positive likelihood ratio (LR+)		1.3	
Negative likelihood ratio (LR−)		0	
Validation cohort	New Orleans criteria defined positive findings on head CT		
Decision rule	Injury	No injury	Totals
Positive (≥ 1 criterion present)	57	640	697
Negative (all criteria absent)	0	212	212
Totals	57	852	909
Sensitivity (CI)		100% (96–100%)	
Specificity (CI)		25% (22–28%)	
Positive likelihood ratio (LR+)		1.3	
Negative likelihood ratio (LR−)		0	

Source: Data from [3].

that the presence of any one of seven factors yielded a decision rule that was 100% sensitive. The final set of clinical criteria (Table 14.1) was then tested on a validation cohort (n = 909). The test results and decision rule performance are shown in Table 14.2.

Within a year of the New Orleans criteria's publication, Canadian researchers, led by Ian Stiell, introduced the Canadian CT head rule.[4] This study examined patients presenting to 10 Canadian EDs within 24 hours of blunt head trauma who had a loss of consciousness, amnesia, or disorientation and an initial GCS ≥ 13 in order to determine two outcome measures: need for neurosurgical intervention (death or neurosurgical procedure) and clinically important brain injury requiring hospital admission and neurological follow-up (abnormal head CT requiring admission). The authors enrolled 3,121 patients who underwent either a head CT or a structured outpatient telephone evaluation (for those who were discharged without a head CT). The overall prevalence of neurosurgical intervention and brain injury on CT was 1.4% and 8.1%, respectively. The study examined 22 clinical factors in each patient, and identified a final set of seven clinical variables, which were categorized according to outcome: five were used to derive a rule that identified patients as high risk for neurosurgical intervention; the addition of two more variables identified additional patients who were at risk for having a clinically important brain injury on CT (Table 14.3). Only patients with complete data were included in the analysis, the results of which are reported in Table 14.4.

Canadian researchers followed their derivation study with a head-to-head study comparing the New Orleans criteria with the Canadian CT head rule.[5] The study was performed in nine Canadian EDs and enrolled 1,822 patients with minor head trauma. To be able to directly compare the two clinical decision rules, only patients with a GCS 15 were included. Treating physicians were asked to complete a data form that included both the New Orleans criteria and Canadian CT head rule prior to ordering a head CT,

Table 14.3 The Canadian CT head rule

CT imaging is indication if any of the following are present:

High risk (for neurosurgical intervention)
1. Glasgow Coma Scale (GCS) score <15 at 2 hours after injury
2. Suspected open or depressed skull fracture
3. Vomiting $\geq$ 2 episodes after injury
4. Any sign of basal skull fracture
5. Age $\geq$ 65 years old.

Medium risk (for brain injury on head CT)
1. Amnesia before impact >30 minutes
2. Dangerous mechanism (pedestrian struck by motor vehicle, ejection from motor vehicle, or fall from >3 foot height or 5 stairs).

Source: Data from [4].

Table 14.4 Test performance of the Canadian CT head rule

Canadian CT head rule: High risk (5 factors)	Injury requiring neurosurgical intervention		
	Injury	No injury	Totals
Positive (≥ 1 criterion present)	44	962	1,006
Negative (all criteria absent)	0	2,115	2,115
Totals	44	3,077	3,121
Sensitivity (CI)	100% (92–100%)		
Specificity (CI)	69% (67–70%)		
Positive likelihood ratio (LR+)	3.2		
Negative likelihood ratio (LR−)	0		
Canadian CT head rule: Medium risk (all 7 factors)	Any clinically important brain injury on head computed tomography (CT)		
	Injury	No injury	Totals
Positive (≥ 1 criterion present)	250	1,446	1,696
Negative (all criteria absent)	4	1,421	1,425
Totals	57	2,867	3,121
Sensitivity (CI)	98% (96–99%)		
Specificity (CI)	50% (47–51%)		
Positive likelihood ratio (LR+)	2.0		
Negative likelihood ratio (LR−)	0.04		

Source: Data from [4].

and the outcomes were the need for neurosurgical intervention and clinically important brain injury seen on head CT, similar to the original Canadian CT head rule. Patients not undergoing head CT were followed up with a 14-day telephone interview. The incidence of neurosurgical intervention and clinically important brain injury on CT was 0.4% and 5.3%, respectively. Table 14.5 shows the test performance of each clinical decision rule.

While both rules performed with very high sensitivities (100%) and did not miss any injuries, application of the New Orleans criteria resulted in significantly more false positives, which yielded a lower specificity. The authors concluded that, given the equivalent sensitivities, using the Canadian CT head rule would result in fewer head CTs being ordered. This finding was confirmed in a recent US study co-authored by some of the same authors as the earlier Canadian studies.[6] They confirmed the 100% sensitivities for both rules as well as the higher specificity for the Canadian CT head rule compared to the New Orleans criteria, both for the need for neurosurgical interventions (81% (CI 76–85%) versus 9.6% (CI 7.0–14%)) and for clinically important brain lesions seen on CT (35% (CI 30–41%) versus 9.9% (CI 7.0–14%)).

Table 14.5 Comparison of the Canadian head CT rule and the New Orleans criteria for patients with Glasgow Coma Scale (GCS) 15

Need for neurosurgical intervention Decision rule	Canadian head CT rule			New Orleans criteria		
	Injury	No injury	Totals	Injury	No injury	Totals
Positive	8	430	438	8	1,595	1,603
Negative	0	1,384	1,384	0	219	219
Totals	8	1,814	1,822	8	1,814	1,822
Sensitivity (CI)	100% (63–100%)			100% (63–100%)		
Specificity (CI)	76% (74–78%)			12% (10–13%)		
Positive likelihood ratio (LR+)	4.2			1.1		
Negative likelihood ratio (LR−)	0			0		
Any clinically important brain injury						
Decision rule	Injury	No injury	Totals	Injury	No injury	Totals
Positive	97	853	950	97	1,506	1,603
Negative	0	872	872	0	219	219
Totals	97	1,725	1,822	97	1,725	1,822
Sensitivity (CI)	100% (96–100%)			100% (96–100%)		
Specificity (CI)	50% (48–53%)			12% (11–14%)		
Positive likelihood ratio (LR+)	2.0			1.1		
Negative likelihood ratio (LR−)	0			0		

Source: Data from [5].

An external validation study of the New Orleans criteria and Canadian CT head rule was performed by a large Dutch study from 2002 to 2004.[7] The multicenter trial included four university hospitals, and a total of 3,181 patients were enrolled after blunt head trauma. Inclusion criteria were presentation within 24 hours after the injury, a GCS ≥13, and at least one of the following risk factors: a reported loss of consciousness, amnesia, short-term memory loss, posttraumatic seizure, severe headache, vomiting, intoxicated appearance, physical evidence of injury above the clavicles, current warfarin use or a history of coagulopathy, or a neurological deficit. Given the differences between the New Orleans criteria and Canadian CT head rule in their GCS inclusion criteria, a separate analysis was performed for each clinical prediction rule. All patients included in the study underwent head CT, and the interpreting radiologist was not blinded to the data being collected. Physician assessment was performed by a neurologist prior to the head CTs being performed. The outcomes were need for neurosurgical intervention within 30 days of the traumatic injury and traumatic injury detected on CT requiring hospitalization.

Table 14.6 External validation results comparing two clinical decision rules performances on a Dutch patient cohort with head injuries

Need for neurosurgical intervention	Canadian head CT rule			New Orleans criteria		
Decision rule	Injury	No injury	Totals	Injury	No injury	Totals
Positive	7	1,269	1,276	2	1,236	1,238
Negative	0	752	752	0	69	69
Totals	7	2,021	2,028	2	1,305	1,307
Sensitivity (CI)	100% (67–100%)			100% (34–100%)		
Specificity (CI)	37% (34–40%)			5.3% (2.5–8.3%)		
Positive likelihood ratio (LR+)	1.6			1.1		
Negative likelihood ratio (LR−)	0			0		

Neurocranial traumatic CT finding

Decision rule	Injury	No injury	Totals	Injury	No injury	Totals
Positive	171	1,105	1,276	115	1,152	1,267
Negative	34	718	752	2	67	69
Totals	205	1,823	2,028	117	1,219	1,336
Sensitivity (CI)	83% (78–88%)			98% (94–100%)		
Specificity (CI)	39% (36–43%)			5.6% (2.7–8.8%)		
Positive likelihood ratio (LR+)	1.4			1.0		
Negative likelihood ratio (LR−)	0.44			0.36		

Source: Data from [7].

The authors concluded that both the New Orleans criteria and Canadian CT head rule performed with 100% sensitivity for the outcome of need for neurosurgical intervention, despite the application in a new setting and with slight differences from the strictly defined inclusion and exclusion criteria and explicit definitions for each criterion in each rule (Table 14.6). The specificities were much lower for each rule and the Canadian CT head rule had a sensitivity of only 83% (CI 78–88%) for the detection of neurocranial traumatic CT findings, compared to a sensitivity of 98% (CI 94–100%) for the New Orleans criteria.

The National Emergency X-Radiography Utilization Study II (NEXUS II) group derived a clinical decision rule to identify patients who are at low risk for having intracranial injuries after blunt trauma in the largest derivation study to date.[8] They performed a multicenter, prospective, observational study in 21 EDs and included patients presenting with blunt trauma for which a head CT was ordered. Detailed clinical and mechanistic information on 19 variables was collected and recorded by physicians prior to head CT. Patients not undergoing head CT at the discretion of the treating physician were not included in the study. The two outcomes examined

Table 14.7 NEXUS II head CT rule

Patients without any of the following are at very low risk of clinically important traumatic brain injury, and CT can routinely be avoided for them:
- Evidence of significant skull fracture
- Scalp hematoma
- Neurological deficit
- Age $\geq$ 65 years old
- Altered level of consciousness
- Abnormal behavior
- Coagulopathy
- Persistent vomiting.

Source: Data from [8].

were the presence of a significant intracranial injury (defined as the need for neurosurgical intervention that might otherwise lead to a precipitous deterioration or long-term neurological impairment) and minor head injury (defined as an intracranial injury in a patient with a GCS 15).

A total of 13,728 patients were enrolled, including 917 (6.9%) patients with intracranial injuries, of whom 330 (2.4%) had a GCS of 15. Eight clinical variables were chosen to derive the NEXUS II head CT rule (Table 14.7), the performance of which is displayed in Table 14.8. As yet, there has not been a published validation study.

Comments

The New Orleans criteria and Canadian CT head rule have both been externally validated. While the studies cited in this chapter verify that the sensitivities of both rules are consistently 100%, the specificity of the New Orleans criteria appears to be significantly lower than that of the Canadian CT head rule, allowing emergency physicians using the Canadian CT head rule to rule out intracranial injuries without obtaining as many head CTs as they would using the New Orleans criteria. It should be noted, however, that the outcomes for the two studies were different; while the New Orleans criteria focused on an outcome of positive findings on CT, the main criteria of the Canadian CT head rule instead focus on injuries requiring neurosurgical intervention, and emergency physicians should feel comfortable with the outcomes of whichever of the two rules they opt to use.

The NEXUS II head CT rule has only been derived and not validated, therefore we cannot comment on its performance beyond the findings in the original study. Readers should take note, however, of the similarities between the three sets of decision rules. All include evidence of head trauma,

Table 14.8 Performance of the NEXUS II head computed tomography (CT) rule

Decision rule	NEXUS II head CT rule–defined clinically important intracranial injury		
	Injury	No injury	Totals
Positive	901	11,059	11,960
Negative	16	1,752	1,768
Totals	917	12,811	13,728
Sensitivity (CI)	98% (97–99%)		
Specificity (CI)	13% (13–14%)		
Positive likelihood ratio (LR+)	1.1		
Negative likelihood ratio (LR−)	0.15		
Decision rule	NEXUS II head CT rule–defined minor head injuries (Glasgow Coma Scale (GCS) 15)		
	Injury	No injury	Totals
Positive	314	8,375	8,689
Negative	16	1,752	1,768
Totals	330	10,127	10,457
Sensitivity (CI)	95% (92–97%)		
Specificity (CI)	17% (16–18%)		
Positive likelihood ratio (LR+)	1.1		
Negative likelihood ratio (LR−)	0.29		

Source: Data from [8].

older patient age, and vomiting as high-risk factors. Therefore, regardless of which rule is ultimately used, it is safe to assume that each of these factors is concerning and not unique to the study from which it emanated.

Given the strengths of both the New Orleans criteria and the Canadian CT head rule, the American College of Emergency Physicians' clinical policy on neuroimaging in adults with mild traumatic brain injury recommends using each for distinct patient populations. Since the New Orleans criteria specifically enrolled patients with loss of consciousness, the policy recommends using the decision rule specifically for those patients. Conversely, since the Canadian CT head rule enrolled both patients with and without loss of consciousness, the clinical policy recommends using it for patients without loss of consciousness.[9] This clinical policy has also been approved by the Emergency Nurses Association and the Centers for Disease Control and Prevention.

Notably, there are still no decision rules that identify which elderly patients with mild head injuries are at low risk of intracranial injury. Instead, all three rules described in this chapter include advanced age as a risk factor for intracranial injury; there is an age criterion in the New Orleans criteria (age > 60 years old), the Canadian CT head rule (≥65 years old), and the NEXUS II head CT rule (≥65 years old), designating elderly patients at high risk in the setting of minor head injury. Until a decision rule for minor head injury includes the elderly population, the decision on whether or not to obtain imaging in these patients will be left to the clinical expertise of their treating physicians.

While the New Orleans criteria and Canadian CT head rule have shown reproducibility and external validity, they have not yet demonstrated that they will be used by clinicians and have an impact in the utilization of head CTs in their target population of patients with minor head injury. Stiell et al performed an impact analysis of the Canadian CT head rule in 2010 but found that head CT utilization at six sites using the Canadian CT head rule actually increased when compared to utilization at six control sites.[10] Given the significant amount of interhospital and interphysician variability that exists around utilization of head CTs,[11,12] future research in this area needs to focus on developing effective methods of implementing these decision rules so that inappropriate imaging can be minimized while patients with minor head injury still receive the best care possible.

References

1. Langlois JA, Rutland-Brown W, Thomas KE. Traumatic brain injury in the United States. Atlanta (GA): US Department of Health and Human Services; 2006.
2. Rutland-Brown W, Langlois JA, Thomas KE, Xi YL. Incidence of traumatic brain injury in the United States, 2003. The Journal of Head Trauma Rehabilitation. 2006; 21(6). Available from: http://journals.lww.com/headtraumarehab/Fulltext/ 2006/11000/Incidence_of_Traumatic_Brain_Injury_in_the_United.9.aspx
3. Haydel MJ, Preston CA, Mills TJ et al. Indications for computed tomography in patients with minor head injury. New England Journal of Medicine. 2000; 343(2): 100–5.
4. Stiell IG, Wells GA, Vandemheen K et al. The Canadian CT head rule for patients with minor head injury. Lancet. 2001; 357(9266): 1391–6.
5. Stiell IG, Clement CM, Rowe BH et al. Comparison of the Canadian CT head rule and the New Orleans criteria in patients with minor head injury. Journal of the American Medical Association. 2005; 294(12): 1511–8.
6. Papa L, Stiell IG, Clement CM et al. Performance of the Canadian CT head rule and the New Orleans criteria for predicting any traumatic intracranial injury on computed tomography in a United States Level I trauma center. Academic Emergency Medicine. 2012; 19(1): 2–10.
7. Smits M, Dippel DWJ, de Haan GG et al. External validation of the Canadian CT head rule and the New Orleans criteria for CT scanning in patients with

minor head injury. Journal of the American Medical Association. 2005; 294(12): 1519–25.

8. Mower WR, Hoffman JR, Herbert M *et al.* Developing a decision instrument to guide computed tomographic imaging of blunt head injury patients. Journal of Trauma. 2005; 59(4): 954–9.

9. Jagoda AS, Bazarian JJ, Bruns JJ Jr *et al.* Clinical policy: Neuroimaging and decision making in adult mild traumatic brain injury in the acute setting. Annals of Emergency Medicine. 2008; 52(6): 714–48.

10. Stiell IG, Clement CM, Grimshaw JM *et al.* A prospective cluster-randomized trial to implement the Canadian CT head rule in emergency departments. Canadian Medical Association Journal. 2010; 182(14): 1527–32.

11. Raja AS, Andruchow J, Zane R, Khorasani R, Schuur JD. Use of neuroimaging in US emergency departments. Archives of Internal Medicine. 2011; 171(3): 260–2.

12. Prevedello LM, Raja AS, Zane RD *et al.* Variation in use of head computed tomography by emergency physicians. The American Journal of Medicine. 2012 125(4): 356–64.

Chapter 15 **Blunt Chest Trauma**

Highlights

- Potential injuries due to blunt chest trauma include cardiac contusion, pneumothorax, hemothorax, lung contusion, diaphragmatic injury, rib fracture, and injuries to the thoracic aorta.
- Chest wall tenderness, hypoxia, and chest pain are sensitive for injury, and a recent decision rule to identify patients at low risk for significant injury has been derived but not validated.
- Chest CT is more sensitive for significant intrathoracic injuries and should be used to evaluate severely injured patients.
- Data on the use of troponin I for detecting cardiac contusion are inconclusive, with some studies reporting high sensitivity and one study reporting very low sensitivity (23%).
- Minor cardiac contusions, while detectable using troponin I, ECG, and echocardiography, are associated with no adverse consequences.
- In pediatric trauma patients with blunt chest injury, one study found that the prevalence of elevated troponin I was 1 in 4; however, this finding was not predictive of significant myocardial injury.

Background

Patients with blunt chest trauma in the emergency department (ED) often require diagnostic testing to exclude potential injuries such as cardiac or pulmonary contusion, pneumothorax, hemothorax, diaphragmatic injury, rib fracture, and injury to the thoracic aorta. For patients with severe thoracic trauma, criterion standard imaging (i.e., computed tomography (CT) angiography) is often performed because, in 70–90% of cases, multiple injuries are present.

There is a clinical divide between multitrauma patients and ambulatory patients with histories of blunt chest trauma and chest pain while both groups

Evidence-Based Emergency Care: Diagnostic Testing and Clinical Decision Rules, Second Edition. Jesse M. Pines, Christopher R. Carpenter, Ali S. Raja and Jeremiah D. Schuur.
© 2013 John Wiley & Sons, Ltd. Published 2013 by John Wiley & Sons, Ltd.

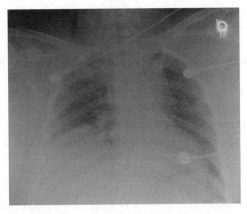

Figure 15.1 Chest X-ray from a patient with a traumatic aortic injury demonstrating a wide mediastinum, blurring of the aortic arch, left apical cap, and deviation of the nasogastric tube.

typically receive screening chest radiography (Figure 15.1), the probabilities of clinically significant injuries in each are considerably different. When a patient is ambulatory or not severely injured, he or she can receive upright posterior-anterior and lateral chest X-rays. In contrast, multitrauma patients typically receive an initial supine anterior-posterior chest X-ray because their presumed critical injuries preclude their receiving upright X-rays safely. Most patients in the United States with severe chest trauma will receive CT scans. The initial screening supine X-ray is less sensitive than an upright chest X-ray for the detection of thoracic injuries, but both can be useful in guiding the initial management of patients with blunt chest trauma.

Clinical question

Which ED patients need diagnostic chest X-rays following blunt chest trauma?
A 2006 study enrolled 507 patients with blunt chest trauma.[1] The investigators' objective was to derive a clinical decision rule able to identify blunt chest trauma patients at low risk for intrathoracic injury. The authors excluded patients <15 years old and those with penetrating trauma, trauma that occurred greater than 72 hours before presentation, isolated head trauma, and Glasgow Coma Scale scores <14. Providers filled out surveys prior to viewing radiographic results and documented the mechanism of injury, vital signs (including oxygen saturation), patient symptoms, intoxication, distracting injuries, and the presence of visible chest wall injury, chest tenderness, pain on

lateral chest compression, crepitus, and abnormal chest auscultation. Significant intrathoracic injuries were defined as pneumothoraces, hemothoraces, aortic injuries, two or more rib fractures, sternal fractures, or pulmonary contusions on blinded plain chest radiography. The prevalence of significant intrathoracic injury was 6% (31 of the 492 who had complete data). Tenderness to palpation and chest pain had the highest sensitivity (90%) as individual criteria to predict significant injuries, and hypoxia (defined as an O_2 saturation <95% on room air) was the most specific (97%). The combination of tenderness to palpation and hypoxia identified all significant injuries: sensitivity 100% (CI 91–100%), specificity 50% (CI 45–54%), positive predictive value 12% (CI 9–17%), and negative predictive value 100% (CI 99–100%).

In a recent follow-up study, the authors derived a decision rule to identify patients with very low risk of significant intrathoracic injury and who therefore do not require any chest imaging. The authors conducted a study at a single Level I trauma center and enrolled patients aged 15 or older with blunt chest trauma. They used the same definition of significant intrathoracic injury as in the earlier study, with the only addition being diaphragmatic rupture. In 2,628 subjects, 271 (10.3%) had a total of 462 significant intrathoracic injuries, with rib fractures (73%), pneumothoraces (38%), and pulmonary contusions (29%) being the most common. Once again, the clinical factors with the highest sensitivities for significant injury were chest pain and chest wall tenderness. Additional high-risk factors in the decision rule included painful distracting injury, intoxication, age >60 years, rapid deceleration, and altered alertness or mental status. If all of the factors were absent, the proposed rule had a sensitivity of 99% (CI 97–100%), a specificity of 14% (CI 13–15%), a negative predictive value if 99% (CI 98–100%), and positive predictive value of 12% (CI 11–13%). When the seven criteria were assessed for interrater reliability (i.e., whether two raters would agree on a factor being present or absent), there was reasonable interrater reliability for all variables, κ (range 0.51–0.81). A multicenter validation study of this decision rule has been completed, and the data are currently being analyzed.

Clinical question

How does chest X-ray compare to CT scan in excluding thoracic injuries in patients with blunt chest trauma?

Most studies addressing this question have been small and retrospective, involving trauma registries and including only severely injured trauma patients seen at large trauma centers. One study of 112 patients with blunt chest trauma found that four of the nine patients with acute aortic rupture had a normal mediastinum on the initial supine chest X-ray while helical CT scan was diagnostic in eight of nine and suggestive in one patient who had a brachiocephalic injury.[3] A study from Australia involved a 2-year retrospective survey of 141 patients with Injury Severity Scores (ISS) >15 (i.e., multitrauma patients) and blunt trauma to the chest.[4] Patients had both a supine chest X-ray and a CT of the chest. In patients with chest wall tenderness, the authors found that the CT was more likely to provide additional diagnostic information compared to plain radiography (OR 6.7, CI 2.6–17.7). Similarly, CT was more likely to add clinical information about patients with reduced air entry (OR 4.5, CI 1.3–15.0) and abnormal respiratory effort (OR 4.1, CI 1.3–12.7). They also found that CT scan was more effective than routine chest X-ray at detecting lung contusions, pneumothoraces, mediastinal injuries, hematomas, and fractures (of the ribs, scapulae, sternums, and vertebrae).

A prospective study of 103 patients with chest trauma and a mean ISS of 30 (severely injured trauma patients) found that, in 67 patients (65%), CT scan detected major chest trauma complications that were missed on chest X-ray; of those, 33 were lung contusions, 27 were pneumothoraces (including seven residual pneumothoraces after tube thoracostomy), 21 were hemothoraces, five were displaced chest tubes, two were diaphragmatic ruptures, and one was a myocardial rupture.[5] In 11 patients, minor additional findings were visualized on CT scan, and in only 14 of the 103 patients did chest X-ray and CT scan show the same results.

Another study followed 93 consecutive trauma patients with blunt chest trauma, all of whom had anterior-posterior chest radiographs and helical chest CTs.[6] Chest radiography was abnormal in 73% of patients. In 13 of the 25 patients with normal radiography (52%), CT demonstrated multiple injuries, including two aortic lacerations and one pericardial effusion.

Clinical question

What is the role of troponin I in excluding myocardial injury in blunt chest trauma?

Patients with blunt chest trauma can sustain myocardial injuries. In severe cases, this can be dramatic, involving hemodynamic instability. In minor cases, however, blunt cardiac injury can be an occult event producing mild symptoms that may be misattributed to musculoskeletal trauma. CT and X-ray are often unhelpful in diagnosing cardiac contusions, unless there is associated great-vessel or other intrathoracic injury. The limited role of CT and X-ray has led to the use of laboratory testing, electrocardiogram, and echocardiogram to detect these injuries. While creatine kinase (CK) levels can be used, their use in the detection of cardiac injury in patients with blunt chest trauma can be difficult because creatine kinase-MB (CK-MB) can be elevated from skeletal muscle injury. Thus, troponin I has emerged as a potential indicator of cardiac contusion.

One study followed 44 patients with blunt chest trauma and suspected cardiac contusion[7] who underwent serial echocardiograms and troponin I testing. Six out of 44 (14%) had evidence of cardiac injury by echocardiography, and all had elevations of CK-MB and troponin I. There was one patient with elevations of both CK-MB and troponin I found to have a pericardial effusion.

Another study followed 32 patients admitted with signs of acute blunt chest trauma.[8] All patients underwent transesophageal echocardiography within 24 hours of injury and had serial troponin I measured. A total of 17 (53%) of patients had abnormal troponin I (>0.4 ng/mL) levels, and 10 had levels of greater than 1 ng/mL. In six out of the 10 with elevated troponins greater than 1 ng/mL, there were segmental wall motion abnormalities consistent with myocardial contusion. None of the patients with troponins between 0.4 ng/mL and 1 ng/mL had abnormal echocardiograms.

Another study followed 96 patients with blunt chest trauma admitted to a trauma center for evaluation.[9] A total of 24/96 (28%) had myocardial contusion diagnosed on echocardiogram, electrocardiogram, or both. Notably, all of the patients survived to admission and were hemodynamically stable. No patients died or had severe in-hospital cardiac complications. There were no differences in the percentage of patients with elevated CK (CK-MB/total CK) ratio, or CK-MB mass concentration among patients with and without cardiac contusion. In patients with cardiac contusion, the percentage of patients with elevated circulating troponin I and troponin T (defined as greater than or equal to 0.1 ug/L) was higher in patients with myocardial contusion (23% versus 3%). The respective sensitivity, specificity, and negative and positive predictive values of troponin I and troponin T in predicting a myocardial contusion in blunt trauma patients were 23%, 97%, 77%, and 75% (for troponin I), and 12%, 100%, 74%, and 100% (for troponin T), respectively. The patients were followed for up to 18 months, and 88% had complete follow-up. There were no deaths from cardiac complications, and no patients had any long-term cardiac complications or myocardial failure related to blunt chest trauma.

A recent study examined this question in pediatric patients.[10] It specifically assessed the prevalence of elevated cardiac troponin I in pediatric trauma patients to determine if elevated TnI correlated with clinically significant myocardial injury, defined as the presence of abnormalities on echocardiogram or ECG. The authors studied a small sample of 59 pediatric trauma patients with an Injury Severity Score (ISS) >12. Both troponin I and CK-MB were measured at admission and then serially until the troponin I had normalized. Patients who had elevated troponin I levels had echocardiograms within 24 hours of admission and underwent daily ECGs. Elevated troponin I was found in 16 patients (27%); all cases had an associated elevated CK-MB. There were abnormal echocardiograms in four out of the 16 patients with elevated troponin I; however, peak troponin I values were not correlated with any echocardiogram abnormality. There was only one patient with a clinically significant reduction in cardiac function. In this small study, all ECGs were normal. The authors concluded that troponin I was a reflection of severity of illness of the patient and that it was frequently elevated with associated clinically significant injuries to the myocardium. However, they cautioned that larger scale studies are needed prior to any definitive conclusions are made.

Comment

The studies on blunt chest trauma reviewed have considerable methodological issues. Most have very small sample sizes and are retrospective. While a clinical decision rule has been derived, it has not yet been validated and there are no other validated decision rules to identify patients who need radiography. In addition, large studies are needed to differentiate patients who require chest X-rays as opposed to CT scans.

Throughout this review a number of clinical themes emerged. In ED patients with blunt chest trauma, the prevalence of clinically significant injuries is relatively low (6%). In these trauma patients, clinical factors such as the presence of chest wall tenderness and chest pain may suggest the need for chest radiography. In patients with severe chest trauma or a high index of suspicion for intrathoracic injury, CT scan seems to be the study of choice given the high miss rate (50%) of chest X-ray in severely injured patients.

The data on myocardial contusion are inconclusive. While some studies have concluded that troponin I is a sensitive marker for myocardial injury, another study found that its sensitivity was only 23%. An interesting finding was that, in patients with these minor contusions (without any hemodynamic instability), there were no clinical complications. Therefore, whether minor contusions are detected electrocardiographically or through laboratory testing, these contusions are not clinically significant. This was confirmed in a recent study in pediatric patients. Certainly a larger study is needed before concluding that objective findings of cardiac contusion are clinically benign.

References

1. Rodriguez RM, Hendey GM, Marek G *et al.* A pilot study to derive clinical variables for selective chest radiography in blunt trauma patients. Annals of Emergency Medicine. 2006; 47: 415–18.

2. Rodriguez RM, Hendey GW, Mower W, Kea B, Fortman J, Merchant G, Hoffman JR. Derivation of a decision instrument for selective chest radiography in blunt trauma. Journal of Trauma. 2011 Sep; 71: 549–53.

3. Demetriades D, Gomez H, Velmahos GC, Asensio JA, Murray J, Cornwell EE *et al.* Routine helical computed tomographic evaluation of the mediastinum in high-risk blunt trauma patients. Archives of Surgery 1998; 133: 1084–8.

4. Traub M, Stevenson M, McEvoy S *et al.* The use of chest computed tomography versus chest X-ray in patients with major blunt trauma. Injury. 2007; 38: 43–7.

5. Trupka A, Waydas C, Hallfeldt KK *et al.* Value of thoracic computed tomography in the first assessment of severely injured patients with blunt chest trauma: Results of a prospective study. Journal of Trauma. 1997; 43: 405–11.

6. Exadaktylos, AK, Sclabas, G, Schmid, SW Do we really need routine computed tomographic scanning in the primary evaluation of blunt chest trauma in patients with "normal" chest radiograph? Journal of Trauma. 2001; 51: 1173–6.

7. Adams JE, Davila-Roman VG, Bessey PQ *et al.* Improved detection of cardiac contusion with cardiac troponin I. American Heart Journal. 1996; 131(2): 308–12.

8. Mori F, Zuppiroli A, Ognibene A *et al.* Cardiac contusion in blunt chest trauma: A combined study of transesophageal echocardiography and cardiac troponin I determination. Italian Heart Journal. 2001; 2: 222–7.

9. Bertinchant JP, Polge A, Mohty, D *et al.* Evaluation of incidence, clinical significance, and prognostic value of circulating cardiac troponin I and T elevation in hemodynamically stable patients with suspected myocardial contusion after blunt chest trauma. Journal of Trauma. 2000; 48: 924–31.

10. Sangha GS, Pepelassis D, Buffo-Sequeira I, Seabrook JA, Fraser DD. Serum troponin-I as an indicator of clinically significant myocardial injury in paediatric trauma patients. Injury. 2011 Nov 25; epub ahead of print.

Chapter 16 **Occult Hip Fracture**

Highlights

- Hip fractures will be missed by plain radiography in up to 10% of patients with hip pain after falls or trauma.
- Advanced imaging (CT or MRI) should be used in cases of suspected occult fracture. MRI is the study of choice if it is available.

Background

Hip fractures are common in the elderly, with an incidence of approximately 250,000 per year in the U.S., a number that is projected to double by 2040.[1] Many of these patients with hip fractures will present to the emergency department (ED) for evaluation and treatment, typically following a fall or other acute traumatic injury. The diagnosis of hip fracture is typically not a diagnostic dilemma because plain radiographs are often diagnostic, particularly in patients with classic anatomic deformities. However, a small proportion of patients with hip fracture (2–9%) will have initially negative plain films.[2] These occult hip fractures are more common in the elderly because of the high prevalence of osteoporosis in this age group.[3] Physicians face a diagnostic dilemma when treating a patient in whom they have a high suspicion for hip fracture based on their physical examination or history and whose plain radiographs are either negative or equivocal. The classic case is an older adult patient who has fallen, has hip tenderness, and cannot bear weight on the affected leg. A missed diagnosis of hip fracture can place elderly patients at substantial risk of fracture displacement, avascular necrosis, and the need for more involved surgical procedures.

Approaches to the diagnosis of occult hip fractures have evolved over the past 10 years. In the past, repeat plain films or bone scans were advocated. Bone scans will typically become positive after 24–72 hours following an

Evidence-Based Emergency Care: Diagnostic Testing and Clinical Decision Rules, Second Edition.
Jesse M. Pines, Christopher R. Carpenter, Ali S. Raja and Jeremiah D. Schuur.
© 2013 John Wiley & Sons, Ltd. Published 2013 by John Wiley & Sons, Ltd.

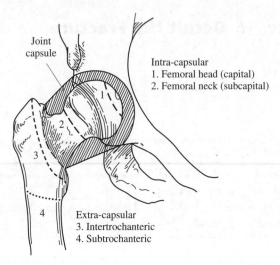

Joint capsule

Intra-capsular
1. Femoral head (capital)
2. Femoral neck (subcapital)

Extra-capsular
3. Intertrochanteric
4. Subtrochanteric

Figure 16.1 Hip fractures. This illustration depicts the different types of proximal hip fractures. (Knoop et al Atlas of Emergency Medicine 2nd edition, Copyright 2002. Reproduced with permission of The McGraw-Hill Companies).

acute fracture. Certain historical factors can predict the presence of hip fractures in patients with acute traumatic hip pain, such as the inability to ambulate. Since their ambulatory status cannot be assessed, these patients all require further imaging to exclude occult hip fracture. However, the choice of which advanced imaging modality to obtain presents another dilemma: computed tomography (CT) or magnetic resonance imaging (MRI)?

Clinical question

What historical and physical examination findings are associated with the presence of a hip fracture among patients with possible occult hip fractures?

A recent study examined the value of various clinical signs in relation to this question.[4] The authors reviewed patients in a single center who had an MRI for suspected hip fracture and also had normal initial X-rays over 6 years. In a retrospective chart review of 57 patients, 35 had occult proximal femoral fractures. Both pain on axial loading of the limb and pre-fracture restricted mobility were associated with fractures ($p < 0.005$), with similar positive predictive values (76%), negative predictive values (69%), and posttest probabilities of disease given a negative test (30%). Predictive values were the same when both factors were combined. Patients who were mobile prior to the fall and without pain on the axial limb were less likely to have fracture; however, these signs alone or in combination were not sufficient to

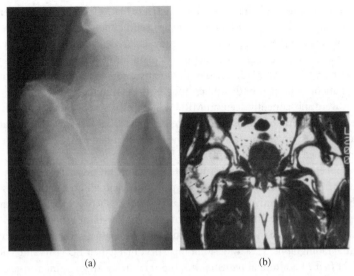

(a)   (b)

Figure 16.2 Occult hip fracture. (a) Anteroposterior radiograph of a 55-year-old patient on steroids who had right hip pain after a fall. No fracture is evident. (b) A T1-weighted coronal MRI of the same hip clearly demonstrates a nondisplaced hip fracture (thin arrows). (Reproduced from Tintanelli et al (2004) Emergency Medicine: A Comprehensive Study Guide 6th edition, with permission of The McGraw-Hill Companies).

exclude fractures. The authors concluded that clinical signs were insufficient to distinguish patients with and without a hip fracture and recommended MRI scanning for all patients with suspected occult fractures.

Clinical question

Which is the optimal diagnostic imaging modality when evaluating the diagnosis of occult hip fracture in the ED?

Since a bone scan can take days to become positive and serial plain films are not practical in the ED setting, these modalities are not efficient strategies to sensitively detect occult hip fractures in the ED.

Once the decision to evaluate a patient for an occult hip fracture has been made, the clinician is faced with the choice of either a MRI or a CT. While there are case series and retrospective studies that address this question indirectly, there are very few studies investigating whether a CT or MRI should be ordered, many of which are referenced throughout this section.[5] The literature primarily describes cases in which MRI has been used to diagnose hip fractures and cases involving a negative CT followed by a

MRI demonstrating a fracture. The concern is that CT scans can miss very small impacted fractures of the femoral head and nondisplaced fractures that run parallel to the axial plane.[6] One study assessed 13 elderly patients who had falls without evidence of fracture on plain film.[7] A total of six patients underwent CT and MRI, and seven patients underwent MRI only. In the six patients who had both studies, four of the CT studies missed fractures that were subsequently seen on MRI. While this is a very small study, this demonstrates that MRI is likely more sensitive than CT scan to evaluate patients with occult hip fracture. In the group that had MRI only, all seven patients had accurate diagnoses of hip fractures.

A recent retrospective study sought to determine the prevalence of hip and pelvic fractures in ED patients with hip pain and negative initial radiographs.[2] This was a retrospective study where plain films and MRIs were ordered at the discretion of the treating physician. Structured follow-up at 1 month after the visit was conducted with 85% follow-up. Of the 545 patients who had negative initial radiographs, 11% underwent hip MRI during their ED visits and MRI identified 24 additional patients with hip fractures with good interobserver agreement among radiologists (kappa = 0.85). There were no patients in the 1-month follow-up period who subsequently had hip fractures identified.

Another study investigated the medical records of patients with suspected occult hip fracture at one hospital over a year (2002–3).[8] A total of 33 patients were enrolled and images were reviewed by two junior and two senior radiologists. Using MRI images, senior radiologists identified occult hip fractures with 100% accuracy and had complete agreement. There was

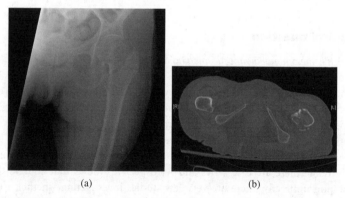

(a)   (b)

Figure 16.3 Intertrochanteric fracture (a) was suspected on the left hip plain X-ray and (b) was confirmed with a noncontrast CT scan.

excellent agreement between junior and senior radiologists (kappa = 0.75). Among the two junior radiologists, MRI was 89% and 96% sensitive for detecting fractures.

Comment

While there is little literature directly addressing whether CT or MRI is the optimal diagnostic test to investigate the occult hip fracture, case series and retrospective studies support the use of MRI. Additionally, the absence of any subsequent diagnoses of hip fracture over 1-month follow-up in patients with negative MRIs in one study reassures us that this modality is close to 100% sensitive for fractures. MRI is also cost-effective compared with CT or bone scans,[7] and also has the advantage of being able to identify alternative diagnoses that may mimic hip fractures, such as hematomas, muscle tears, degenerative joint diseases, and osteonecrosis.[9] MRI, however, may not be available at all EDs, particularly during off-hours. For these patients, other strategies may also be considered, such as using CT (knowing that it is not as sensitive as MRI) or hospital admission for delayed MRI when available.

A recent algorithm was proposed as an approach to the evaluation of patients with suspected hip fractures.[3] The first step in ED care should include pain control, assessing comorbid conditions, and X-ray imaging. If a fracture is identified on X-ray, then initiate appropriate fracture care. If not, the patient should be tested for safe weight bearing. If the patient can safely bear weight, then discharge the patient home if there is no other reason to admit. If the patient is unable to weight bear, then an MRI should be the test of choice.

References

1. Cummings SR, Rubin SM, Black D. The future of hip fractures in the United States: Numbers, costs, and potential effects of postmenopausal estrogen. Clinical Orthopaedics and Related Research. 1990;(252): 163–6.
2. Dominguez S, Liu P, Roberts C *et al.* Prevalence of traumatic hip and pelvic fractures in patients with suspected hip fracture and negative initial standard radiographs: A study of emergency department patients. Academic Emergency Medicine 2005; 12: 366–9.
3. Carpenter CR, Stern ME. Emergency orthogeriatrics: Concepts and therapeutic alternatives. Emergency Medicine Clinics of North America. 2010; 28: 927–49.
4. Hossain M, Barwick C, Sinha AK, Andrew JG. Is magnetic resonance imaging (MRI) necessary to exclude occult hip fracture? Injury. 2007; 38(10): 1204–8.

5. Mlinek EJ, Clark KC, Walker C. Limited magnetic resonance imaging in the diagnosis of occult hip fracture. American Journal of Emergency Medicine. 1998; 16: 390–3.
6. Perron AD, Miller MD, Brady WJ. Orthopedic pitfalls in the ED: Radiographically occult hip fracture. American Journal of Emergency Medicine. 2002; 20: 234–7.
7. Lubovsky O, Liebergall M, Mattan Y et al. Early diagnosis of hip fractures: MRI versus CT scan. Injury. 2005; 36: 788–92.
8. Verbeeten KM, Hermann KL, Hasselqvist M et al. The advantages of MRI in the detection of occult hip fractures. European Radiology. 2005; 15(1): 165–9.
9. Oka M, Monu JU. Prevalence and patterns of occult hip fractures and mimics revealed by MRI. American Journal of Roentgenology. 2004; 182(2): 283–8.

Chapter 17 **Blunt Soft Tissue Neck Trauma**

Highlights

- Blunt cerebrovascular injury is a rare but potentially severe outcome of blunt trauma.
- While no definitive evidence exists to determine which asymptomatic patients should be screened for blunt cerebrovascular injury, we recommend considering screening in otherwise asymptomatic patients with blunt neck trauma who have associated cervical spine injuries, basilar skull or severe facial injuries, or ligature mechanisms.
- While cerebral angiography remains the criterion standard for the diagnosis of blunt cerebrovascular injury, modern CT angiography (>16 slice) has similar test characteristics and should be considered an acceptable screening modality.

Background

Blunt neck trauma is a rare event, accounting for 5–10% of all trauma to the neck. It occurs most commonly following motor vehicle accidents, although clothesline mechanisms and strangulation can also cause blunt injury to the aerodigestive tract and cervical vasculature. While blunt esophageal injuries are exceptionally rare (a 1988 review found only 96 cases reported since 1900),[1] airway and vascular injuries are far more common.

The most common mechanism for blunt neck trauma, motor vehicle accidents, typically occurs due to impact with the steering column or dashboard. The "padded dash syndrome" primarily causes crushing of the trachea and the cricoid ring, although it can lead to esophageal compression against the cervical vertebral bodies. The next most common mechanism, clothesline injuries, is usually the result of motorcycle, all-terrain vehicle, or snowmobile riders and unseen wire fences or tree branches. Since the force involved is

Evidence-Based Emergency Care: Diagnostic Testing and Clinical Decision Rules, Second Edition.
Jesse M. Pines, Christopher R. Carpenter, Ali S. Raja and Jeremiah D. Schuur.
© 2013 John Wiley & Sons, Ltd. Published 2013 by John Wiley & Sons, Ltd.

applied to a much smaller area, the injuries are usually more localized but also more severe. Crushed laryngeal cartilage and even cricotracheal separation can be seen with these clothesline injuries. The third most commonly seen blunt neck injury, strangulation, includes several distinct mechanisms. Manual strangulation can occlude and traumatize the carotid arteries, and the blunt force involved can result in delayed laryngeal edema. Ligature strangulation results in injuries typical of clothesline mechanisms. Lastly, suicidal strangulation typically leads to jugular venous compression and occlusion, leading to increased intracranial pressure, loss of consciousness, and eventual airway occlusion.

Blunt trauma patients in extremis with obvious airway compromise should be emergently intubated with a well-thought-out rescue plan in case direct or video laryngoscopy is unsuccessful, and those with any stridor or dysphonia should undergo bronchoscopy and observation. Patients with neurologic deficits, neck hematomas, or new carotid bruits should undergo imaging of both the cervical spine and cervical vasculature. However, the evaluation of stable patients with the potential for blunt cerebrovascular injury is more controversial. Although these injuries are rare, with an incidence of approximately 1% with blunt trauma, they are associated with mortality rates between 23% and 28%.[2-4] In addition, there is commonly a delay in symptom onset; 25–50% of patients develop symptoms more than 12 hours after the traumatic event, prompting evaluation for blunt cerebrovascular injury in patients who are initially asymptomatic.[4] While the mainstay of less severe blunt cerebrovascular injury treatment, antithrombotic therapy, may be contraindicated in some patients with blunt trauma, more severe blunt cerebrovascular injuries are typically treated endovascularly or surgically, necessitating screening in patients with suspected disease.

Clinical question

Which stable patients with no apparent blunt cerebrovascular injury should undergo screening with an imaging test?

A number of studies have demonstrated that blunt cerebrovascular injury can present in a delayed fashion, sometimes days after the initial injury, making diagnosis of these injuries extremely difficult.[5,6] However, given their potentially devastating nature and the fact that treatment in this "silent period" before the onset of neurologic symptoms can improve outcomes, some authors have advocated for standardized screening protocols based on mechanism of injury and associated injuries.[4] While there are no published clinical decision rules applicable to blunt cerebrovascular injuries, a recent meta-analysis by Franz et al evaluated studies with proposed screening criteria for blunt cerebrovascular injury to determine which mechanisms or associated findings were most associated with the diagnosis of blunt cerebrovascular injury.

The authors included 10 studies in their meta-analysis, all of which used either four-vessel digital subtraction angiography (DSA) or computed tomography (CT) angiography as the criterion standard and seven of which used routine diagnostic screening based on specified protocols. These studies included 24,435 patients and had incidences of blunt cerebrovascular injury between 0.2% and 2.7%. In the pooled analysis, no specific mechanisms of injury (including head injury, basilar skull fracture, "seatbelt sign," and facial fracture) were significantly associated with blunt cerebrovascular injury, while both cervical spine injuries and thoracic injuries were significantly associated with blunt cerebrovascular injury.

The meta-analysis is limited by the fact that some centers used specified protocols that mandated screening for blunt cerebrovascular injury, which may have biased the results, and the fact that extremely broad definitions may have led to increased weight being given to certain associated injuries ("thoracic injury," e.g., included all injuries of any severity to the thorax). While national guidelines do exist,[7,8] they do not yet include data from this recent study. However, given the limitations of the study, we would not advocate for changing practice based on its results.

Clinical question

In patients requiring screening for blunt cerebrovascular injury after blunt trauma, which imaging modality has the best test characteristics?
Four-vessel DSA has long been the criterion standard for the diagnosis of blunt cerebrovascular injury. However, Willinsky et al found a 1.3% neurologic complication rate for DSA, with 0.5% of all patients undergoing DSA having a permanent neurologic impairment.[9] In addition, it is not rapidly available in all centers and so other imaging modalities have been studied for screening these patients. While no systematic reviews or meta-analyses exist, a number of studies have directly compared duplex ultrasound, CT angiography, and MRI/MR angiography (MRA) to DSA.

Mutze et al evaluated 1,471 patients who were screened for blunt cerebrovascular injury using duplex ultrasound and found a sensitivity of 38.5% (CI 13.9–68.4%) and a specificity of 100% (CI 99.7–100%).[10] Sturzenegger et al found higher (86%) sensitivity for duplex ultrasound, but noted that the sensitivity was still too low for an appropriate screening modality.[11]

CT angiography (CTA) is much more widely available than duplex sonography in the emergency department (ED) and has become the screening modality of choice for blunt cerebrovascular injury. However, early reports indicated that CT scanners with 1–4 slices were not sensitive enough to detect blunt cerebrovascular injury; a 2002 study by Biffl et al found that, in 46 symptomatic blunt trauma patients undergoing screening with both DSA and early CTA, CTA had a sensitivity of 68%, a specificity of 67%, a PPV of 65%, and a NPV of 70%.[12] More recent reports using 16-slice CT scanners have shown more promising results, although only one study to date has directly compared 16-slice CTA to DSA. Eastman et al evaluated 162 patients at risk for blunt cerebrovascular injury, 146 of whom had both CTA and DSA. Test characteristics for CTA in this study were a sensitivity of 97.7%, a specificity of 100%, a PPV of 100%, and a NPV of 99.3%. In addition, a recent cost-effective analysis found CTA to be a cost-effective method for screening patients for blunt cerebrovascular injury after blunt trauma.[13]

A few studies have evaluated the use of MRI or MRA in patients being screened for blunt cerebrovascular injury. While MRA is more expensive and time-consuming than CTA, MRA avoids both the risks of contrast as well as radiation. However, its test characteristics have demonstrated that, like duplex ultrasound, it is not appropriate for screening these patients. Biffl et al in their 2002 study also evaluated MRA and found that it had a sensitivity of 75%, a specificity of 67%, a PPV of 43%, and a NPV of 89%.[12] These results were supported by a study by Miller et al who found that MRA had a sensitivity of 50% for carotid injury and only 47% for vertebral injury.[14]

Comments

Patients with blunt neck trauma can have airway, vascular, and esophageal injuries. While esophageal injuries are extremely rare and airway injuries are typically apparent or easily evaluated by direct visualization in patients stable enough for bronchoscopy, the evaluation of blunt cerebrovascular injury is much more controversial.

While there are no large randomized trials regarding treatment for blunt cerebrovascular injury, the mainstay of therapy involves anticoagulation even in asymptomatic patients, based on small prospective and database studies.[14–16] Given both the potential for delayed symptoms, as well as the fact that earlier treatment during the asymptomatic period may improve outcomes, we recommend using CTA for asymptomatic patients thought to be at risk for blunt cerebrovascular injury. The recent meta-analysis by Franz et al found that the presence of any cervical spine injury or any thoracic injury was significantly associated with blunt cerebrovascular injury;

however, their study has a number of limitations. Instead, we recommend imaging otherwise asymptomatic patients with blunt neck trauma who have associated cervical spine injuries, basilar skull or severe facial injuries, or ligature mechanisms with CTA to evaluate for blunt cerebrovascular injury.

References

1. Beal SL, Pottmeyer EW, Spisso JM. Esophageal perforation following external blunt trauma. Journal of Trauma. 1988; 28(10): 1425–32.
2. Biffl WL, Moore EE, Ryu RK *et al.* The unrecognized epidemic of blunt carotid arterial injuries: Early diagnosis improves neurologic outcome. Annals of Surgery. 1998; 228(4): 462–70.
3. Fabian TC, Patton JH Jr, Croce MA *et al.* Blunt carotid injury: Importance of early diagnosis and anticoagulant therapy. Annals of Surgery. 1996; 223(5): 513–22; discussion 522–5.
4. Berne JD, Norwood SH, McAuley CE *et al.* The high morbidity of blunt cerebrovascular injury in an unscreened population: More evidence of the need for mandatory screening protocols. Journal of the American College of Surgeons. 2001; 192(3): 314–21.
5. Fakhry SM, Jaques PF, Proctor HJ. Cervical vessel injury after blunt trauma. Journal of Vascular Surgery. 1988; 8(4): 501–8.
6. Batnitzky S, Price HI, Holden RW, Franken EA Jr. Cervical internal carotid artery injuries due to blunt trauma. American Journal of Neuroradiology. 1983; 4(3): 292–5.
7. Biffl WL, Cothren CC, Moore EE *et al.* Western Trauma Association critical decisions in trauma: Screening for and treatment of blunt cerebrovascular injuries. Journal of Trauma. 2009; 67(6): 1150–3.
8. Bromberg WJ, Collier BC, Diebel LN *et al.* Blunt cerebrovascular injury practice management guidelines: The Eastern Association for the Surgery of Trauma. Journal of Trauma. 2010; 68(2): 471–7.
9. Willinsky RA, Taylor SM, TerBrugge K *et al.* Neurologic complications of cerebral angiography: Prospective analysis of 2,899 procedures and review of the literature. Radiology. 2003; 227(2): 522–8.
10. Mutze S, Rademacher G, Matthes G, Hosten N, Stengel D. Blunt cerebrovascular injury in patients with blunt multiple trauma: Diagnostic accuracy of duplex Doppler US and early CT angiography. Radiology. 2005; 237(3): 884–92.
11. Sturzenegger M, Mattle HP, Rivoir A, Rihs F, Schmid C. Ultrasound findings in spontaneous extracranial vertebral artery dissection. Stroke. 1993; 24(12): 1910–21.
12. Biffl WL, Ray CE Jr, Moore EE *et al.* Noninvasive diagnosis of blunt cerebrovascular injuries: A preliminary report. Journal of Trauma. 2002; 53(5): 850–6.
13. Kaye D, Brasel KJ, Neideen T, Weigelt JA. Screening for blunt cerebrovascular injuries is cost-effective. Journal of Trauma. 2011; 70(5): 1051–6; discussion 1056–7.

14. Miller PR, Fabian TC, Croce MA *et al*. Prospective screening for blunt cerebrovascular injuries. Annals of Surgery. 2002; 236(3): 386–95.
15. Biffl WL, Ray CE Jr, Moore EE *et al*. Treatment-related outcomes from blunt cerebrovascular injuries: Importance of routine follow-up arteriography. Annals of Surgery. 2002; 235(5): 699–706; discussion 706–7.
16. Cothren CC, Moore EE, Biffl WL *et al*. Anticoagulation is the gold standard therapy for blunt carotid injuries to reduce stroke rate. Archivesof Surgery. 2004; 139(5): 540–5; discussion 545–6.

Chapter 18 **Occult Scaphoid Fractures**

Highlights

- Suspicion for a scaphoid fracture should be raised based on the mechanism of injury (fall on an outstretched hand) and physical examination findings.
- Physical exam findings concerning for scaphoid fracture include pain with longitudinal compression (axial loading) of the thumb, tenderness over the scaphoid tubercle, and anatomical snuffbox tenderness.
- Initial plain radiography will not detect 5–20% of scaphoid fractures in the ED.
- Missed scaphoid fractures are associated with poor outcomes, including non-union, delayed union, and avascular necrosis.
- Patients with normal x-rays but suspicious physical exam findings should be splinted using a thumb spica splint.
- MRI is the most sensitive test for occult scaphoid fractures, but CT and ultrasound show promising early results.

Background

The scaphoid, also known as the carpal navicular, is the most frequently fractured carpal bone, accounting for 70–80% of all carpal fractures.[1] Suspicion of a scaphoid fracture is based largely on a patient's mechanism of injury that, in most cases, is a fall on an outstretched hand. While they do not occur only in adolescents and young adults, scaphoid fractures have their highest incidence in these age groups.[1] Physical examination findings of tenderness in the anatomic snuffbox (Figure 18.1), pain with axial loading of the ipsilateral thumb, and tenderness over the scaphoid tubercle have all been used as signs associated with scaphoid fractures. Clinicians should maintain a high level of suspicion either when a compatible mechanism is

---

Evidence-Based Emergency Care: Diagnostic Testing and Clinical Decision Rules, Second Edition. Jesse M. Pines, Christopher R. Carpenter, Ali S. Raja and Jeremiah D. Schuur. © 2013 John Wiley & Sons, Ltd. Published 2013 by John Wiley & Sons, Ltd.

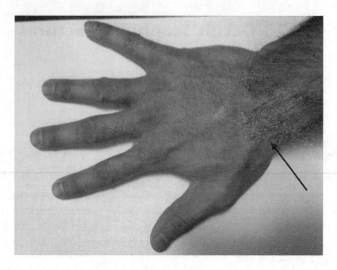

Figure 18.1 Location of anatomic snuffbox.

described (i.e., a fall on an outstretched hand) or if any of the associated signs are elicited on exam. As the scaphoid bone has a retrograde blood supply, failure to diagnose a scaphoid fracture in the emergency department (ED) can result in avascular necrosis, non-union, and delayed union, all of which can lead to varying degrees of degenerative osteoarthritis and arthrosis.

While plain radiography is typically used as the initial imaging modality for suspected scaphoid fractures (Figure 18.2), it is only 80–95% sensitive, regardless of whether four or six image series are obtained. In patients with a suspected fracture despite negative initial x-rays, follow-up x-rays (typically in 5–14 days) reveal an initially occult fracture in approximately 10–15% of cases. In addition to x-ray imaging, computed tomography (CT), bone scintigraphy (BS), and magnetic resonance imaging (MRI) can all be considered for patients with suspected occult scaphoid fractures.

Once a scaphoid fracture has been documented, referral to a hand surgeon and prompt immobilization of the wrist are imperative. Treatment in the ED should include immobilizing the suspected injury with a thumb spica (or other similar) splint.

Clinical question

Which physical exam finding is most sensitive and specific for scaphoid fractures?
As the appropriate management of a potentially occult scaphoid fracture is dependent on a high clinical suspicion of injury without, by definition,

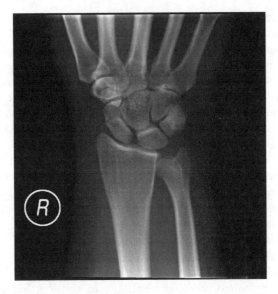

Figure 18.2 Scaphoid fracture on wrist X-ray.

any radiographic correlation, specific physical examination findings must be evaluated in patients with the appropriate mechanism. Parvezi et al examined 215 consecutive patients with suspected scaphoid fractures and determined that pain with longitudinal compression of the thumb, tenderness over the scaphoid tubercle, and anatomical snuffbox tenderness all had sensitivities of 100% for detecting scaphoid fractures.[2] While the signs had low individual specificities (48%, 30%, and 9%, respectively), when combined their specificity increased to 74%. Given their sensitivities, the lack of these signs essentially rules out scaphoid fracture while their presence necessitates further investigation.

More recently, Rhemrev et al developed a decision rule for the evaluation of scaphoid fractures.[3] However, given that the rule necessitates the use of a dynamometer to assess supination strength (a device not typically available in the ED), it is not clinically relevant to emergency medicine.

Clinical question

Which diagnostic imaging modality is preferred for the evaluation of a clinically suspected scaphoid fracture when x-rays are negative or nondiagnostic?
Studies of the optimal diagnostic modality for a suspected occult scaphoid fracture with negative initial x-rays initially compared MRI and BS. The

largest of the studies, by Fowler et al involved 61 patients with wrist injuries with negative initial and 7–10-day follow-up x-rays. BS and MRI each detected four additional scaphoid fractures.[4] Kitis et al compared MRI and BS results performed 2–4 weeks after initial assessment in 22 patients with suspected scaphoid injuries but negative plain films.[5] Scaphoid fractures were identified in three patients by both MRI and BS; bone scan also detected one scaphoid fracture that MRI missed. Ten other nonscaphoid injuries were detected on MRI but not BS. The authors concluded that both modalities were sensitive tests but that MRI had greater specificity for nonscaphoid injuries. Thorpe et al in the United Kingdom studied 59 patients with suspected occult scaphoid fractures using both MRI and BS.[7] All four scaphoid fractures identified on BS were also identified on MRI, which also detected additional non-scaphoid fractures. Three significant ligamentous injuries were diagnosed by MRI but not seen on BS.

Given the comparative test characteristics of MRI and BS, two cost-effectiveness analyses were performed to determine whether the increased cost of MRI was balanced by the decreased time to diagnosis and increased sensitivity of the test. Both found MRI to be cost-effective, despite its additional expense.[8,9] McCullough et al recently published their experience with early MRI and found it to be feasible in their Scottish ED.[10]

However, MRI is not easily obtainable in most EDs, whereas CT imaging typically is. A number of studies have evaluated the test characteristics of CT for evaluation of scaphoid fracture, finding mixed sensitivities (67–100%) and generally high specificities (96–100%).[11–13] A 2010 meta-analysis by Yin et al analyzed data from 26 studies and determined pooled test characteristics for BS, MRI, and CT that are displayed in Table 18.1, essentially finding no significant differences between the sensitivities of BS and MRI and the specificities of MRI and CT.[14] However, given the inherent difficulties in interpreting the results of pooled data (which, in this case, included results

Table 18.1 Test performance summaries of BS, MRI, and CT to detect scaphoid fractures

Test	Sensitivity	Specificity	LR+	LR−
BS	97%	89%	8.82	0.03
MRI	96%	99%	96	0.04
CT	93%	99%	93	0.07

Note: BS = bone scintigraphy; MRI = magnetic resonance imaging; CT = computed tomography; LR+ = likelihood ratio positive; and LR− = likelihood ratio negative.
Source: Data from [14].

from studies with widely disparate criterion standards), these data should be confirmed by prospective studies before changing the standard of care.

Finally, a 2011 study by Platon et al determined that ultrasound was highly sensitive for scaphoid fractures when compared to a criterion standard of CT.[15] Of the 13 fractures detected by CT in 28 patients, ultrasound was positive in 12. More importantly, of the eight fractures thought to have the highest potential for complications (fractures of the proximal scaphoid or scaphoid waist), ultrasound detected all eight.

Comments

While plain x-rays detect the majority of scaphoid fractures during an initial evaluation, the long-term disability and the complications that arise from non-union or avascular necrosis necessitate concern for occult scaphoid fractures. While the initial management remains similar for confirmed fractures and suspected occult scaphoid injuries, there is debate over the next appropriate diagnostic study to order.

Based on the studies presented in this chapter, we recommend initial plain x-ray or CT, with immobilization with a thumb spica splint and follow-up for patients with pain on axial loading, tenderness over the scaphoid tubercle, or anatomical snuffbox tenderness. While CT imaging has high specificity and can rule in fractures, its sensitivity is not high enough to prevent the need for immobilization and it should not be used to rule out scaphoid fractures.

Given the results of the series of small studies examining both MRI and BS, it appears that MRI is as sensitive as, and more specific than, BS for detecting occult scaphoid fractures. Given its additional benefit of discretely differentiating soft tissue and ligamentous injury from true bony injury, we recommend early outpatient MRI as the follow-up modality of choice, noting that either x-ray or BS is appropriate when early MRI is unavailable.

References

1. Adams JE, Steinmann SP. Acute scaphoid fractures. Orthopedic Clinics of North America. 2007; 38(2): 229–35.
2. Parvizi J, Wayman J, Kelly P, Moran CG. Combining the clinical signs improves diagnosis of scaphoid fractures. Journal of Hand Surgery, British and European Volume. 1998; 23(3): 324–7.
3. Rhemrev SJ, Beeres FJP, van Leerdam RH, Hogervorst M, Ring D. Clinical prediction rule for suspected scaphoid fractures: A prospective cohort study. Injury. 2010; 41(10): 1026–30.
4. Fowler C, Sullivan B, Williams LA et al. A comparison of bone scintigraphy and MRI in the early diagnosis of the occult scaphoid waist fracture. Skeletal Radiology. 1998; 27(12): 683–7.

5. Kitsis C, Taylor M, Chandey J *et al*. Imaging the problem scaphoid. Injury. 1998; 29(7): 515–20.

6. Tiel-van Buul MM, Roolker W, Verbeeten BW, Broekhuizen AH. Magnetic resonance imaging versus bone scintigraphy in suspected scaphoid fracture. European Journal of Nuclear Medicine. 1996; 23(8): 971–5.

7. Thorpe AP, Murray AD, Smith FW, Ferguson J. Clinically suspected scaphoid fracture: A comparison of magnetic resonance imaging and bone scintigraphy. British Journal of Radiology. 1996; 69(818): 109–13.

8. Hansen TB, Petersen RB, Barckman J, Uhre P, Larsen K. Cost-effectiveness of MRI in managing suspected scaphoid fractures. Journal of Hand Surgery, European Volume. 2009; 34(5): 627–30.

9. Dorsay TA, Major NM, Helms CA. Cost-effectiveness of immediate MR imaging versus traditional follow-up for revealing radiographically occult scaphoid fractures. American Journal of Roentgenology. 2001; 177(6): 1257–63.

10. McCullough NP, Smith FW, Cooper JG. Early MRI in the management of the clinical scaphoid fracture. European Journal of Emergency Medicine. 2011; 18(3): 133–6.

11. Rhemrev SJ, de Zwart AD, Kingma LM *et al*. Early computed tomography compared with bone scintigraphy in suspected scaphoid fractures. Clinical Nuclear Medicine. 2010; 35(12): 931–4.

12. Ilica AT, Ozyurek S, Kose O, Durusu M. Diagnostic accuracy of multidetector computed tomography for patients with suspected scaphoid fractures and negative radiographic examinations. Japanese Journal of Radiology. 2011; 29(2): 98–103.

13. Mallee W, Doornberg JN, Ring D *et al*. Comparison of CT and MRI for diagnosis of suspected scaphoid fractures. Journal of Bone and Joint Surgery, American Volume. 2011; 93(1): 20–8.

14. Yin Z-G, Zhang J-B, Kan S-L, Wang X-G. Diagnosing suspected scaphoid fractures: A systematic review and meta-analysis. Clinical Orthopaedics and Related Research. 2010; 468(3): 723–34.

15. Platon A, Poletti P-A, Van Aaken J *et al*. Occult fractures of the scaphoid: The role of ultrasonography in the emergency department. Skeletal Radiology. 2011; 40(7): 869–75.

Chapter 19 **Penetrating Abdominal Trauma**

Highlights

- Patients with penetrating stab wounds to the abdomen and high-risk clinical signs, including unstable vital signs, evisceration, or peritonitis, should be taken for immediate laparotomy.
- In patients with penetrating thoraco-abdominal injuries, CT can miss diaphragmatic injuries, so additional testing (thorascopy or laparoscopy) should be considered.
- In patients with penetrating back and flank wounds, fewer than 5% will have intraperitoneal injury, and the absence of apparent injury on CT scan can rule out these injuries.
- In patients with penetrating anterior abdominal trauma, both CT and focused assessment with sonography in trauma (FAST) have imperfect sensitivity and specificity in detecting intraperitoneal injuries and should not be used as the only basis to rule out injuries. In these patients, local wound exploration (LWE), when done properly, is highly sensitive and can rule out peritoneal violation.
- Diagnostic peritoneal lavage (DPL) is not useful to rule in or rule out injuries. Because of its invasiveness and the availability of other diagnostic strategies, it should not be a part of the evaluation of stable abdominal stab wounds.

Background

Over the past 150 years, there has been a major revolution in the management of penetrating abdominal injuries. Prior to the Civil War and into the latter 19th century, penetrating injuries were managed with observation; significant organ injuries that led to peritonitis, or other serious infections, were almost universally fatal. During World Wars I and II, early laparotomy became

Evidence-Based Emergency Care: Diagnostic Testing and Clinical Decision Rules, Second Edition.
Jesse M. Pines, Christopher R. Carpenter, Ali S. Raja and Jeremiah D. Schuur.
© 2013 John Wiley & Sons, Ltd. Published 2013 by John Wiley & Sons, Ltd.

the treatment of choice. Laparotomy involves surgical exploration of intra-abdominal injuries and repair or removal of damaged structures. Early exploration has led to dramatic improvements in survival. However, not all patients with penetrating abdominal injuries have serious injuries. Using early laparotomy or potentially less invasive laparoscopy for all cases of penetrating abdominal trauma may be the most conservative strategy, but it is not always necessary. In certain subsets of patients with penetrating wounds, such as stab wounds, the rate of negative laparotomy can approach 70%.[1]

In the past 20 years, there has been a proliferation of availability of rapid diagnostic testing in emergency departments (EDs). In hemodynamically stable patients with abdominal stab wounds, management strategies have been developed to provide more rapid and less invasive ways to risk-stratify intra-abdominal injuries.[2] It is important to distinguish stab wounds from penetrating gunshot wounds (GSWs). Because of the high prevalence of peritoneal penetration in abdominal GSWs, most surgeons will perform immediate laparotomy in GSW cases.[3] It is also important to distinguish which patients can be managed conservatively and the importance of the physiology and anatomy of the injury. This is particularly true in high-volume trauma centers where the presence of multiple patients with severe injuries at once (i.e., multiple GSW cases) can overwhelm operating room resources. Indications for immediate surgical exploration include signs of evisceration, unstable vital signs such as hypotension and tachycardia, and clinical signs of peritonitis, all of which are evidence of significant injury to the intra-abdominal organs or vasculature.

By contrast, patients with abdominal stab wounds with otherwise stable vital signs and without peritonitis present a diagnostic challenge. Some patients will have injuries requiring immediate repair, others can be managed expectantly without invasive laparotomy. Anterior abdominal wounds can be explored locally with local wound exploration (LWE). In addition, contrast-enhanced computed tomography (CT) and the focused assessment with sonography in trauma (FAST) and serial clinical assessment (SCA) have emerged as modalities to help risk-stratify stable patients with penetrating abdominal injuries. Historically, diagnostic peritoneal lavage (DPL) performed at the bedside in the ED has been used to risk-stratify these injuries; however, this modality is becoming much less common.

Clinical question

What is the sensitivity of different types of diagnostic testing and management strategies (including CT, ultrasound, LWE, DPL, and SCA) to detect important injuries in stable patients with penetrating abdominal stab wounds?

Because management strategies can vary by body site, it is important to divide injuries into three separate regions, the anterior abdomen, the thoraco-abdomen, and the flank and back region.

Thoraco-abdominal injuries

Thoraco-abdominal stab wounds can damage structures in the chest and abdomen, including the diaphragm (Figure 19.1). Diaphragmatic injuries due to stab wounds frequently do not result in specific signs and symptoms, leaving clinicians in need of diagnostic tests. Diaphragmatic injuries can sometimes go unnoticed during an initial hospitalization and can cause delayed sequelae. Using radiography to diagnose these injuries alone can be a problem because even small injuries can go undetected using advanced radiography. In a case series at the University of Maryland Shock Trauma Center, 50 patients had CT findings of potential diaphragmatic injuries and only 40% were termed as "specific," including contiguous organ injury and/or herniation of abdominal fat through a diaphragmatic defect.[4] In that study, patients' nonspecific findings included wound tracts extending to the diaphragm, thickening of the diaphragm from blood or edema, and an apparent diaphragmatic defect. About one-third (34%) had surgical

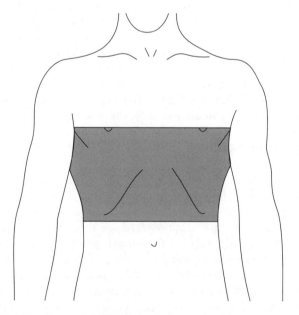

Figure 19.1 The thoraco-abdominal region for penetrating injuries.

evaluations of the diaphragm; of those 31%, 71% had confirmed diaphragmatic injuries. Importantly, there were two cases where the CT demonstrated a diaphragmatic injury that was not present on surgical evaluation.

Historically, another helpful modality for detecting diaphragmatic wounds was DPL. In previous work, a red blood cell (RBC) threshold of 5000 RBCs/mm^3 was positive for diaphragmatic injury after instillation of 1 L of normal saline because peritoneal aspirate cell counts above 5000 RBCs/mm^3 are thought to likely not be caused by the procedure.[5] More recent data have studied other ways to assess the diaphragm, including thorascopy and laparoscopy. In 28 patients with penetrating thoraco-abdominal trauma, nine had diaphragmatic injuries on thorascopy, and eight of those nine had concomitant intra-abdominal injuries and laparotomy.[6] In another series of 110 patients with left lower chest penetrating trauma, 24% had diaphragmatic injuries on laparoscopy.[7] A more recent study confirmed these findings in 34 patients with penetrating thoraco-abdominal trauma – eight (24%) had diaphragmatic injuries.

Recently, a management strategy has been proposed for stable patients with penetrating thoraco-abdominal injuries; however, the strategy has not been formally studied. The authors suggested that an initial upright chext X-ray and FAST should be performed on stable patients with penetrating thoraco-abdominal trauma.[2] If the FAST is positive, laparoscopy or laparotomy should be performed. In the case of a hemo- or pneumothorax with a negative FAST, thoracoscopy is performed because it will result in no additional invasive treatment – tube thoracostomy will already be required. In the case of diaphragmatic injury on thoracostomy, a laparoscopy or laparotomy should performed. If both X-ray and FAST are negative, then a DPL should be performed, and if positive (by the threshold of 5000/mm^3), then laparoscopy or laparotomy would be the next step.

Back and flank injuries

Penetrating injuries to the back and the flank (Figure 19.2) have a lower likelihood of intraperitoneal injury than thoraco-abdominal or anterior abdominal injuries. However, these injuries can be challenging because of the difficulty in assessing injuries with FAST, which detects intraperitoneal blood only and does not adequately evaluate the retroperitoneum. Two studies have evaluated the use of CT scanning in penetrating flank injuries.[8,9] One study investigated 88 stable patients; of those, 78 received a DPL before CT scan.[8] A total of 9/88 (10%) had high-risk CT scans, and two had significant injuries identified on laparotomy. Of the 79 patients with non-high-risk scans, 77 were observed without complication, and no high-risk lesions were found in the two patients with non-high-risk scans and

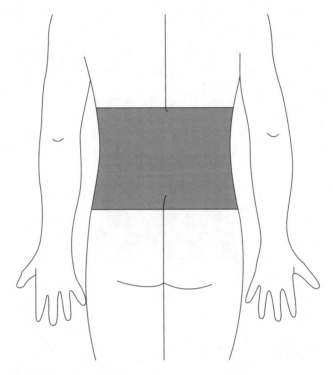

Figure 19.2 The back and flank region for penetrating injuries.

positive DPLs. The authors concluded that the negative predictive value of a non-high-risk scan was close to 100%.

Anterior abdominal injuries

There is currently a debate over how best to manage stable patients with penetrating anterior abdominal injuries without obvious signs of peritonitis, evisceration, or hemodynamic instability (Figure 19.3). A recent study was conducted that observed the management of these injuries across 11 medical centers in the Western Trauma Association (WTA) Multicenter Clinical Trials Group.[10] Over a 2-year period, 359 patients were enrolled, of whom 77% did not have an immediate indication for laparotomy. Of those 278 patients, 61 (22%) required a therapeutic laparotomy (the main study outcome). There were several management strategies employed, including CT, FAST, LWE, DLP, and SCA. The sensitivities and specificities of each of these modalities are summarized in Table 19.1, where the criterion standard was a therapeutic laparotomy.

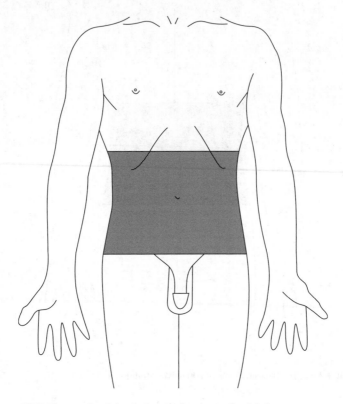

Figure 19.3 The anterior abdominal region for penetrating injuries.

Table 19.1 Test characteristics of various diagnostic modalities in detecting serious intra-abdominal injuries in stable patients with penetrating abdominal trauma

Test	N	Prevalence	Sensitivity, %	Specificity, %	Positive predictive value, %	Negative predictive value, %
Computed tomography	145	35 (24%)	77	73	47	91
Focused assessment with sonography in trauma (FAST)	132	29 (22%)	21	94	50	81
Local wound exploration	125	25 (20%)	100	54	35	100
Diagnostic peritoneal lavage	45	11 (24%)	82	88	69	94
Serial clinical examinations	26	2 (8%)	100	96	67	100

Source: Data from [10].

These data were notably limited by spectrum and incorporation bias (Chapter 6) and the fact that these are observational data; however, this was the largest study on the topic to date. The study is also limited by non-uniform follow-up of patients. In addition, determining if someone needs a laparotomy is not accurately assessed in analyzing whether the surgeon provided a therapeutic intervention because in many cases, some of these injuries may have been managed non-operatively.

The authors also calculated the proportion of patients with negative test results who underwent a therapeutic laparotomy as an additional value of the test. This could be calculated for tests that were not 100% sensitive. For CT the rate was 7%, for DPL it was 6%, and for FAST it was higher at 19%.

A recent Cochrane review has investigated the sensitivity and specificity of FAST to detect either intraperitoneal or pericardial fluid.[11] This was different from the WTA study because the outcome was therapeutic laparotomy. The authors found in eight observational studies (n = 565 patients) that the prevalence of an abnormal FAST exam after penetrating trauma was low (24–56%). FAST is highly specific (94–100%), but demonstrated low sensitivity (28–100%). The Cochrane review authors concluded that a positive FAST should prompt immediate laparotomy, but a negative FAST requires additional testing.

Comment

Patients with abdominal stab wounds and high-risk signs or symptoms (instability, evisceration, and peritonitis) should be taken to the operating room immediately. In stable patients, several diagnostic strategies can be undertaken, depending upon the site of the injury. In thoraco-abdominal injuries, advanced radiography is not sensitive. Therefore, even in cases where the initial chest X-ray and FAST are normal, patients should still receive a DPL because of the possibility for occult diaphragmatic injuries. In flank and back penetrating trauma, patients have a low prevalence of intra-abdominal injury that can be ruled out if stable with a negative CT.

In penetrating anterior abdominal stab wounds, FAST is a useful test to rule in significant injuries, but not to rule out injuries. In the WTA study, it was performed in almost half of the cases; however, it affected the management in only 5% of cases. In addition, a positive FAST was associated with either a nontherapeutic laparotomy or no laparotomy performed in 28% of the cases. In addition, a negative FAST can also be deceiving in that 19% of patients with negative FASTs went on to have a therapeutic laparotomy. Therefore, in the case of stable penetrating trauma to the abdomen, FAST should not be used to exclude important injuries.

Similar to FAST, CT is poorly sensitive and specific in predicting the need for therapeutic laparotomy. CT often identifies patients with injuries of questionable significance since 24% of patients with positive CT findings ultimately have a negative laparotomy. In addition, a negative CT scan can be falsely reassuring. Therefore, CT should not be the only determinant of laparotomy in stable anterior abdominal stab injuries.

Local wound exploration (LWE) was performed in about half of the WTA patients. The primary value of LWE is to assess if the stabbing object violated the peritoneal cavity. Positive local wound explorations should not be the only indicator for laparotomy because more than half (57%) of the laparotomies performed were nontherapeutic. These studies use a variety of definitions of a positive LWE across the sites in the WTA (some defining it as violation of the anterior fascia – which is not necessarily intraperitoneal – while others defined it as violation of the posterior fascia). However, given the high sensitivity and negative predictive value of LWE, it may be suggested that negative LWE patients can be discharged home if explored properly by a surgeon. Patients with a positive LWE may be admitted and observed with serial exams.

Data on DPL demonstrated low sensitivity and specificity, which are dependent upon the cutoff for DPL positivity. In most centers the cutoff for a positive DPL is $>100,000\,RBC/mm^3$, $>500\,WBC/mm^3$, or elevated alkaline phosphatase and bilirubin in the effluent in addition to grossly positive blood, succus, bile, or food. Reducing the cutoffs for these numbers would increase sensitivity but result in greater false positives. The WTA authors calculated that reducing the DPL cutoff to $10,000\,RBC/mm^3$ would result in two additional nontherapeutic laparotomies for every therapeutic laparotomy. Given the shortcomings of DPL, and the reduction in the volume of training in these procedures that can cause iatrogenic injury, it has been suggested that DPL be removed from management pathways in stable patients with anterior abdominal stab wounds.

References

1. Shaftan GW. Indications for operation in abdominal trauma. American Journal of Surgery. 1960; 99: 657–64.
2. Biffl WL, Moore EE. Management guidelines for penetrating abdominal trauma. Current Opinion in Critical Care. 2010 Sep 16; epub ahead of print.
3. Moore EE, Moore JB, Van Duzer-Moore S, Thompson JS. Mandatory laparotomy for gunshot wounds penetrating the abdomen. American Journal of Surgery. 1980; 140: 847–51.

4. Shanmuganathan K, Mirvis SE, Chiu WC *et al.* Penetrating torso trauma: Triple-contrast helical CT in peritoneal violation and organ injury: A prospective study in 200 patients. Radiology. 2004; 231: 775–84.

5. Moore EE, Marx JA. Penetrating abdominal wounds: Rationale for exploratory laparotomy. Journal of the American Medical Association. 1985; 253: 2705–8.

6. Uribe RA, Pachon CE, Frame SB *et al.* A prospective evaluation of thoracoscopy for the diagnosis of penetrating thoracoabdominal trauma. Journal of Trauma. 1994; 37: 650–4.

7. Murray JA, Demetriades D, Asensio JA *et al.* Occult injuries to the diaphragm: Prospective evaluation of laparoscopy in penetrating injuries to the left lower chest. Journal of the American College of Surgeons. 1998; 187: 626–630.

8. Himmelman RG, Martin M, Gilkey S, Barrett JA. Triple-contrast CT scans in penetrating back and flank trauma. Journal of Trauma. 1991; 31: 852–6.

9. Boyle EM Jr, Maier RV, Salazar JD *et al.* Diagnosis of injuries after stab wounds to the back and flank. Journal of Trauma. 1997; 42: 260–5.

10. Biffl WL, Kaups KL, Cothren CC *et al.* Management of patients with anterior abdominal stab wounds: A Western Trauma Association Multicenter Trial. Journal of Trauma. 2009; 66: 1294–1301.

11. Quinn AC, Sinert R. What is the utility of the focused assessment with sonography in trauma (FAST) exam in penetrating torso trauma? Injury. 2011; 42: 482–7.

Chapter 20 **Penetrating Trauma to the Extremities and Vascular Injuries**

> **Highlights**
>
> - Penetrating injuries of the extremities are a leading cause of vascular injuries.
> - "Hard signs" of vascular injury are reliable to rule in arterial injury and proceed directly to the operating room, depending on the clinical status of the patient and the time of warm ischemia.
> - "Soft signs" of vascular injury do not increase diagnostic accuracy and should not be used.
> - Arterial pressure indices (APIs) can be used to rule out arterial injury and identify those patients who do not need additional evaluation.
> - Compared to traditional angiography, multidetector CT angiography (CTA) is more reliable and carries lower morbidity when used for the detection and characterization of traumatic extremity arterial injuries.

Background

Penetrating injuries to the extremities can damage the major arteries or veins, threatening the limb's viability and risking death by exsanguination. In the United States (US), 70–90% of peripheral vascular injuries are due to penetrating injuries,[1] with the majority occurring in men and as a result of the high rates of gunshot and knife wounds. While the incidence of low-velocity (i.e., handgun) injuries has decreased in recent years, nearly 70,000 people were treated in US emergency departments (EDs) for nonfatal gunshot wounds in 2007.[2] In 2008, firearms were the third leading cause of injury-related death overall and the second leading cause for those between 10 and 24 years of age.[3] The incidence of iatrogenic vascular injuries has also increased, in parallel with the rising use of endovascular procedures.[4]

Evidence-Based Emergency Care: Diagnostic Testing and Clinical Decision Rules, Second Edition. Jesse M. Pines, Christopher R. Carpenter, Ali S. Raja and Jeremiah D. Schuur.
© 2013 John Wiley & Sons, Ltd. Published 2013 by John Wiley & Sons, Ltd.

Trauma care of extremity vascular injuries has evolved over the last 60 years; rather than resulting in simple amputations, the majority of extremity vascular injuries can now be identified and repaired. Since the beginning of the Vietnam War, routine angiography and improved surgical techniques have decreased amputation rates to as low as 5–15%, and recent reports show limb salvage rates of over 95%.[5] As operative repair has improved, the role of the diagnostic evaluation has also evolved. The physical examination (especially examination for "hard signs" of vascular injury) and arterial pressure indices (APIs) can both be used to identify patients at risk for vascular injury. Since traditional angiography is invasive and carries risks that outweigh its benefits in routine use, noninvasive diagnostic techniques have emerged as accurate alternatives to angiography or surgical exploration. While Doppler ultrasonography was used previously, multidetector CT angiography has emerged as the imaging modality of choice for identifying the presence or absence of an extremity vascular injury. Many centers have developed diagnostic algorithms that utilize all these diagnostic modalities to avoid invasive angiography and surgical exploration while still maximizing limb salvage and patient outcomes. For example, Dennis followed 3,218 patients with penetrating trauma and potential vascular injuries and found that only six operations were required (1.8%).[6] For this chapter, we reviewed studies of civilian penetrating extremity trauma, as military injuries typically involve much higher energy trauma than typical civilian injuries caused by knives and handguns.

Clinical question

What clinical signs and symptoms reliably predict a penetrating vascular injury?
The physical examination remains the mainstay of the evaluation of penetrating extremity wounds in the modern era. Physical findings that are highly suggestive of vascular injury are labeled "hard signs" (Table 20.1). Some authors have described other findings as "soft signs" of vascular injury – meaning that they are less accurate than the hard signs. Soft signs include: stable hematomas, unexplained hypotension, transient history of hemorrhage, and adjacent nerve injury. Soft signs should not be used to rule in or rule out the possibility of penetrating vascular injury, as they do not add diagnostic value.[6,7]

Several studies of varying quality have examined the diagnostic characteristics of physical findings. Frykberg et al prospectively studied all cases of penetrating extremity trauma seen at an urban trauma center.[7] Of 2,674 trauma patients evaluated during the 1-year study period, 310 (11.6%) had 366 penetrating extremity wounds. Every patient taken immediately to surgery for

Table 20.1 Hard signs of arterial injury after penetrating trauma

---

- Absent distal pulses
- Pulsatile bleeding
- Expanding or pulsatile hematoma
- Audible bruit or palpable thrill
- Distal ischemia (6 Ps)
  - Pain
  - Paresthesia
  - Pallor
  - Poikilothermia – cool limb
  - Pulselessness
  - Paralysis (a late finding)

---

hard signs had major arterial injury requiring repair. There were two missed vascular injuries, both of which were asymptomatic and proximal vessels (0.7% false negatives). Gonzalez and Falimirski studied 406 patients with 489 injured extremities secondary to proximal penetrating extremity trauma over a 30-month period in one center. All of the patients were admitted and categorized into three groups: (i) no hard signs of vascular injury present, and admitted for 24-hour observation; (ii) presence of at least one hard sign of vascular injury, and taken immediately to the operating room; and (iii) positive soft sign of arterial injury, and angiography performed.[8] Inaba prospectively studied 635 patients with penetrating extremity trauma, evaluating hard signs of vascular injury and multidetector CT angiography (MDCTA).[9]

The diagnostic test characteristics of the hard signs are listed in Table 20.2. These studies are limited by variable inclusion criteria as well as differential application of the criterion standard (e.g., only performing angiography on patients with a higher clinical suspicion). In aggregate, the presence of a hard sign of vascular injury in a patient with penetrating extremity trauma has a high specificity and is reliable for ruling in vascular injury. Thus, hard signs of vascular injury mandate surgical exploration.

Clinical question

Can arterial pressure indices (APIs) be used to rule out penetrating vascular injury?

The arterial pressure index (API) is a test to compare arterial pressures and is used for both acute and chronic vascular evaluation. The API is the ratio between systolic blood pressures measured distal to a penetrating injury in one extremity and measured at the same location on the contralateral uninjured extremity. The API is valid for injuries distal to the "shoulder"

Table 20.2 Diagnostic characteristics of the physical exam

Author	Test	N	Prevalence (%)	Sensitivity (%)	Specificity (%)	PPV (%)	NPV (%)	LR+	LR−
Frykberg, 1991	Hard signs	2,674	12	99	100	100	100	994	0
Gonzalez, 2009	Hard signs	489	10	73	100	95	97	159	0.3
Inaba, 2011	Hard signs	635	9	60	100	97	96	345	0.4
Lynch 1991	API <0.9	100	21	95	97	91	99	32	0.1
Nassoura, 1996	API <0.9	258	9	73	100	100	96	730	0.3
Kurtoğlu, 2009	API <1	1,489	3	85	93	27	100	12	0.2

Note: API = arterial pressure indices; PPV = positive predictive value; NPV = negative predictive value; LR+ = positive likelihood ratio; and LR− = negative likelihood ratio. Source: Data from [7–12].

and "groin." These are inexact terms, so the more proximal the injury, the less valid the use of API becomes. Generally, pressures are obtained using a Doppler vascular probe and a blood pressure cuff. The injured limb's pressure is divided by the non-injured limb's pressure, and the resulting proportion is the API.

The findings from three studies are described in Table 20.2. A study by Lynch and Johansen evaluated APIs in 93 consecutive trauma patients with 100 consecutive injured limbs, using an API <0.9 as the definition of a vascular injury.[10] Nassoura et al prospectively studied the role of APIs in penetrating proximity extremity trauma. A total of 258 patients with 323 penetrating proximity extremity traumas were evaluated by physical examination and Doppler pressure determination. An API of <0.9 was considered abnormal. The findings were compared with those of arteriography in all patients.[11] A Turkish study by Kurtoğlu et al evaluated the API as a screening tool, using an API of <1 as the criterion standard for vascular injury.[12] They enrolled and prospectively collected data for 1,772 patients with the suspicion of peripheral arterial injury. Two hundred eighty-three patients (16%) with any hard sign underwent immediate surgery. APIs were calculated in 1,489 patients with soft signs of injury. Patients with APIs <1 were evaluated by duplex ultrasonography and/or angiography, and if arterial injury was detected, they underwent surgery. Patients with APIs ≥ 1 were treated conservatively. All authors concluded that APIs are useful to rule out a penetrating vascular injury.

Clinical question

Can CT angiography rule out vascular injury?
A number of studies have evaluated multidetector computed tomography angiography (MDCT) for the diagnosis of penetrating vascular injury. The

Table 20.3 Diagnostic characteristics of multidetector computed tomography angiography (MDCT)

Author	Test	N	Prevalence (%)	Sensitivity (%)	Specificity (%)	PPV (%)	NPV (%)	LR+	LR−
Soto, 1999	MDCT	43	44	89	100	100	92	895	0.1
Soto, 2001	MDCT	137	45	95	99	98	96	72	0
Busquets, 2004	MDCT	97	26	100	100	100	100	1000	0
Inaba, 2006	MDCT	82	28	100	98	96	100	59	0
Peng, 2008	MDCT	38	45	100	100	100	100	1000	0
Seamon, 2009	MDCT	21	52	100	100	100	100	1000	0
Wallin, 2011	MDCT	53	36	100	100	100	100	1000	0
Inaba, 2011	MDCT	82	29	100	100	100	100	1000	0

Note: MDCT = multidetector computed tomography angiography; PPV = positive predictive value; NPV = negative predictive value; LR+ = positive likelihood ratio; and LR− = negative likelihood ratio.
Source: Data from [9, 13–19].

test characteristics of these studies are listed in Table 20.3. The studies of MDCT for vascular injury have similar features and weaknesses. First, most are small studies performed at a single center. Second, most studies evaluate MDCT in patients of intermediate risk who have no hard signs and have at least one soft sign. Third, they generally exclude the 3% to 10% of MDCTs that are indeterminate or nondiagnostic. Finally, the choice of criterion standard varies, both between studies and within certain studies. Many studies use a composite criterion standard of surgical findings, other imaging, and follow-up. Most studies allowed MDCT to serve as its own criterion standard, thereby significantly inflating both sensitivity and specificity.

Comments

There is a robust literature on diagnostic testing for penetrating extremity wounds with the risk of vascular injury, but the studies are limited by studying only a single center, having variable inclusion criteria, and differentially applying their criterion standards. Of note, we found no studies of these injuries in children.

There are several reasonable approaches to the diagnosis of major-vessel injuries following penetrating extremity injury. We think every ED should create a standard protocol in collaboration with their trauma and vascular surgeons. We present one well-designed algorithm in Figure 20.1.

The physical exam remains critically important in the evaluation of these injuries. Hard signs of vessel injury (Table 20.2) can reliably rule in vascular

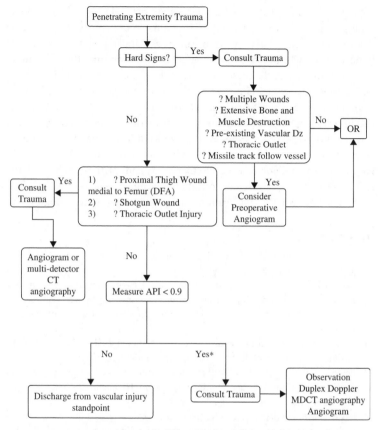

Figure 20.1 Management algorithm for evaluation of vascular injury due to penetrating extremity trauma. (Reprinted from [1] Manthey DE, Nicks BA. Penetrating trauma to the extremity. J Emerg Med. 2008; 34:187–193. Copyright (2008), with permission from Elsevier).
Note: Dz = disease; DFA = deep femoral artery; CT = computed tomography; US = ultrasound; API = arterial pressure indices; and MDCT angiography = multidetector computed tomography angiography.

injury and are an indication for operative repair. The posttest probability with a hard sign is too high for any diagnostic test to rule out injury, and the risk of delay with angiogram is greater than the benefit of preventing unnecessary operations. In a select group of cases with hard signs, an angiogram may be useful preoperatively to guide operative management, but the decision to activate surgical resources should not be predicated on the angiogram's results. Factors which necessitate surgical intervention include: multiple sites of injury, such as a shotgun wound; preexisting vascular disease in the injured extremity; missile track parallel to a vessel; extensive bone and muscle injury mimicking arterial injury; and thoracic outlet injury. Hard signs in the presence of high-risk features are an indication for an intraoperative angiogram to assess the extent and location of the injury.

In the absence of hard signs, one of two approaches should be taken. High-risk injuries (e.g., shotgun) and injuries in proximal locations (e.g., proximal thigh and thoracic outlet) should undergo MDCT and trauma or vascular surgeon consultation. Distal injuries can be evaluated using an API. If the API is ≥ 0.9, one can reliably rule out vascular injury and end the evaluation. If the API is <0.9, trauma or vascular consultation is indicated and further evaluation can include MDCT, observation, duplex ultrasonography, or angiogram.

References

1. Manthey DE, Nicks BA. Penetrating trauma to the extremity. Journal of Emergency Medicine. 2008; 34: 187–93.
2. National Center for Injury Prevention & Control, Centers for Disease Control & Prevention. Web-based injury statistics query & reporting system (WISQARS) nonfatal injury reports. Available from: http://www.cdc.gov/injury/wisqars/index.html
3. National Center for Health Statistics (NCHS), National Vital Statistics System. 10 leading causes of injury deaths by age group highlighting violence-related injury deaths, United States – 2008. Available from: http://www.cdc.gov/Injury/wisqars/pdf/Leading_Causes_Injury_Deaths_Age_Group_Highlighting_Violence-Related%20Injury_Deaths_US_2008-a.pdf
4. Giswold ME, Landry GJ, Taylor LM *et al.* Iatrogenic arterial injury is an increasingly important cause of arterial trauma. American Journal of Surgery. 2004; 187: 590–2; discussion 592–3.
5. Applebaum R, Yellin AE, Weaver FA *et al.* Role of routine arteriography in blunt lower-extremity trauma. American Journal of Surgery. 1990; 160: 221–4; discussion 224–5.
6. Dennis JW, Frykberg ER, Crump JM *et al.* New perspectives on the management of penetrating trauma in proximity to major limb arteries. Journal of Vascular Surgery. 1990; 11: 84–92; discussion 92–3.
7. Frykberg ER, Dennis JW, Bishop K *et al.* The reliability of physical examination in the evaluation of penetrating extremity trauma for vascular injury: Results at one year. Journal of Trauma. 1991; 31: 502–11.
8. Gonzalez RP, Falimirski ME. The utility of physical examination in proximity penetrating extremity trauma. American Surgeon. 1999; 65: 784–9.
9. Inaba K, Branco BC, Reddy S *et al.* Prospective evaluation of multidetector computed tomography for extremity vascular trauma. Journal of Trauma. 2011; 70: 808–15.

10. Lynch K, Johansen K. Can Doppler pressure measurement replace "exclusion" arteriography in the diagnosis of occult extremity arterial trauma? Annals of Surgery. 1991; 214: 737–41.

11. Nassoura ZE, Ivatury RR, Simon RJ et al. A reassessment of Doppler pressure indices in the detection of arterial lesions in proximity penetrating injuries of extremities: A prospective study. American Journal of Emergency Medicine. 1996; 14: 151–6.

12. Kurtoglu M, Dolay K, Karamustafaoglu B et al. The role of the ankle brachial pressure index in the diagnosis of peripheral arterial injury. Ulusal Travma ve Acil Cerrahi Dergisi. 2009; 15: 448–52.

13. Soto JA, Munera F, Cardoso N et al. Diagnostic performance of helical CT angiography in trauma to large arteries of the extremities. Journal of Computer Assisted Tomography. 1999; 23: 188–96.

14. Soto JA, Munera F, Morales C et al. Focal arterial injuries of the proximal extremities: Helical CT arteriography as the initial method of diagnosis. Radiology. 2001; 218: 188–94.

15. Busquets AR, Acosta JA, Colon E et al. Helical computed tomographic angiography for the diagnosis of traumatic arterial injuries of the extremities. Journal of Trauma. 2004; 56: 625–8.

16. Inaba K, Potzman J, Munera F et al. Multi-slice CT angiography for arterial evaluation in the injured lower extremity. Journal of Trauma. 2006; 60: 502–6; discussion 506–7.

17. Peng PD, Spain DA, Tataria M et al. CT angiography effectively evaluates extremity vascular trauma. American Surgeon. 2008; 74: 103–7.

18. Wallin D, Yaghoubian A, Rosing D et al. Computed tomographic angiography as the primary diagnostic modality in penetrating lower extremity vascular injuries: A level I trauma experience. Annals of Vascular Surgery. 2011; 25: 620–3.

19. Seamon MJ, Smoger D, Torres DM et al. A prospective validation of a current practice: The detection of extremity vascular injury with CT angiography. Journal of Trauma. 2009; 67: 238–43; discussion 243–4.

SECTION 3
Cardiology

Chapter 21 **Heart Failure**

Highlights

- The incidence of heart failure is high, with nearly half a million new cases in the United States each year.
- Overall clinical impression is specific but insensitive for heart failure, as are the presence of a S3 heart sound, abdominojugular reflux, jugular venous distension, and chest X-ray findings of pulmonary venous congestion and interstitial edema.
- An elevated brain natriuretic peptide (BNP) level can be informative, but it is not a definitive test for heart failure.

Background

Heart failure is a widespread disease that accounts for more than 1 million hospitalizations annually in the United States, and nearly a half a million new cases arise each year. A number of models of the pathophysiologic paradigms of cardiac decompensation have been described and include cardiorenal, cardiocirculatory, and neurohormonal models.[1] Briefly, the cardiorenal model describes heart failure as a process of peripheral edema resulting from decreased renal blood flow as a result of cardiac dysfunction. The cardiocirculatory model is based on a cascade of events beginning with peripheral vasoconstriction and resulting in reduced preload, ventricular wall stress, and arterial vasoconstriction, eventually leading to increased afterload. In turn, cardiac output and renal perfusion decrease, resulting in sodium retention and edema. Finally, the neurohormonal model acknowledges the role that neurohormones play in the development of decreased cardiac function, increased vascular tone, and fluctuating volume retention, all of which are found to some degree in most patients with heart failure.

Heart failure is a syndrome with a number of possible etiologies, and it manifests clinically as a spectrum of signs and symptoms. As

Evidence-Based Emergency Care: Diagnostic Testing and Clinical Decision Rules, Second Edition.
Jesse M. Pines, Christopher R. Carpenter, Ali S. Raja and Jeremiah D. Schuur.
© 2013 John Wiley & Sons, Ltd. Published 2013 by John Wiley & Sons, Ltd.

emergency physicians, we must overcome the challenge of using limited information–history, physical exam, and diagnostic tests when available–to make a diagnosis and begin treatment. Since the most common presentation of a patient with heart failure is new or progressive dyspnea, most of us aim to differentiate between heart failure and primary pulmonary processes like chronic obstructive pulmonary disorder (COPD) or severe asthma. This review will focus on the physical exam finding of a S3 (ventricular filling gallop), the routine chest X-ray findings seen with heart failure, and brain natriuretic peptide (BNP) levels and their utilities in making or ruling out the diagnosis of heart failure.

Clinical question

Which elements of the history and physical exam can predict or exclude heart failure? Are the chest X-ray or electrocardiogram (ECG) able to rule in or rule out the disease? What is the role of BNP in making the diagnosis?

A 2005 meta-analysis examined the diagnostic accuracy of a number of factors from the history and physical exam as well as results of diagnostic studies and laboratory tests in making the diagnosis of heart failure among ED patients with acute dyspnea.[2] The pooled analysis examined only studies with original data in which patients were 18 years or older, and in which there was a criterion standard that included a panel of physician reviewers who examined clinical data and cardiac studies to determine the presence of heart failure. Studies were excluded if they were population based or review articles, used only echocardiography or computed tomography (CT) scans as criterion standards, did not report clinical examination data, or did not specifically state that patients with dyspnea were enrolled. Out of a total of 815 citations, 18 studies were included in the analysis.

The "overall clinical impression" was found to be moderately specific (86%) but insensitive (61%). Summary likelihood ratios for the initial treating physician's overall clinical impression of the diagnosis of heart failure were LR+ 4.4 (CI 1.8–10) and LR- 0.45 (CI 0.28–0.73). Pooled test characteristics for elements of the history, physical examination, chest X-ray, and ECG are listed in Table 21.1. Given the number of findings tested, we have included only those LRs greater than 2.0 or less than 0.5.

An update of this meta-analysis noted that all post-MI patients should have formal echocardiographic assessment of their ejection fraction, since history and physical exam are inaccurate.[3] However, the presence of an anterior Q-wave, radiographic vascular congestion, or a third heart sound identifies most patients with an ejection fraction of 40% or less. In addition, the presence of multiple symptoms and signs probably increases the posttest

Table 21.1 Summary of diagnostic accuracy of findings on history and physical examination, chest X-ray, and electrocardiogram (ECG)

Finding	Sensitivity	Specificity	LR+ (CI)	LR− (CI)
History				
Heart failure	0.60	0.90	5.8 (4.1–8.0)	0.45 (0.38–0.53)
Myocardial infarction	0.40	0.87	3.1 (2.0–4.9)	0.69 (0.58–0.82)
Symptoms				
Paroxysmal nocturnal dyspnea	0.41	0.84	2.6 (1.5–4.5)	0.70 (0.54–0.91)
Orthopnea	0.50	0.77	2.2 (1.2–3.9)	0.65 (0.45–0.92)
Edema	0.51	0.76	2.1 (0.92–5.0)	0.64 (0.39–1.1)
Dyspnea on exertion	0.84	0.34	1.3 (1.2–1.4)	0.48 (0.35–0.67)
Physical examination				
Third heart sound	0.13	0.99	11 (4.9–25)	0.88 (0.83–0.94)
Abdominojugular reflux	0.24	0.96	6.4 (0.81–51.0)	0.79 (0.62–1.0)
Jugular vein distension	0.39	0.92	5.1 (3.2–7.9)	0.66 (0.57–0.77)
Rales	0.60	0.78	2.8 (1.9–4.1)	0.51 (0.37–0.70)
Any murmur	0.27	0.90	2.6 (1.7–4.1)	0.81 (0.73–0.90)
Lower extremity edema	0.50	0.78	2.3 (1.5–3.7)	0.64 (0.47–0.87)
Valsalva maneuver	0.73	0.65	2.1 (1.0–4.2)	0.41 (0.17–1.0)
Chest X-ray				
Pulmonary venous congestion	0.54	0.96	12 (6.8–21)	0.48 (0.28–0.83)
Interstitial edema	0.34	0.97	12 (5.2–27)	0.68 (0.54–0.85)
Alveolar edema	0.06	0.99	6.0 (2.2–16)	0.95 (0.93–0.97)
Cardiomegaly	0.74	0.78	3.3 (2.4–4.7)	0.33 (0.23–0.48)
Pleural effusion	0.26	0.92	3.2 (2.4–4.3)	0.81 (0.77–0.85)
Any edema	0.70	0.77	3.2 (0.60–16)	0.38 (0.11–1.3)
ECG				
Atrial fibrillation	0.26	0.93	3.8 (1.7–8.8)	0.79 (0.65–0.96)
New T-wave changes	0.24	0.92	3.0 (1.7–5.3)	0.83 (0.74–0.92)
Any abnormal finding	0.50	0.78	2.2 (1.6–3.1)	0.64 (0.47–0.88)

Source: Data from [2].

probability of congestive heart failure (CHF) more than previously believed since existing studies suffer from verification bias.

BNP is a neurohormone secreted by cardiac ventricles under conditions of increased ventricular volumes and pressures. An international multicenter prospective study examined ED patients with acute dyspnea to determine the use of BNP levels in making the diagnosis of BNP analysis. Patients with a history of myocardial infarction or advanced renal failure were

Table 21.2 BNP levels for ED patients with acute dyspnea

	No heart failure (n = 770)	Non-heart-failure dyspnea (n = 72)	Heart failure (n = 744)
BNP (pg/mL), (SD)	110 (225)	346 (390)	675 (450)

Source: Data from [4].

Table 21.3 BNP levels and heart failure severity

	New York Heart Association Class			
	I	II	III	IV
BNP (pg/mL), (SD)	244 (286)	389 (374)	640 (447)	817 (435)

Source: Data from [4].

excluded based on the known elevations of BNP associated with these conditions. Patients with blunt or penetrating chest trauma or the presence of a pneumothorax were excluded. Final determination of heart failure was decided by two cardiologists who were blinded to the BNP levels. Heart failure history, reported by patients, was dichotomized into acute exacerbations of heart failure or dyspnea from other causes. A total of 1,586 patients were enrolled and included 744 patients with a final diagnosis of heart failure (47%). Non-heart-failure causes of dyspnea were present in 72 patients (5%). Table 21.2 shows the BNP levels for each group of patients. Table 21.3 demonstrates increasing levels of BNP with higher classifications of the New York Heart Association Classification system.

Additional analysis showed that a BNP level ≥ 100 pg/mL was independently associated with heart failure (OR 29.6 (CI 18–49)). This threshold of 100 pg/mL resulted in a sensitivity of 90% (CI 88–92), a specificity of 76% (CI 73–79), a positive predictive value of 79% (CI 76–81), a negative predictive value of 89% (CI 87–91), and an accuracy of 83%. Other factors that were strongly independently associated with heart failure were a history of heart failure (OR 11 (CI 7–19)), and cephalization of vessels on chest X-ray (OR 11 (CI 5–21)). Notably, the test characteristics of a BNP cutoff of 100 pg/mL are approximately similar to those of a NT-proBNP value of 300 pg/mL.[5]

A subset analysis of the Breathing Not Properly Multinational Study examined the accuracy of the chest radiograph in diagnosing heart failure.[6] Eight hundred and eighty patients with complete data were included, and heart failure was the final diagnosis in 51% of patients. Assessments of the chest radiographs were performed by radiologists who were blinded to clinical findings. Specific chest radiograph findings of alveolar edema, interstitial

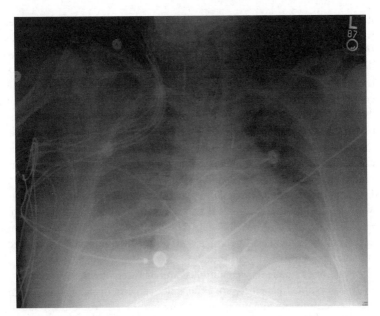

Figure 21.1 Interstitial edema seen on the chest X-ray of a patient with decompensated heart failure.

edema (Figure 21.1), cephalization, and cardiomegaly were present in 4%, 15%, 23%, and 50% of the patients, respectively. The authors also included data on the presence of a third heart sound, which was present in 7% of patients. Table 21.4 shows the univariate performance characteristics of the chest radiograph and S3 findings. Multivariate logistic modeling performed using all of the clinical, historic, radiographic, and BNP data found that

Table 21.4 Diagnostic performance of variable for predicting heart failure

	Odds ratio (95% CI)	Sensitivity, %	Specificity, %	LR+	LR−
Chest x-ray findings					
Alveolar edema	7.1 (2.5–20.6)	6	99	7.0	1.0
Cephalization	15.4 (9.4–25.3)	41	96	9.4	0.6
Cardiomegaly	15.4 (11.1–21.3)	79	80	4.0	0.3
Interstitial edema	17.1 (8.6–34.2)	27	98	12.7	0.7
Clinical findings					
S3	9.1 (4.1–20)	13	98	8.1	0.9

Source: Data from [6].

three chest X-ray findings were significantly associated with heart failure: interstitial edema had an OR of 7.0 (CI 2.9–17), cephalization an OR of 6.4 (CI 3.3–12.5), and cardiomegaly an OR of 2.3 (CI 1.4–3.7).

Collins et al examined physician auscultation of heart sounds with electronically detected heart sounds in order to assess both the ability of emergency physicians to assess the third heart sound as well as the utility of the third heart sound in diagnosing heart failure.[7] Using a convenience sample of patients in four EDs presenting with signs or symptoms of heart failure, the authors compared prospectively recorded physician determination of the presence or absence of a third heart sound with electronically recorded heart sounds that were analyzed in a blinded fashion after the patient encounter. The final diagnosis of heart failure was made by two senior cardiologists who had copies of the complete patient charts that had been edited to remove all heart sound and BNP data. The electronic heart sound was taken as the criterion standard in comparison against the physician-determined auscultation of the third heart sound.

A total of 439 patients were enrolled and 343 were included in the final analysis. Excluded patients were either pilot subjects or patients in whom there were problems obtaining or interpreting the electronic heart sound data. Acute heart failure was the final diagnosis in 133 (39%) of patients. Table 21.5 shows the performance characteristics of both auscultation and electronically detected S3s.

Limitations of this study included patient enrollment method, which was a convenience sample, leaving the possibility of selection bias, as well as the

Table 21.5 Test parameters for auscultated and electronically detected S3s

	Auscultated			Electronic		
	Acute heart failure (HF) (+)	Acute HF (−)	Totals	Acute HF (+)	Acute HF (−)	Totals
S3 Present (+)	21	7	28	45	14	59
S3 Absent (−)	107	200	307	88	196	284
Totals	128	207	335	133	210	343
Sensitivity, % (95% CI)	16 (11–24)			34 (26–43)		
Specificity, % (95% CI)	97 (93–99)			93 (89–96)		
Positive predictive value, % (95% CI)	84 (76–89)			66 (57–74)		
Negative predictive value, % (95% CI)	3 (2–7)			7 (4–11)		
Diagnostic accuracy, % (95% CI)	66 (61–71)			70 (65–75)		

Source: Data from [7].

fact that a significant number of patients were excluded due to problems with the electronically detected heart recorder. Failure to blind the examining physician to the rest of the clinical information and findings could have also led to incorporation bias in the reporting of auscultated heart sounds.

Comment

Specific elements of the history, physical examination, ECG, and chest X-ray are valuable in evaluating patients with suspected heart failure. In addition to the initial clinician's clinical judgment, patient histories of heart failure and myocardial infarction are both useful for increasing the likelihood of heart failure when present and decreasing its likelihood when absent. On physical exam, the presence of a third heart sound (ventricular filling gallop) is able to rule in heart failure, while the presence of either abdominojugular reflux or jugular venous distension makes the diagnosis of heart failure more likely.

The plain chest radiograph can contribute additional data about the likelihood of acute heart failure. Findings of pulmonary venous congestion, interstitial and alveolar edema, vascular redistribution in the form of cephalization, and cardiomegaly are all highly specific for the diagnosis of acute heart failure. The abysmally low sensitivity of these findings, however, should deter clinicians from total reliance on chest radiography in the setting of a normal or nondiagnostic X-ray. Similarly, while ECG findings of atrial fibrillation and new T-wave changes can increase the likelihood of heart failure, they cannot rule in or rule out the disease due to their insensitivity.

An elevated BNP level can further help diagnose acute heart failure, especially when an elevated level is found in conjunction with other factors, such as the presence of an S3 or findings on X-ray. A word of caution about BNP levels; an elevation in BNP can be associated with conditions that elevate right-heart pressures. In the acute setting, these might include acute myocardial infarction or pulmonary embolism and in the chronic setting these might include pulmonary hypertension and systemic conditions of volume overload (as in the case of end stage renal disease necessitating hemodialysis). Therefore, an elevated BNP should be interpreted with these other conditions in mind. In addition, awareness of BNP levels in ED patients with suspected heart failure may not improve their outcomes. Carpenter et al recently reviewed the literature on this subject, including five trials that randomized clinicians to either knowledge or no knowledge of BNP or NT-proBNP levels in patients with suspected heart failure.[8] They found that there did not appear to be any benefit of knowledge of BNP or NT-proBNP levels in terms of overall health care costs, length of stay, or rate of return visits. They note that BNP levels may be more helpful in the dyspneic patient in whom there is not a high suspicion of heart failure, since an elevated level may prompt consideration of the diagnosis in a patient otherwise thought to have another pulmonary disease (e.g., asthma or COPD).

Lastly, rapid assessment of the acutely dyspneic patient using a physical exam, plain chest X-ray, and BNP level can allow clinicians to tailor appropriate therapies for acute heart failure patients. While a number of decision rules allow risk stratification of patients with heart failure, they were designed to prognosticate outcomes after the diagnosis of heart failure has been made and were not developed or validated specifically in ED patients.[9,10] We recommend additional testing to establish left ventricular function and to rule out proximal causes of acute heart failure, prompting inpatient admission for most patients with acute decompensated heart failure.

References

1. Chung P, Hermann L. Acute decompensated heart failure: Formulating an evidence-based approach to diagnosis and treatment (part I). Mount Sinai Journal of Medicine. 2006; 73(2): 506–15.
2. Wang CS, FitzGerald JM, Schulzer M, Mak E, Ayas NT. Does this dyspneic patient in the emergency department have congestive heart failure? Journal of the American Medical Association. 2005; 294(15): 1944–56.
3. Badgett RG, Lucey CR. Update: Congestive heart failure. In: The rational clinical examination: Evidence-based clinical diagnosis. New York: McGraw-Hill; 2008.
4. Maisel AS, Krishnaswamy P, Nowak RM *et al*. Rapid measurement of B-type natriuretic peptide in the emergency diagnosis of heart failure. New England Journal of Medicine. 2002; 347(3): 161–7.
5. Collins S, Storrow AB, Kirk JD *et al*. Beyond pulmonary edema: Diagnostic, risk stratification, and treatment challenges of acute heart failure management in the emergency department. Annals of Emergency Medicine. 2008; 51(1): 45–57.
6. Knudsen CW, Omland T, Clopton P *et al*. Diagnostic value of B-type natriuretic peptide and chest radiographic findings in patients with acute dyspnea. American Journal of Medicine. 2004; 116(6): 363–8.
7. Collins SP, Lindsell CJ, Peacock WF *et al*. The combined utility of an S3 heart sound and B-type natriuretic peptide levels in emergency department patients with dyspnea. Journal of Cardiac Failure. 2006; 12(4): 286–92.
8. Carpenter CR, Keim SM, Worster A, Rosen P. Brain natriuretic peptide in the evaluation of emergency department dyspnea: Is there a role? Journal of Emergency Medicine. 2012; 42(2): 197–205.
9. Fonarow GC, Adams KF, Abraham WT, Yancy CW, Boscardin WJ. Risk stratification for in-hospital mortality in acutely decompensated heart failure. Journal of the American Medical Association. 2005; 293(5): 572–80.
10. Lee DS, Austin PC, Rouleau JL *et al*. Predicting mortality among patients hospitalized for heart failure. Journal of the American Medical Association. 2003; 290(19): 2581–7.

Chapter 22 **Syncope**

Highlights

- Patients with syncope can appear clinically benign in the ED, but a small proportion will have a life-threatening precipitant.
- Several clinical decision rules have been developed to differentiate patients who can safely be discharged from the ED.
- While the decision rules can be useful guides for clinicians to identify risk factors for serious diagnoses or death in ED patients with syncope, no current ED-based syncope rules are sufficiently sensitive and specific for broad use.

Background

Syncope is a transient loss of consciousness associated with a return to preexisting neurological function. A chief complaint of "syncope" accounts for up to 2% of all emergency department (ED) visits. Syncope is a symptom and has a wide variety of causes, ranging from the benign to the life threatening. The evaluation of patients with "unstable" syncope where there is a clear etiology (e.g., ongoing chest pain, gastrointestinal bleeding, or cardiac rhythm disturbances) can typically be focused on correcting or treating the underlying cause. The evaluation of syncope that is "stable" poses a greater diagnostic conundrum to the emergency physician because in approximately half of these cases, the cause for syncope is unclear, even after a thorough ED evaluation.[1-3] Even in stable patients with syncope, there are several potentially lethal causes including cardiac arrhythmias, myocardial infarction, ruptured ectopic pregnancy, stroke, subarachnoid hemorrhage, and pulmonary embolism. However, it should be mentioned that the clinical presentation can sometimes be confused with other conditions where there is a loss of consciousness. This can include seizures (see Chapter 51), vertigo, dizziness, coma, or shock and can be the result of trauma, alcohol intoxication, or other toxic substances.

Evidence-Based Emergency Care: Diagnostic Testing and Clinical Decision Rules, Second Edition.
Jesse M. Pines, Christopher R. Carpenter, Ali S. Raja and Jeremiah D. Schuur.
© 2013 John Wiley & Sons, Ltd. Published 2013 by John Wiley & Sons, Ltd.

As a result of the diagnostic uncertainty and the multiple potentially serious etiologies of syncope, patients are frequently admitted to the hospital for further evaluation, monitoring, and additional testing. As an inpatient, patients may receive further diagnostic testing such as echocardiogram, electroencephalogram, cardiac monitoring, and cardiac stress testing.[4] Specific treatments, such as pacemakers or defibrillators, can be used if a cardiac arrhythmia is determined as the cause for syncope (see Chapter 24), or changes in medication that impact blood pressure, heart rate, or underlying rhythm disturbances may be made to reduce the risk of syncope in the future. Over the last decade, numerous studies across several continents have been performed to identify lower risk syncope patients who may be safe for discharge after ED evaluation.

Clinical question

What are current clinical decision rules for syncope in the ED, and how do their sensitivities and specificities compare?

To answer this question, we will consider four clinical decision rules in various stages of derivation and validation: the Osservatorio Epidemiologico sulla Sincope nel Lazio (OESIL) risk score, the San Francisco syncope rule, the risk stratification of syncope in the ED (ROSE) rule, and the Boston syncope rule. The earliest decision rule was the OESIL, where the Italian study group followed a consecutive sample of patients who presented to the ED with syncope to determine risk factors for all-cause mortality at 1 year.[5] These investigators included patients as young as 12 years old. The OESIL rule is listed in Table 22.1.

In the OESIL rule, each risk factor is given 1 point. Patients with 0 or 1 point had a mortality rate of 0 at 1 year. The authors have concluded that patients with a score of 0 or 1 are low risk; however, the authors did not measure interventions such as the placement of pacemakers or defibrillators or any further diagnostic testing that was performed on these patients. Validation studies have been conducted that failed to demonstrate that patients with an OESIL score of 0 or 1 were low risk because the mortality rates varied from 5% to as high as 13%.[6,7]

Table 22.1 The OESIL rule*

- Age older than 65 years
- Cardiovascular disease in the history
- Syncope with prodrome
- Abnormal electrocardiogram

---

*Each element is given one point. A score of 0 or 1 points is considered "low risk."

Table 22.2 San Francisco syncope rule

- Abnormal electrocardiogram
- A complaint of shortness of breath
- Hematocrit less than 30%
- A triage systolic blood pressure of less than 90 mm Hg
- A history of congestive heart failure

Quinn et al derived and, two years later, validated the San Francisco syncope rule.[8] In comparison to the OESIL study, the authors used outcomes at 7 days as the standard by which to assess whether a patient with syncope requires hospital admission. The outcomes included mortality, myocardial infarction, arrhythmia, pulmonary embolism, stroke, subarachnoid hemorrhage, significant hemorrhage, or return to the ED. In the derivation study, the authors followed 684 patients with syncope or near syncope who were evaluated in the ED. Of the 684, there were 79 serious outcomes. They performed a kappa analysis (test of interrater agreement) and only used variables with good agreement (0.5 to 1.0) for the decision rule. The rule, which required the absence of all the risk factors listed in Table 22.2, was 96% sensitive and 62% specific for identifying serious outcomes at 7 days. If the rule had been applied to the derivation cohort, it could have safely decreased admission rates for syncope by 10%.

The validation of the San Francisco syncope rule conducted by the same group included 791 consecutive ED visits, with 53 serious reported outcomes.[9] The authors found that the rule was 98% sensitive (CI 89–100%) and 56% specific (CI 52–60%). Some limitations of the study included that they were all from one hospital. Because they used a composite outcome that included multiple serious outcomes, the study was not powered to detect any outcome (such as pulmonary embolism) individually. The authors advocated that the rule should be used as a risk stratification instrument rather than as an admission guideline, citing the fact that there are many reasons for admission to the hospital.

Another group performed an independent validation study of the San Francisco rule in an ED population in a single academic center.[10] At the time of care, physicians recorded the elements of the San Francisco syncope rule. They contacted patients at 14 days with a structured interview. The primary outcome of the study was the sensitivity of the San Francisco syncope rule to predict serious events at 7 days. A secondary outcome of the study was the prediction of any serious clinical events that were not detected during the initial ED visits. They enrolled 477 patients and obtained full follow-up records (either from the admission or through telephone follow-up). The serious event prevalence was 12%, and 3% had a serious diagnosis that was not identified at the initial ED valuation. They reported a sensitivity of 89% (CI 81–97%) and specificity of 42% (CI 37–48%) for the San Francisco syncope rule to predict 7-day serious outcomes. They also reported a sensitivity of 69% (CI 46–92%) and specificity of 42% (CI 37–48%) for a serious diagnosis that was not identified during the initial ED evaluation. The authors concluded that the San Francisco syncope rule had a lower sensitivity and specificity than had been previously reported. A recent systematic review pooled 12 studies and found that the sensitivity and specificity of the San Francisco syncope rule were 87% (79–93%) and 52% (43–62%), respectively.[11] Among those studies, the authors reported substantial between-study heterogeneity that resulted in a 95% prediction interval for sensitivity of 55–98%. In patients with all high-risk factors absent, the probability of a serious outcome was 5% or lower, and it was 2% or lower when the rule was used for patients where no cause of syncope was identified after initial ED evaluation.

In 2007, Grossman and colleagues derived the Boston syncope rule.[12] They conducted a prospective observational study that included patients 18 and older with syncope from a single, academic hospital. The primary outcome was a critical intervention or adverse outcome that occurred during the ED stay or subsequent hospitalization, within 30 days after the initial visit. Critical interventions were the placement of a pacemaker or implantable cardiac defibrillator, coronary intervention, surgery, blood transfusion, cardiopulmonary resuscitation (CPR), alterations in antiarrhythmic therapy, endoscopy with intervention, or intervention for carotid stenosis. Adverse outcomes were death, pulmonary embolism, stroke, severe infection or sepsis, ventricular dysrhythmia, atrial dysrhythmia, intracranial hemorrhage, myocardial infarction, cardiac arrest, or life-threatening sequelae of syncope (e.g., rhabomyolysis or long-bone or cervical spine fractures). They included consecutive ED patients aged 18 years or older presenting with syncope. The Boston syncope rule is described in Table 22.3.

Among 362 patients enrolled with syncope, there was complete follow-up in 293 (81%) patients at 30 days. A total of 68 patients (23% of 293) had either a critical intervention or adverse outcome. The derived rule identified 66/68 patients with a sensitivity of 97% (CI 93–100%) and a specificity of 62% (CI 56–69%). Notably, the rule was not derived using standard decision rule methods such as recursive partitioning (see Chapter 4). Instead, according to the authors, the Boston syncope rule was developed using previous work such as the San Francisco syncope rule, clinical guidelines, and clinical judgment.

In the same ED, the authors conducted a before-after study to assess the effectiveness of implementing the Boston syncope rule.[13] They conducted an in-service training of the rule and implemented it as a clinical guideline

Table 22.3 Boston syncope rule

- Signs and symptoms of acute coronary syndrome (e.g., chest pain, ischemic ECG, or other significant arrhythmia)
- Worrisome cardiac history (e.g., history of coronary disease, heart failure, or significant arrhythmia)
- Family history of sudden death in first-degree relative
- Valvular heart disease (murmur noted in history or on ED examination)
- Signs of conduction disease
- Volume depletion (gastrointestinal bleeding, hematocrit <30, and dehydration not corrected in the ED)
- Persistence (>15 min) of abnormal vital signs in the ED without the need of concurrent interventions such as oxygen, pressors, and temporary pacemakers
- Primary central nervous system event (stroke or subarachnoid hemorrhage)

---

that encouraged emergency physicians to make admission decisions based on the criteria. In the "before" phase, 69% of patients with syncope were admitted (which was the original cohort for the derivation), while in the "after" phase 58 were admitted (an 11% reduction in admission rate). In the 160 patients admitted in the "after" phase, 64 (40%) had adverse events during hospitalization, compared to none in the discharged group. When follow-up was conducted at 30 days, 6 additional patients (4%) had adverse outcomes, all of whom were admitted initially. The authors concluded that a real-time application of the Boston syncope rule had a sensitivity of 100% (CI 94–100%) and a specificity of 57% (CI 50–63%).

In 2010, another group out of the United Kingdom aimed to derive and validate a clinical decision rule for syncope, called the *risk stratification of syncope in the ED* (ROSE).[14] They conducted the study in a single center, and used a split derivation and validation cohort, both consisting of 550 patients. The authors defined their outcome as all-cause death, or serious outcomes (acute myocardial infarction, life-threatening arrhythmia, decision to implant a pacemaker or cardiac defibrillator, pulmonary embolism, stroke, intracranial hemorrhage, subarachnoid hemorrhage, hemorrhage requiring a blood transfusion of ≥ 2 units, acute surgical procedure, or endoscopic intervention). In the derivation cohort, 1-month serious outcome or all-cause death happened in 40 (7.3%) patients. Predictors included an elevated BNP (OR 7.3), fecal occult blood (OR 13.2), a low hemoglobin (OR 6.7), an oxygen saturation $\leq 94\%$ (OR 3.0), and a Q-wave on the presenting electrocardiogram (OR 2.8). In the validation cohort, 1-month serious outcome or all-cause death occurred in 39 (7.1%) patients. The ROSE rule that was derived is listed in Table 22.4.

Table 22.4 The ROSE rule

Admit if any of the following are present:
B   Bradycardia (heart rate ≤ 50 beats per minutes in the ED) or
    prehospital BNP level ≥ 300 pg/mL
R   Rectal exam showing fecal occult blood
A   Anemia – hemoglobin ≤ 90 g/L
C   Chest pain associated with syncope
E   ECG showing a Q wave (not in lead III)
S   Saturation of oxygen ≤ 94% on room air

Table 22.5 Sensitivities and specificities of ED-based clinical decision rules for PE

	Sensitivity	Specificity
OESIL	95% (CI 88–98%)	31% (CI 29–34%)
San Francisco syncope rule	86% (CI 83–89%)	49% (CI 48–51%)
Boston syncope criteria*	97% (CI 93–100%)	62% (CI 56–69%)
ROSE*	90% (CI 81–95%)	70% (CI 67–72%)

*Both of these are based on only a single study.
Source: Data from [15].

In the validation cohort, the ROSE rule had a sensitivity of 87% and a specificity of 66%. The negative predictive value of the rule was 99%. The authors noted that an elevated BNP alone was the major predictor of serious cardiovascular outcomes (i.e., it predicted 36% of the events) and deaths (i.e., 89% of the deaths). To date, the ROSE rule has not been validated in an external cohort.

A recent systematic review of clinical decision rules for syncope has provided pooled sensitivities and specificities of the four decision rules[15] (Table 22.5). Notably, the calculated sensitivity and specificity for the San Francisco syncope rule are slightly different from those listed from the 2011 CJEM study because the 2011 study included more recent data.

Comment

The current decision rules available for syncope in the ED do provide good risk stratification schemes to identify patients at low risk for serious outcomes in the short or long term (up to 1 year). That is, clinicians can look at the factors that were significant across the four rules (many of which were the same) and make their own decisions regarding the risk of a serious diagnosis. However, no rule has been rigorously derived and validated sufficiently to provide a definitive guide for which patients should be admitted or discharged. The most widely tested rule is the San Francisco syncope rule, which was validated in a population similar to that in which it was derived; however, it did not perform sufficiently well to be used as a definitive clinical rule when tested on an external ED population. Other decision rules are in earlier phases of development and may ultimately be validated. While considerable preliminary work has been conducted to help differentiate patients with high-risk causes for syncope, there is no current decision rule that can be broadly recommended.

References

1. Martin GJ, Adams SL, Martin HG et al. Prospective evaluation of syncope. Annals of Emergency Medicine. 1984; 13(7): 499–504.
2. Kapoor WN, Hanusa BH. Is syncope a risk factor for poor outcomes? Comparison of patients with and without syncope. American Journal of Medicine. 1996; 100(6): 646–55.
3. Sarasin FP, Pruvot E, Louis-Simonet M et al. Stepwise evaluation of syncope: A prospective population-based controlled study. International Journal of Cardiology. 2008; 127(1): 103–11.
4. Strickberger SA, Benson DW, Biaggioni I et al. AHA/ACCF scientific statement on the evaluation of syncope. Circulation. 2006; 113: 316–27.
5. Colivicchi F, Ammirati F, Melina D, et al. Development and prospective validation of a risk stratification system for patients with syncope in the emergency department: The OESIL risk score. European Heart Journal. 2003; 24: 811–19.
6. Dipaola F, Costantino G, Perego F et al. San Francisco syncope rule, Osservatorio Epidemiologico sulla Sincope nel Lazio risk score, and clinical judgment in the assessment of short-term outcome of syncope. American Journal of Emergency Medicine. 2010; 28: 432–9.
7. Numeroso F, Mossini G, Spaggiari E et al. Syncope in the emergency department of a large northern Italian hospital: Incidence, efficacy of a short-stay observation ward and validation of the OESIL risk score. Emergency Medicine Journal. 2010; 27: 653–8.
8. Quinn JV, Steill IG, McDermott DA et al. Derivation of the San Francisco syncope rule to predict patients with short-term serious outcomes. Annals of Emergency Medicine. 2004; 43: 224–32.
9. Quinn J, McDermott D, Stiell I et al. Prospective validation of the San Francisco syncope rule to predict patients with serious outcomes. Annals of Emergency Medicine. 2006; 47: 448–54.
10. Sun BC, Mangione CM, Merchant G et al. External validation of the San Francisco syncope rule. Annals of Emergency Medicine. 2007; 49: 420–7.
11. Saccilotto RT, Nickel CH, Bucher HC et al. San Francisco syncope rule to predict short-term serious outcomes: A systematic review. CMAJ. 2011; 183(15): E1116–26.

12. Grossman SA, Fischer C, Lipsitz LA *et al*. Predicting adverse outcomes in syncope. Journal of Emergency Medicine. 2007; 33: 233–9.
13. Grossman SA, Bar J, Fischer C *et al*. Reducing admissions utilizing the Boston syncope criteria. Journal of Emergency Medicine. 2011 Mar 19:epub ahead of print.
14. Reed MJ, Newby DE, Coull AJ *et al*. The ROSE (risk stratification of syncope in the emergency department) study. Journal of American College of Cardiology. 2010; 55: 713–21.
15. Serrano LA, Hess EP, Bellolio MF *et al*. Accuracy and quality of clinical decision rules for syncope in the emergency department: A systematic review and meta-analysis. Annals of Emergency Medicine. 2010; 56: 362–73.

Chapter 23 **Acute Coronary Syndrome**

Highlights

- Acute coronary syndrome (ACS) is a spectrum of conditions ranging from acute myocardial infarction (AMI) to stable angina.
- History and physical exam characteristics increasing the likelihood of AMI include chest pain that radiates to both arms or the right arm, a third heart sound, and hypotension, while chest pain that is pleuritic, positional, sharp or stabbing, or reproducible by palpation is less likely to be caused by AMI.
- Troponin I is poorly sensitive but highly specific as an initial test for ACS, but its sensitivity increases considerably with serial testing, typically 6 hours.
- Highly sensitive troponin assays can decrease the time interval between serial tests to 3 hours.
- Exercise ECG stress testing is widely available but lacks sensitivity or specificity.
- Pharmacologic agents can increase sensitivity when combined with myocardial perfusion imaging, and when combined with echocardiography or MRI their specificity is maximized.
- Stress echocardiography with dobutamine has higher specificity compared to stress nuclear scintigraphy in women.
- CT coronary angiography may be useful for low-risk ED patients and appears to be at least as sensitive and specific as stress myocardial perfusion imaging.

Background

Coronary artery disease (CAD) is a leading cause of death, both in the United States and worldwide, and patients with symptomatic CAD frequently present directly to the emergency department (ED) for evaluation of their acute chest pain. The term *acute coronary syndrome* (ACS) covers the entire spectrum of myocardial ischemia, which ranges from acute myocardial

---

Evidence-Based Emergency Care: Diagnostic Testing and Clinical Decision Rules, Second Edition. Jesse M. Pines, Christopher R. Carpenter, Ali S. Raja and Jeremiah D. Schuur. © 2013 John Wiley & Sons, Ltd. Published 2013 by John Wiley & Sons, Ltd.

infarction (AMI) with myocardial necrosis to reversible ischemic damage or unstable angina (UA).

The first step in the ED evaluation and management of patients who present with chest pain or other symptoms concerning for ACS is a 12-lead electrocardiogram (ECG). While findings on the initial ECG may be diagnostic or suggestive of ACS, the initial ECG can also be normal or nondiagnostic, underscoring the need for additional monitoring and testing of patients with suspected ACS. Evaluation of the initial ECG in patients with suspected ACS should focus on the presence of ST-segment elevations, new left bundle branch blocks, or new dynamic ST changes, all indicative of AMI. In patients with known left bundle branch blocks, the Sgarbosa criteria (ST-segment elevation of 1 mm or more concordant with the QRS complex; ST-segment depression of 1 mm or more in lead V1, V2, or V3; and ST-segment elevation of 5 mm or more discordant with the QRS complex) can still be used to diagnose ACS.[1] However, while the standard ECG is the single best test to identify patients with AMI upon their presentation to the ED, it has relatively low sensitivity. In patients with AMI, ST segments may be elevated in only 50% of initial ECGs.[2,3] Due to this insensitivity, distinguishing AMI and UA from other noncardiac chest pain in patients at risk for ACS typically involves serial ECGs and/or serial serum biomarkers of myocardial injury, also with diagnostic imaging (stress tests or CT imaging) or cardiac catheterization.

Clinical questions relevant to the assessment of a patient with suspected ACS involve the test characteristics of history and physical examination findings, cardiac biomarkers, non-invasive stress testing, and cardiac CT imaging.

Clinical question

Which elements of the history and physical examination make the diagnosis of AMI more or less likely?
A large meta-analysis by Panju et al reviewed historical and physical examination findings of patients with suspected AMI and was subsequently updated in 2008.[4,5] Fourteen studies met their inclusion criteria, most of which used the World Health Organization (WHO) definition of AMI as the criterion standard, which includes evolving changes on serial ECGs, a rise in serial biomarkers, and either chest pain with an abnormal ECG or other symptoms with evolving changes on serial ECGs.[6] The analysis of the pooled data in the meta-analysis (Table 23.1) demonstrates a number of historical and physical exam characteristics that increase and decrease the likelihood of AMI. For the sake of clarity, the authors chose to only report LRs that were either greater than 2.0 or less than 0.5.

Table 23.1 History and physical examination characteristics associated with either a greater or lesser risk of acute myocardial infarction

Clinical feature	Positive likelihood ratio (LR+) (CI)	Negative likelihood ratio (LR−) (CI)
Chest or center arm pain*	2.7	–
Chest pain radiation to:		
Right shoulder	2.2 (1.4–3.4)	–
Right arm	7.3 (3.9–14)	–
Left arm	2.2 (1.6–3.1)	–
Both left and right arms	9.7 (4.6–20)	–
Chest pain most important symptom*	2.0	–
History of myocardial infarction**	1.5–3.0	–
Nausea or vomiting	1.9 (1.7–2.3)	–
Diaphoresis	2.0 (1.9–2.2)	–
Third heart sound on auscultation	3.2 (1.6–6.5)	–
Hypotension***	3.1 (1.8–5.2)	–
Pulmonary crackles on auscultation	2.1 (1.4–3.1)	–
Pleuritic chest pain	–	0.2 (0.2–0.3)
Sharp or stabbing chest pain	–	0.3 (0.2–0.5)
Positional chest pain	–	0.3 (0.2–0.4)
Chest pain reproducible by palpation**	–	0.2–0.4

*Data not available to calculate confidence intervals.
**Reported as a range due to heterogeneity of the pooled studies.
***Defined as systolic blood pressure ≤ 80 mm Hg.
Source: Data from [4].

Serum biomarkers

For over 30 years, serum biomarkers have been used for the assessment of patients with suspected ACS who do not have ECG signs of ST-elevation MI or dynamic ECG changes. Advances in the technology of laboratory testing have led to a move away from nonspecific biomarkers, such as lactate dehydrogenase (LDH) and aspartate aminotransferase (AST), to more sensitive and specific cardiac-specific biomarkers, including creatine kinase (CK)-MB, troponin-T, and troponin-I.[7] The biokinetic properties of the cardiac troponins are similar in terms of the rate of rise in serum concentrations (usually within 4–6 hours of AMI) to that of CK-MB, but the levels remain elevated for over a week. The I and T subunits are both part of the striated cardiac muscle contractile unit; while the I subunit is a smaller inhibitory protein not found in the serum without myocardial injury, the T subunit is larger and is not found in the serum of patients without complaints or heart disease. Troponin-T releases slightly more slowly into the serum and is elevated in patients with reversible ischemic injury, resulting in more false positives in the setting of UA.

Clinical question

What are the performance characteristics of the cardiac troponins (I and T) for the diagnosis of acute cardiac ischemia? Do these differ when initial biomarker levels are compared to serial biomarkers? How can highly sensitive troponin assays decrease the time necessary between serial biomarker evaluations?

One systematic review and three meta-analyses were found that examined the diagnostic performance of biomarkers for ACS, including AMI and unstable angina.[8–11] While a number of more recent meta-analyses focus on biomarkers' performance in specific populations (after bypass grafting, diabetics, etc.), the only systematic reviews or meta-analyses of their performance in all patients with suspected ACS were published in 2001 and therefore do not incorporate more recent data.

Two studies published by the New England Medical Center Evidence–Based Practice Center provide summary data on the accuracy of diagnostic performance of cardiac biomarkers in ED populations of adult patients aged 18 years and older.[8,9] The results were an effort to consolidate and interpret the explosion of publications evaluating various diagnostic technologies since 1994, but include relevant studies dating to 1966. Non-ED studies were included when there were not studies that included ED patients. Criterion standards varied (as might be expected given the time interval included) and included final hospital diagnosis, WHO criteria for AMI, or angiography. The time between serial biomarker evaluations also varied, between 1 and 16 hours after symptom onset. Table 23.2 shows the summary diagnostic

Table 23.2 Summary performance characteristics of biomarker studies in the diagnosis of acute myocardial infarction in ED patients from published studies from 1966 to 1998

Cardiac biomarker	Number of studies (number of patients)	Sensitivity, % (95% CI)	Specificity, % (95% CI)	Positive likelihood ratio (LR+)	Negative likelihood ratio (LR−)
		Initial presentation			
Troponin-I*	4 (1,149)	39 (10–78)	93 (88–97)	5.6	0.7
Troponin-T	5 (1,171)	44 (32–56)	92 (88–95)	5.5	0.6
CK-MB	10 (2,504)	44 (35–53)	96 (94–97)	11	0.6
		Serial evaluation			
Troponin-I*	2 (1,393)	90–100	83–96	5.3–25	0–0.10
Troponin-T*	3 (904)	93 (85–97)	85 (76–91)	6.2	0.1
CK-MB	7 (3,229)	80 (61–91)	96 (94–98)	20	0.2

*Includes all studies, not ED-specific studies.
**Not reported.
Source: Data from [8,9].

performances of CK-MB, troponin-I, and troponin-T. Data for ED specific patients are shown separately when possible.

A single set of biomarkers obtained upon presentation to the ED has low sensitivity but high specificity for detecting AMI. Serial measurement greatly increases the sensitivity and maintains high specificities. These data indicate that troponin-I and troponin-T, when compared to each other, have similar performance characteristics, both at initial presentation and when assessed serially for the diagnosis of AMI.

Another meta-analysis examined the predictive value of troponin-I and troponin-T for adverse events at 30 days including death and AMI without ST-elevation in ACS.[10] The authors included published articles in MEDLINE that included 30-day outcomes and serial biomarker assessments, and excluded patients who received thrombolytics. The meta-analysis presents summary performances for each of the cardiac troponins, in addition to a comparison of performances of clinical trials and cohort studies. Seven studies that included 3,579 patients were found that reported both troponin-I and troponin-T data. Two hundred and sixty patients (7.2%) had an adverse event. The summary predictive sensitivity and specificity were 65% (CI 59–71%) and 74.5% (CI 73–76%), respectively, for troponin-I and 57% (CI 51–63%) and 77% (CI 75–78%), respectively, for troponin-T. The summary negative predictive values, reflecting the prevalence of the outcomes, were 97% (CI 96–97%) for troponin-I and 96% (CI 95–97%) for troponin-T. There were no meaningful differences in the performance characteristics of either troponin biomarker when these studies were compared.

Heidenreich et al examined the prognostic performance of troponin-T and troponin-I in clinical trials and cohort studies of patients with acute coronary syndrome.[11] A total of seven clinical trials and 19 cohort studies were found in their MEDLINE search. Studies that included only AMIs were excluded, and the outcomes of death and death or AMI were reported. Two trials and two cohort studies directly compared troponin-I and troponin-T values, and the summary odds ratios for predicting mortality were similar (troponin-I: OR 3.9, CI 2.3–6.6; troponin-T: OR 5.2, CI 3.1–8.5). When deaths following positive troponin-I or troponin-T tests were compared between clinical trials and cohorts, the cohort studies had higher summary odds ratios than the clinical trials regardless of troponin subtype (troponin-I: clinical trials summary OR 2.6, CI 1.8–3.6, and cohort studies OR 8.5, CI 3.5–21.1, p<0.01; troponin-T: clinical trials summary OR 3.0, CI 1.6–5.5, and cohort studies OR 5.1, CI 3.2–8.4, p<0.2).

A number of recent trials have evaluated highly sensitive troponin assays to determine whether the time interval between serial cardiac biomarker evaluations might be decreased from 6 hours.[12–14] The most recent, by

Keller et al enrolled 1,818 patients, 23% of whom were diagnosed as having a final diagnosis of AMI based on all clinical, laboratory, and imaging findings, including 30-day follow-up and review of the civil death records.[14] They found that, using a cutoff concentration representing the 99th percentile of a reference population, highly sensitive troponin-I had a sensitivity of 98% (96–99%), a specificity of 90% (88–92%), a LR+ of 10, and a LR− of 0.02 at 3 hours for AMI. They also found similar test characteristics for contemporary sensitive troponin-I, which had a sensitivity of 98% (96–99%), a specificity of 90% (88–92%), a LR+ of 9.6, and a LR− of 0.02 at 3 hours for AMI.

Non-invasive cardiac testing

There are several non-invasive tests commonly used during the assessment of patients with chest pain to evaluate for underlying CAD. Exercise ECG stress testing involves assessment of a continuous ECG under an exercise protocol, often using a treadmill or bicycle. Dynamic ECG changes over time during exercise yield important and useful diagnostic information about the presence of underlying CAD, and the test is both low cost and widely available. Myocardial perfusion imaging with single-photon emission computed tomography (SPECT) uses a safe nuclear tracer (thallium-201 or technetium-99 sestamibi) that permits an evaluation of ventricular function, coronary artery perfusion, and regional blood flow. It is often coupled with a pharmacologic stressing agent with vasodilatory effects, usually adenosine or dipyridamole, to enhance its diagnostic accuracy. Stress echocardiography, either with exercise alone or with exercise and a pharmacological stressor (commonly dobutamine), permits assessment of global cardiac and regional biventricular function, transient regional wall motion abnormalities, and valvular dysfunction. Lastly, stress cardiac magnetic resonance imaging (MRI) couples MRI with exercise or pharmacologic (adenosine, dipyridamole, or dobutamine) stress and provides information regarding wall motion and thickness as well as perfusion. Since SPECT imaging, echocardiography testing, and cardiac MRI require specialized facilities for both preparation for and execution of the studies, determining which stress test to use is based on patient characteristics, exercise capacity, and study availability.

Clinical question

What are the performance characteristics for diagnosing coronary artery disease of the following forms of non-invasive stress testing: exercise ECG stress, stress echocardiography (exercise and pharmacologic), stress myocardial perfusion imaging with SPECT, and cardiac MRI?

A number of studies have examined the performance of the various non-invasive stress-testing techniques. A meta-analysis of 147 studies on exercise

EGC testing was conducted by Gianrossi et al[15] The exercise ECG was compared to coronary angiography for 24,074 patients in whom the prevalence of CAD was 66% based on the angiographic definition of >50% stenosis of a major coronary artery. There was wide variability of the performance characteristics across the studies. The summary sensitivity of the exercise ECG stress test was 68% (CI 36–100%) and the summary specificity was 77% (CI 43–100%), with a predictive accuracy of 73%. More recent data from another meta-analysis with exercise ECG stress information from 24 studies from 1990 to 1997 (that included 2,456 patients with corresponding coronary angiography data) showed a summary sensitivity of 52% (CI 50–55%) and summary specificity of 71% (CI 68–74%) for detecting CAD.[16] The prevalence of CAD in this study was 69%.

Data extracted from several meta-analyses permit side-by-side comparisons of exercise and vasodilator echocardiography studies (Table 23.3). The data show higher sensitivity of stress echocardiography when used with SPECT imaging, and that the use of vasodilators (adenosine or dipyridamole) maximizes specificity for the diagnosis of CAD.

Kim et al compared the different pharmacologic agents used in combination with either echocardiography or SPECT stress testing in a meta-analysis for the diagnosis of CAD (Table 23.4).[18] Patients had to have undergone one of the types of stress test as well as a coronary angiography. Studies that included patients imaged following known AMI, post-angioplasty, or post–coronary artery bypass grafting were excluded. Dobutamine was most commonly used in combination with echocardiography and had higher sensitivity but lower specificity compared to adenosine and dipyridamole studies. Conversely, dipyridamole was most commonly used together with SPECT imaging and had a higher sensitivity but a lower specificity compared to dobutamine.

Table 23.3 Summaries of performance characteristics of stress echocardiography results from meta-analyses

	Reference	Number of patients	Number of studies	Coronary artery disease prevalence (%)	Sensitivity, % (95% CI)	Specificity, % (95% CI)
Exercise stress echo	17	533	8	74	79	82
	16	2,637	24	66	85 (83–87)	77 (74–80)
Dipyridamole stress echo	17	533	8	74	72	92
	18	1,835	20	67	70 (66–74)	93 (90–95)
Adenosine stress echo	18	516	6	73	72 (62–79)	91 (88–93)

Table 23.4 Summary performance test characteristics of different pharmacologic agents coupled with echocardiography or SPECT stress testing

	Number of studies (number of patients)	Coronary artery disease prevalence, %	Sensitivity, % (95% CI)	Specificity, % (95% CI)
Echocardiography stress				
Adenosine	6 (516)	73	72 (62–79)	91 (88–93)
Dipyridamole	20 (1,835)	67	70 (66–74)	93 (90–95)
Dobutamine	40 (4,097)	70	80 (77–83)	84 (80–86)
SPECT stress				
Adenosine	9 (1,207)	80	90 (89–92)	75 (70–79)
Dipyridamole	21 (1,464)	71	89 (84–93)	65 (54–74)
Dobutamine	14 (1,066)	66	82 (77–87)	75 (70–79)

Source: Data from [18]

Women have been underrepresented in the majority of noninvasive stress-testing studies throughout the 20th century.[19] Because the majority of studies examined middle-aged men (who have an overall higher prevalence of CAD), there have been concerns about the application of the various stress-testing modalities to women. Fortunately, once CAD is recognized, treatments and interventions are similar for both sexes. However, for the emergency physician, the concern about gender bias in the literature is a reasonable clinical question.

Kwok et al examined studies published from 1966 to 1995 that included at least 50 women who underwent at least one type of exercise stress test and who had corresponding coronary angiography information.[20] Studies that did not present female-specific data were not included, nor were non-English studies or studies done for post-MI or post-angioplasty evaluations. A total of 21 studies involving 4,113 patients were included in the meta-analysis with a mean CAD prevalence of 39% (Table 23.5).

Table 23.5 Summary performance characteristics of various exercise stress tests

	Number of studies (number of patients)	Sensitivity, % (95% CI)	Specificity, % (95% CI)	Positive likelihood ratio (LR+), % (95% CI)	Negative likelihood ratio (LR−), % (95% CI)
Electrocardiogram	19 (3,721)	61 (54–68)	70 (64–75)	2.3 (1.8–2.7)	0.6 (0.5–0.6)
Radionuclide (thallium)	5 (842)	78 (72–83)	64 (51–77)	2.9 (1.0–5.0)	0.4 (0.3–0.4)
Echocardiography	3 (296)	86 (75–96)	79 (72–86)	4.3 (2.9–5.7)	0.2 (0.1–0.3)

Source: Data from [20]

These data demonstrated that none of the non-invasive exercise stress tests were highly sensitive or specific in women. Stress echocardiography yielded the highest sensitivity and specificity, but also was the least studied modality in this report.

Dutch researchers examined dobutamine stress echocardiography among women in a meta-analysis of 14 studies from 1992 to 2002 in which there was corresponding coronary angiography data.[21] For six studies, direct comparisons between male and female subjects could be made. The researchers were also able to compare dobutamine stress echocardiography with stress nuclear scintigraphy in six studies. The results from the meta-analysis are shown in Table 23.6.

Performance of dobutamine stress echocardiography was similar among men and women in the studies reviewed. Interestingly, dobutamine stress echo had substantially higher specificity in women compared with stress nuclear scintigraphy. It has been postulated that breast tissue attenuation artifact, smaller ventricle size in women, and estrogen-related effects on endothelial tissues may all contribute to the false-positive tests in women (and hence the lower specificity).[19]

Nandalur et al published a recent meta-analysis of studies evaluating the use of stress MRI as a diagnostic test for CAD (defined as >50% diameter stenosis). The 37 studies included all used angiography as the criterion standard and included 2,191 total patients. As stress MRI can be performed

Table 23.6 Summary weighted test characteristics of stress tests

	Number of studies (number of patients)	Coronary artery disease prevalence, %	Sensitivity, %*	Specificity, %*
All dobutamine stress echo	14 (901)	48	72	88
Studies comparing dobutamine stress echo by sex				
Females	7 (482)	59	77	81
Males	7 (966)	73	77	77
Studies comparing dobutamine stress echo to stress nuclear scintigraphy in women				
Echocardiography	6 (379)	**	77	90
Nuclear	6 (372)	**	73	70

*95% confidence intervals not provided.
**Data not provided.
Source: Data from [21]

Table 23.7 Summary performance characteristics of both techniques of cardiac MRI

	Number of studies (number of patients)	Sensitivity, % (95% CI)	Specificity, % (95% CI)	Positive likelihood ratio (LR+) (95% CI)	Negative likelihood ratio (LR−) (95% CI)
Perfusion imaging	14 (1,183)	91 (88–94)	81 (77–85)	5.10 (3.92–6.28)	0.11 (0.07–0.15)
Wall motion imaging	13 (735)	83 (79–88)	86 (81–91)	5.24 (3.28–7.21)	0.19 (0.15–0.24)

Source: Data from [22]

with two different techniques (perfusion imaging and wall motion imaging), studies of both types were included.[22] Results from the meta-analysis are listed in Table 23.7.

Computed tomography coronary angiography

Computed tomography (CT) angiography of the coronary vessels for the purposes of identifying potential ACS is one of the newest diagnostic modalities available to emergency physicians for the evaluation of patients with chest pain in the ED. Advances in CT technology with improved spatial and temporal resolution have permitted acquisition of detailed pictures of the coronary anatomy, allowing detection of coronary artery stenosis as well as calcified and noncalcified coronary artery plaques.

Clinical question

How do the test characteristics of multidetector computed tomography angiography (MDCT) compare with conventional invasive coronary angiography (CA)?
Four meta-analyses have examined this question. The first, a Dutch study, examined original studies published between 2000 and 2005, all of which included at least 20 patients with native coronary arteries on whom both MDCT and CA were performed.[23] Fifteen studies were found totaling 944 patients (range 27–153). The mean prevalence of CAD in the studies was 59% (range 31–81%). Pooled patient-based sensitivity for the 10 studies reporting patient-based data was 89% (CI 85–92%), and the pooled LR- was 0.16 (CI 0.10–0.26).

Another meta-analysis by European researchers evaluated studies from 2002 to 2006 reporting results with at least 30 patients who had undergone both MDCT and CA studies.[24] The MDCTs had to employ newer generation CT technology (≥ 16 slices) and a total of 27 studies were included in

Table 23.8 Pooled performance characteristics of multidetector computed tomography angiography compared to coronary angiography

	Level of analysis		
	Coronary segment (n = 22,789)	Coronary vessel (n = 2,726)	Patient (n = 1,570)
Sensitivity, % (CI)	81 (72–89)	82 (80–85)	96 (94–98)
Specificity, % (CI)	93 (90–97)	91 (90–92)	74 (65–84)
Positive likelihood ratio (LR+) (CI)	22 (13–35)	12 (7–21)	5 (3–8)
Negative likelihood ratio (LR−) (CI)	0.11 (0.06–0.21)	0.08 (0.02–0.32)	0.05 (0.03–0.09)

Source: Data from [24]

Table 23.9 Pooled performance characteristics of multidetector computed tomography angiography compared to coronary angiography

	Level of analysis		
	Coronary segment (n = 34 studies)	Coronary vessel (n = 16 studies)	Patient (n = 21 studies)
Sensitivity % (95% CI)	83 (79–89)	90 (87–94)	91 (88–95)
Specificity % (95% CI)	93 (91–96)	87 (80–93)	86 (81–92)

Source: Data from [25]

the analysis, permitting analysis at the coronary segment (evaluating each segment separately), vessel (pooling all segments of each coronary artery together), and patient (pooling all segments for a patient together) levels. The results are summarized in Table 23.8.

The largest meta-analysis comes from Sun and Jiang, who examined 47 studies from 1998 to 2006.[25] The studies included reports with 10 or more patients who underwent MDCT and CA. The included studies used CTs with between four and 64 detectors. Table 23.9 summarizes the results. The prevalence of CAD was 74% (CI 64–84%).

The most recent study by Takakuwa et al includes nine studies published between 2005 and 2011, all of which used 64-detector MDCT to evaluate ED patients with chest pain, with CA as the criterion standard.[26] Overall, 1,559 low- to intermediate-risk patients were included, and the pooled analysis calculated a sensitivity of 93% (CI 88–97%), a specificity of 90% (CI 88–91%), a LR+ of 9.2, and a LR- of 0.07. Overall, 7.5% of the patients had CAD on CA.

Comments

Non-invasive cardiac testing

Non-invasive stress testing is currently recommended in patients suspected of having CAD when there is no ECG or enzymatic evidence of AMI or UA. While exercise stress testing is the most widely available testing modality, it suffers from insufficient sensitivity and specificity. However, exercise stress testing is a reasonable first step when evaluating patients with a low to very low suspicion of CAD. If the facilities and resources for exercise imaging are available, additional information can be obtained with better test performance. Pharmacologic additions to the stress tests enhance diagnostic accuracy and can be used in those patients incapable of exercising. Vasodilator drugs such as adenosine and dipyridamole can maximize sensitivity when combined with SPECT imaging, whereas when combined with echocardiography the specificity is maximized. For women, stress echocardiography with dobutamine appear to have better specificity compared to stress nuclear scintigraphy methods. Cardiac MRI test characteristics rival other stress imaging modalities; perfusion MRI is more sensitive, and wall motion MRI more specific, for CAD.

Serum biomarkers

Cardiac biomarkers are an integral part of the assessment of patients presenting with acute chest pain concerning for ACS. However, cardiac biomarkers should not be the sole determinant for detecting the presence of ACS. The studies we reviewed show poor sensitivity and high specificity for initial cardiac troponins, and increased sensitivity with serial testing. The presence of any positive troponin indicates higher short-term risks of the adverse outcomes of death and/or AMI. Results from cohort studies using either troponin-I or troponin-T show worse short-term outcomes when compared to clinical trials, indicating that study-specific subject selection, study patient heterogeneity, or trial conditions impact outcome.

Most EDs and hospital laboratories will run cardiac panels that typically include CK-MB and either troponin-I or troponin-T. In the absence of ST-elevations, new left bundle branch blocks, or dynamic ST segment changes on the initial ECG, cardiac troponins for the initial assessment of suspected ACS should be obtained. A positive troponin should result in a cardiology evaluation, depending on the patient's medical history and presentation, and often will necessitate an evaluation of the coronary arteries, either invasively or non-invasively. However, due to the biokinetic properties of the troponins, patients presenting acutely for the evaluation of chest pain may have non-elevated initial cardiac biomarkers. In these patients, the emergency physician should obtain serial ECGs and serial cardiac biomarkers. Among patients presenting with reliably longer episodes of chest pain (beyond the period after which a second set of biomarkers would be obtained) and who have normal or nondiagnostic ECGs, the strategy of using of a single troponin assessment for risk stratification may be appropriate.

Of note, while serial biomarkers are typically obtained at 6 hours, the recent publication by Keller et al confirmed that highly sensitive troponin-I and contemporary troponin-I are both very sensitive and very specific for AMI at 3 hours.[14]

Computed tomography coronary angiography

While none of the three early meta-analyses presented included patients presenting to the ED with chest pain, the most recent meta-analysis by Takakuwa et al not only included ED patients but also used modern 64-detector CT scanners. In a low- to intermediate-risk population, the authors found that MDCT angiography had significantly better test characteristics than demonstrated in the earlier meta-analyses, with a near-perfect NPV of 99%. Given MDCT's potential to decrease overall evaluation time and its favorable test characteristics, it has the potential to change the way that these patients are evaluated in the ED. Nevertheless, these advantages must be weighed against the risks of radiation-induced malignancy and contrast-induced nephropathy, both of which should be discussed with individual patients when deciding upon their optimal cardiac risk stratification technique.

Clinical prediction rules for ED patients with chest pain

The evaluation of ED patients with chest pain is an area ripe for a validated clinical decision rule, but many of the decision rules published in this area have been poorly developed or are not suitable for ED patients. However, a recently developed decision rule by Hess et al was developed using only ED patients and aimed to identify those who were at very low risk for 30-day cardiac events and could be discharged, provided that outpatient follow-up could be arranged within that time period.[27] They enrolled 2,718 patients (12% of whom had a cardiac event within 30 days) and used recursive partitioning to develop their decision rule (Figure 23.1). While their rule has not yet undergone prospective validation and is similar to what is commonly being practiced already, if validated it may give emergency physicians a solid evidence base for the identification of patients at very low risk for ACS who can be safely discharged home without further inpatient or observation unit testing.

A patient with chest pain and possible acute coronary syndrome can be safely discharged from the ED without additional diagnostic testing if NONE of the following four criteria are met:

1. New ischemia in initial ECG*
2. History of coronary artery disease
3. Pain is typical for acute coronary syndrome**
4. Initial cardiac troponin is positive
         AND
5. Age ≤ 40 years
         OR
6. Age 41-50 years and repeat troponin ≥ 6 hours from symptom onset is negative

*Defined as ST-segment deviation ≥ 1mm or T-wave inversion ≥ 0.2mm in at least 2 contiguous leads.

**As determined by the attending emergency physician.

Figure 23.1 The North American chest pain rule (Source 27).

References

1. Sgarbossa EB, Pinski SL, Barbagelata A *et al*. Electrocardiographic diagnosis of evolving acute myocardial infarction in the presence of left bundle-branch block: GUSTO-1 (Global Utilization of Streptokinase and Tissue Plasminogen Activat or for Occluded Coronary Arteries) Investigators. New England Journal of Medicine. 1996; 334(8): 481–7.

2. Rude RE, Poole WK, Muller JE *et al*. Electrocardiographic and clinical criteria for recognition of acute myocardial infarction based on analysis of 3,697 patients. American Journal of Cardiology. 1983; 52(8): 936–42.

3. Gibler WB, Young GP, Hedges JR *et al*. Acute myocardial infarction in chest pain patients with nondiagnostic ECGs: Serial CK-MB sampling in the emergency department. Annals of Emergency Medicine. 21(5): 504–12.

4. Panju AA, Hemmelgarn BR, Guyatt GH, Simel DL. The rational clinical examination. Is this patient having a myocardial infarction? Journal of the American Medical Association. 1998; 280(14): 1256–63.

5. Simel DL. Update: Myocardial infarction. In: The rational clinical examination: Evidence-based clinical diagnosis. New York: McGraw-Hill; 2008.

6. Tunstall-Pedoe H, Kuulasmaa K, Amouyel P *et al*. Myocardial infarction and coronary deaths in the World Health Organization MONICA Project. Registration procedures, event rates, and case-fatality rates in 38 populations from 21 countries in four continents. Circulation. 1994; 90(1): 583–612.

7. Jaffe AS, Ravkilde J, Roberts R *et al*. It's time for a change to a troponin standard. Circulation. 2000; 102(11): 1216–20.

8. Lau J, Ioannidis JP, Balk EM *et al*. Diagnosing acute cardiac ischemia in the emergency department: A systematic review of the accuracy and clinical effect of current technologies. Annals of Emergency Medicine. 2001; 37(5): 453–60.

9. Balk EM, Ioannidis JP, Salem D, Chew PW, Lau J. Accuracy of biomarkers to diagnose acute cardiac ischemia in the emergency department: A meta-analysis. Annals of Emergency Medicine. 2001; 37(5): 478–94.

10. Fleming SM, Daly KM. Cardiac troponins in suspected acute coronary syndrome: A meta-analysis of published trials. Cardiology. 2001; 95(2): 66–73.

11. Heidenreich PA, Alloggiamento T, Melsop K *et al.* The prognostic value of troponin in patients with non-ST elevation acute coronary syndromes: A meta-analysis. Journal of the American College of Cardiologists. 2001; 38(2): 478–85.

12. deFilippi CR, de Lemos JA, Christenson RH *et al.* Association of serial measures of cardiac troponin T using a sensitive assay with incident heart failure and cardio-vascular mortality in older adults. Journal of the American Medical Association. 2010; 304(22): 2494–502.

13. Saunders JT, Nambi V, de Lemos JA *et al.* Cardiac troponin-T measured by a highly sensitive assay predicts coronary heart disease, heart failure, and mortality in the Atherosclerosis Risk in Communities Study. Circulation. 2011; 123(13): 1367–76.

14. Keller T, Zeller T, Ojeda F *et al.* Serial Changes in highly sensitive troponin I assay and early diagnosis of myocardial infarction. Journal of the American Medical Association. 2011; 306(24): 2684–93.

15. Gianrossi R, Detrano R, Mulvihill D *et al.* Exercise-induced ST depression in the diagnosis of coronary artery disease: A meta-analysis. Circulation. 1989; 80(1): 87–98.

16. Fleischmann KE, Hunink MGM, Kuntz KM, Douglas PS. Exercise echocardiography or exercise SPECT imaging? A meta-analysis of diagnostic test performance. Journal of Nuclear Cardiology. 2002; 9(1): 133–4.

17. Fonseca Lde A, Picano E. Comparison of dipyridamole and exercise stress echocardiography for detection of coronary artery disease (a meta-analysis). American Journal of Cardiology. 87(10): 1193–6.

18. Kim C, Kwok YS, Heagerty P, Redberg R. Pharmacologic stress testing for coronary disease diagnosis: A meta-analysis. American Heart Journal. 2001; 142(6): 934–44.

19. Shaw L, Peterson E, Johnson L. Non-invasive stress testing. In: Coronary artery disease in women: What all physicians need to know. Philadelphia (PA): American College of Physicians; 1999: 327–50.

20. Kwok Y, Kim C, Grady D, Segal M, Redberg R. Meta-analysis of exercise testing to detect coronary artery disease in women. American Journal of Cardiology. 1999; 83(5): 660–6.

21. Geleijnse ML, Krenning BJ, Soliman O II *et al.* Dobutamine stress echocardiography for the detection of coronary artery disease in women. American Journal of Cardiology. 2007; 99(5): 714–17.

22. Nandalur KR, Dwamena BA, Choudhri AF, Nandalur MR, Carlos RC. Diagnostic performance of stress cardiac magnetic resonance imaging in the detection of coronary artery disease: A meta-analysis. Journal of the American College of Cardiologists. 2007; 50(14): 1343–53.

23. van der Zaag-Loonen HJ, Dikkers R, de Bock GH, Oudkerk M. The clinical value of a negative multi-detector computed tomographic angiography in patients suspected of coronary artery disease: A meta-analysis. European Radiology. 2006; 16(12): 2748–56.

24. Hamon M, Biondi-Zoccai GGL, Malagutti P *et al*. Diagnostic performance of multislice spiral computed tomography of coronary arteries as compared with conventional invasive coronary angiography: A meta-analysis. Journal of the American College of Cardiologists. 2006; 48(9): 1896–910.

25. Sun Z, Jiang W. Diagnostic value of multislice computed tomography angiography in coronary artery disease: A meta-analysis. European Journal of Radiology. 2006; 60(2): 279–86.

26. Takakuwa KM, Keith SW, Estepa AT, Shofer FS. A meta-analysis of 64-section coronary CT Angiography findings for predicting 30-day major adverse cardiac events in patients presenting with symptoms suggestive of acute coronary syndrome. Academic Radiology. 2011; 18(12): 1522–8.

27. Hess EP, Brison RJ, Perry JJ *et al*. Development of a clinical prediction rule for 30-day cardiac events in emergency department patients with chest pain and possible acute coronary syndrome. Annals of Emergency Medicine. 2012; 59(2): 115–25.e1.

Chapter 24 **Palpitations**

Highlights

- The epidemiology of palpitations and diagnostic accuracy of history, physical exam, and ancillary testing in palpitation patients seen in the emergency setting have not been described.
- History and physical exam do not accurately distinguish clinically significant dysrhythmias as the etiology of palpitations.
- Psychiatric etiologies of palpitations are diagnoses of exclusion and frequently delay definitive diagnostic testing.
- Unless a patient's physical condition precludes it, patient-triggered event recorders are generally superior to auto-activated devices.

Background

Palpitations are the subjectively unpleasant awareness of heartbeats. In this chapter, we will review palpitations without syncope because syncope is discussed in Chapter 22. In the absence of syncope, there has been no established association between palpitations and sudden cardiac death. In fact, most individuals with cardiac dysrhythmias do not report palpitations, and only 35% of palpitation patients who present for evaluation are found to have a dysrhythmia.[1,2] Sudden cardiac death has been reported in 1.6% of patients investigated for palpitations.[1] The incidence of palpitations in emergency department (ED) populations has not been well described.

The differential diagnosis for palpitations is broad (Table 24.1).[3] Some elements of the history may provide clues as to the etiology of palpitations, allowing focused additional diagnostic testing to be obtained. Patients who present with new-onset palpitations at a younger age are likely to have developed paroxysmal supraventricular tachycardia (PSVT), while atrial fibrillation and ventricular tachycardia (VT) are more often associated with structural heart diseases that afflict aging adults.[4] The onset

Evidence-Based Emergency Care: Diagnostic Testing and Clinical Decision Rules, Second Edition.
Jesse M. Pines, Christopher R. Carpenter, Ali S. Raja and Jeremiah D. Schuur.
© 2013 John Wiley & Sons, Ltd. Published 2013 by John Wiley & Sons, Ltd.

Table 24.1 Differential diagnosis of palpitations

Dysrhythmia
   Supraventricular
      Atrial fibrillation or atrial flutter
      AV node re-entry
      Premature atrial complex
   Ventricular
      Ventricular tachycardia
      Premature ventricular complex
Sinus tachycardia
   Hyperthyroidism
   Hypovolemia
   Stimulants
   Hypoglycemia
   Pheochromocytoma
   Medications
Anxiety or panic disorder

Source: Data from [3].

of symptoms with exercise or stress (due to catecholamine surges) can implicate VT or sinus tachycardia,[5] while symptoms that occur during periods of increased vagal tone or while sleeping can be associated with atrial fibrillation or prolonged QT syndrome (an inherited abnormality of myocardial repolarization).[6,7] Medications associated with prolonged QT and subsequent torsades de pointes include antiarrhythmics, antimicrobials, antihistamines, psychotropics, diuretics, protease inhibitors, and gastrointestinal motility agents.[8,9] Inappropriate sinus tachycardia is characterized by atypical increases in sinus rates and occurs most frequently in young women during minimal exertion or with emotional stress, possibly due to a hypersensitivity to beta-adrenergic stimulation.[10]

Although anxiety and panic disorders can be associated with palpitations, these psychiatric conditions must remain diagnoses of exclusion in the ED. One investigation of 107 consecutive PSVT patients found that 67% fulfilled DSM (*Diagnostic and Statistical Manual of Mental Disorders*) criteria for panic disorder and that true dysrhythmias were misdiagnosed for a median of 3.3 years.[11] About half of patients referred for Holter monitoring will have at least one anxiety or depressive disorder if tested using DSM criteria.[12] At 6 months, 84% of palpitation patients have recurrent palpitations with significantly higher rates of psychosocial morbidity and physician visits.[13] A 10-item screening instrument has been derived to distinguish patients whose palpitations are more likely to result from panic disorder and in whom monitoring might be avoided, but this decision aid still requires validation and has not been tested in emergency medicine settings.[14]

Table 24.2 Electrocardiographic clues to palpitation etiology

ECG finding	Possible etiology
Complete heart block	PVC, VT
LVH (Q$_I$, aVL, V4-V6)	Hypertropic cardiomyopathy with VT
P-mitrale	Atrial fibrillation
Premature ventricular complexes	PVC, VT
Prolonged QT	VT
Q-waves	PVC, VT
Short PR interval, delta waves	WPW, other re-entrant tachycardia

Source: Data from [15].

Multiple diagnostic tests have been used to identify the etiology of palpitations and distinguish clinically significant sources. The initial study is generally a standard 12-lead electrocardiogram (ECG) (Table 24.2). If electrical or structural abnormalities are identified on the ECG, additional cardiac evaluation may be warranted. A Holter monitor simultaneously records two or three electrocardiographic leads and may record continuously (loop recorders) or be triggered at the time of symptoms (event recorders). Stored events on the Holter monitor can be transmitted through a telephone for physician review. Electrophysiological studies are more invasive tests of cardiac conduction that require a cardiology lab, and exercise treadmill testing may be useful if palpitations are precipitated by exercise or thought to be associated with subendocardial ischemia.[16] Echocardiography is indicated to evaluate suspected structural heart disease that may be associated with palpitations; however, identifying structural heart disease does not establish a causal relationship with palpitations.

Clinical question

What is the diagnostic accuracy of the history and physical exam in distinguishing clinically significant dysrhythmia from insignificant palpitations?
Six studies have evaluated the diagnostic accuracy of history for significant dysrhythmias.[3] The only useful clinical finding is the sensation of rapid pounding in the neck, which has a positive likelihood ratio of 177 (CI 25–1251) and a negative likelihood ratio of 0.07 (CI 0.03–0.19) for AV nodal re-entry (Table 24.3).[17]

None of these trials were conducted in ED settings. Summerton et al evaluated 139 adults patients with new-onset palpitations from 36 primary care practices in the United Kingdom over 9 months using an event recorder as the criterion standard.[18] Hoefman et al evaluated 127 consecutive patients with palpitations and lightheadedness from 41 general practice clinics in the

Table 24.3 Diagnostic accuracy of signs and symptoms to identify clinically significant dysrhythmia in palpitations

	Positive likelihood ratio (LR+)	Negative likelihood ratio (LR−)
History		
Family history palpitations	1.07	0.98
Panic disorder	1.0	1.0
Any psychiatric disorder	0.67	1.12
Description		
Continuous	0.93	1.20
Duration > 5 minutes	0.79	1.23
Duration > 1 minute	1.17	0.63
Heart rate > 100	1.08	0.86
Regular	1.38	0.55
Precipitants		
Alcohol	1.94	0.90
Breathing	0.52	1.20
Caffeine	2.06	0.89
Exercise	0.78	1.07
Holiday	0.79	1.04
Lying in bed	1.02	0.97
Resting	1.02	0.97
Sleeping	2.44	0.63
Weekend	0.72	1.08
Working	1.54	0.86
Associated symptoms		
Chest pain	0.92	1.02
Dizzy	1.34	0.67
Dyspnea	0.27	1.12
Neck fullness	0.85	1.04
Neck pounding	177	0.07
Presyncope	1.04	0.95
Vasovagal	1.72	0.63
Visible neck pulsations	2.68	0.87

Source: Data from [3].

Netherlands using a continuous event recorder as the criterion standard.[19] Barsky studied two cohorts of 131 and 145 patients who had been evaluated for palpitations using a 24-hour Holter monitor and DSM criteria as the criterion standard for dysrhythmia and psychiatric disorder, respectively.[12,20] Gürsoy assessed 244 patients referred for electrophysiology to assess AV nodal re-entry tachycardia.[17] Sakhuja evaluated 239 patients referred for electrophysiology studies, cardiac ablation, or cardioversion using a combination of the EP studies, Holter monitoring, telemetry, and ECG for the criterion standard.[21]

Clinical question

What is the diagnostic accuracy of ancillary testing (ECG, Holter, or labs) to distinguish clinically significant dysrhythmias from insignificant palpitations?
The initial diagnostic test of choice during symptomatic palpitations is a 12-lead ECG, but in primary care this is possible for only one-third of patients.[22] If an ECG is performed while palpitations are being reported, 48% have a rhythm abnormality, including 19% with clinically relevant dysrhythmia.[22] The diagnostic yield of ECG in the ED evaluation of palpitations has not been described, nor has the diagnostic accuracy of laboratory testing.

One systematic review evaluated six diagnostic devices for the evaluation of palpitations.[23]

1. Holter monitor: Records an ECG continuously for up to 72 hours with palpitations linked to the electrical rhythm via a patient diary.[24–26]
2. External event recorders without a loop (PER): Patient-activated ECG transmitted via telephone to a receiving center for interpretation.[27–30]
3. Event recorders with looping memory (CER): Continuous one-lead recording with pre- and post-event electrical rhythm saved when patients activate the device.[18,31–34]
4. Auto-triggered event monitors with looping memory (Auto-CER): Automatically recognizes prespecified brady- or tachy-dysrhythmias via continuous monitoring. Transmit ECG data to a monitor at the patient's home when triggered by prespecified criteria or patient activation. If appropriate, the rhythm is then transmitted to a monitoring center for interpretation and therapeutic intervention.
5. Implantable auto-triggered loop recorder (ILR): Same capability as 4 without the requirement of external electrodes. Generally, reserved for longer periods of monitoring (12–24 months).
6. Pacemakers and cardiac defibrillators: Can be programmed to detect, store, and send rhythm data to remote receiving facilities.

Twenty-eight studies have evaluated these diagnostic instruments, including 12 simple descriptive studies.[23] Since the descriptive studies suffer from numerous diagnostic biases (e.g., the criterion standard is the reference device, or an unequal distribution of patients with preexisting structural heart disease or device-guided interventions), the comparative studies assessing the diagnostic performance for one device against another are more informative. These comparative trials demonstrate the following:

- CER versus Holter: CER is superior at establishing a diagnosis with a range of 21–62% definitive diagnoses (vs. 30% maximum for Holter) in six studies. CER was also superior at excluding a significant dysrhythmia (34% excluded by CER vs. 2% for Holter).[35–40]

- CER versus ECG: Within 30 days, the CER is diagnostic in 37% versus 10% with only the initial ECG.[41]
- CER versus routine primary care physician gestalt: At 6 months, relevant dysrhythmias were diagnosed in 22% of CER versus 7% of patients using gestalt alone, while primary care physicians had no explanation for symptoms in 17% of CER and 38% of gestalt patients. CER did not alter referral rates or ancillary diagnostic testing, but cardiology referrals in the CER group may have been more productive since a cardiac problem was identified in 92% (vs. 57% of gestalt patients) of referrals.[42]
- Auto-CER versus PER: Both modes established a diagnosis in >80% of patients, although Auto-CER found an additional 11–17% of relevant diagnoses.[43–46]
- Auto-ILR versus patient-triggered ILR: A dysrhythmia occurred with symptoms in 16% of patient-triggered ILR. Auto-ILR had an 83% inappropriate activation rate, and no relevant dysrhythmias were detected by auto-ILR that were not detected by patient-triggered ILR.[47]
- ILR versus conventional strategy (24-hour Holter, 4-week CER, or electrophysiology testing if the first two strategies were nondiagnostic): At 1 year a dysrhythmia diagnosis was obtained in 21% via the conventional strategy and 73% with the ILR.[48]

The cost-effectiveness of outpatient CER has been reported as $98 per new diagnosis at 1 week, rising to $5,832 per new diagnosis at 3 weeks.[32] The optimal duration of PER is 2 weeks during which 75% of all diagnoses are established, including 83% of all clinically relevant diagnoses.[49]

Comment

The history and physical exam are not accurate enough to distinguish clinically significant dysrhythmias from benign etiologies in patients with palpitations. Current evidence is limited by significant selection biases and may not be representative of ED patients presenting with palpitations. In addition, the criterion standards for clinically significant or diagnostic dysrhythmias are not well accepted and suffer from incorporation bias that often includes the index test within the decision to label a rhythm as abnormal and diagnostic. Figure 24.1 provides one ED protocol to begin standardizing the diagnostic approach for palpitations based upon the available evidence. High-risk patients may require additional testing even if history, physical exam, and electrocardiogram do not delineate a clear etiology for palpitations. High-risk patients are defined as follows:[15]

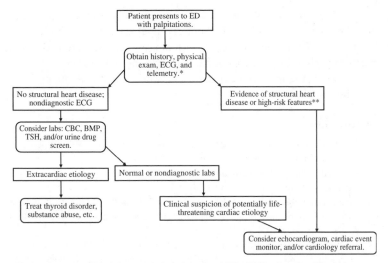

*If palpitations occur while on telemetry, obtain rhythm strip and 12-lead ECG to formulate differential diagnosis and diagnostic or therapeutic decision making.
**High-risk = Known structural heart disease or family history of dysrhythmia, sudden death, prolonged QT syndrome, or cardiomyopathy.

Figure 24.1 Evaluation of palpitations in the emergency department.

1. Abnormal heart structure including scar formation from myocardial infarction, idiopathic dilated cardiomyopathy, clinically significant valvular regurgitation or stenosis, or hypertrophic cardiomyopathy
2. Family history of dysrhythmia, syncope, cardiomyopathy, long-QT syndrome, or sudden death.

Optimally, an ECG should be obtained while palpitations are being reported. Since the ECG and the initial evaluation of patients presenting to the ED for evaluation of palpitations will usually be nondiagnostic, emergency providers will have to decide upon the role of ancillary outpatient testing in conjunction with primary care physicians. Several general considerations can aid effective decision making. The frequency of palpitations is the first factor, as daily symptoms are congruent with Holter monitoring, while weekly symptoms make an event recorder more appropriate. Another factor is patient awareness of his or her symptoms. If patients are unaware of palpitation-inducing dysrhythmias (paroxysmal atrial fibrillation) or are unable to trigger a device (due to comorbidities or age), then an auto-triggered device is more appropriate. However, patient-triggered devices have been shown to be superior in the detection of clinically significant dysrhythmias.

Future ED-based trials are needed to assess the prevalence, incidence, and short-term sequelae of palpitations without syncope. In addition, the diagnostic and prognostic properties, including the accuracy and reliability of the history, physical exam, labs, and ECG, need to be evaluated in ED patients while defining the appropriate risk strata for whom outpatient monitoring is most beneficial.

References

1. Weber BE, Kapoor WN. Evaluation and outcomes of patients with palpitations. American Journal of Medicine. 1996; 100(2): 138–48.
2. Barsky AJ. Palpitations, arrhythmias, and awareness of cardiac activity. Annals of Internal Medicine. 2001; 139(9Pt 2): 832–7.
3. Thavendiranathan P, Bagai A, Khoo C, Dorian P, Choudhry N. Does this patient with palpitations have a cardiac arrhythmia? Journal of the American Medical Association. 2009; 302(19): 2135–43.
4. Porter MJ, Morton JB, Denman R, Lin AC, Tierney S, Santucci PA et al. Influence of age and gender on the mechanism of supraventricular tachycardia. Heart Rhythm. 2004; 1(4): 393–6.
5. Lampert R, Joska T, Burg MM, Batsford WP, McPherson CA, Jain D. Emotional and physical precipitants of ventricular arrhythmia. Circulation. 2002; 106(14): 1800–5.
6. Coumel P. Clinical approach to paroxysmal atrial fibrillation. Clinical Cardiology. 1990; 13(3): 209–12.
7. Hansson A, Madsen-Härdig B, Olsson SB. Arrhythmia-provoking factors and symptoms at the onset of paroxysmal atrial fibrillation: A study based on interviews with 100 patients seeking hospital assistance. BMC Cardiovascular Disorders. 2004; 4: 13.
8. De Ponti F, Poluzzi E, Cavalli A, Recanatini M, Montanaro N. Safety of non-antiarrhythmic drugs that prolong the QT interval or induce torsade de pointes: An overview. Drug Safety. 2002; 25(4): 263–86.
9. Roden DM. Drug-induced prolongation of the QT interval. New England Journal of Medicine. 2004; 350(10): 1013–22.
10. Morillo CA, Klein GJ, Thakur RK, Li H, Zardini M, Yee R. Mechanism of "inappropriate" sinus tachycardia: Role of sympathovagal balance. Circulation. 1994; 90(2): 873–7.
11. Lessmeier TJ, Gamperling D, Johnson-Liddon V, Fromm BS, Steinman RT, Meissner MD et al. Unrecognized paroxysmal supraventricular tachycardia: Potential for misdiagnosis as panic disorder. Archives of Internal Medicine. 1997; 157(5): 537–43.
12. Barsky AJ, Cleary PD, Coeytaux RR, Ruskin JN. Psychiatric disorders in medical outpatients complaining of palpitations. Journal of General Internal Medicine. 1994; 9(6): 306–13.
13. Barsky AJ, Cleary PD, Coeytaux RR, Ruskin JN. The clinical course of palpitations in medical outpatients. Archives of Internal Medicine. 1995; 155(16): 1782–8.

14. Barsky AJ, Ahern DK, Delamater BA, Clancy SA, Bailey ED. Differential diagnosis of palpitations: Preliminary development of a screening instrument. Archives of Family Medicine. 1997; 6(3): 241–5.
15. Zimetbaum P, Josephson ME. Evaluation of patients with palpitations. New England Journal of Medicine. 1998; 338(19): 1369–73.
16. Abbott AV. Diagnostic approach to palpitations. American Family Physician. 2005; 71(4): 743–50.
17. Gürsoy S, Steurer G, Brugada J, Andries E, Brugada P. Brief report: The hemodynamic mechanism of pounding in the neck in atrioventricular nodal reentrant tachycardia. New England Journal of Medicine. 1992; 327(11): 772–4.
18. Summerton N, Mann S, Rigby A, Petkar S, Dhawan J. New-onset palpitations in general practice: Assessing the discriminant value of items within the clinical history. Family Practice. 2001; 18(4): 383–92.
19. Hoefman E, Boer KR, van Weert HCPM, Reitsma JB, Koster RW, Bindels PJE. Predictive value of history taking and physical examination in diagnosing arrhythmias in general practice. Family Practice. 2007; 24(6): 636–41.
20. Barsky AJ, Cleary PD, Sarnie MK, Ruskin JN. Panic disorder, palpitations, and the awareness of cardiac activity. Journal of Nervous and Mental Disease. 1994; 182(2): 63–70.
21. Sakhuja R, Smith LM, Tseng ZH, Badhwar N, Lee BK, Lee RJ et al. Test characteristics of neck fullness and witnessed neck pulsations in the diagnosis of typical AV nodal reentrant tachycardia. Clinical Cardiology. 2009; 32(8): E13–E8.
22. Zwietering PJ, Knottnerus JA, Rinkens PE, Kleijne MA, Gorgels AP. Arrhythmias in general practice: Diagnostic value of patient characteristics, medical history and symptoms. Family Practice. 1998; 15(4): 343–53.
23. Hoefman E, Bindels PJE, van Weert HCPM. Efficacy of diagnostic tools for detecting cardiac arrhythmias: Systematic literature search. Netherlands Heart Journal. 2010; 18(11): 543–51.
24. Eriksson L, Pahlm O. The clinical impact of long-term ECG recording: A retrospective study of 150 patients. Acta Medica Scandinavica. 1980; 208(5): 355–8.
25. Rana MZ, Dunstan EJ, Allen SC. Ambulatory electrocardiography in the elderly: An audit. British Journal of Clinical Practice. 1989; 43(9): 341–2.
26. McClennen S, Zimetbaum PJ, Ho KK, Goldberger AL. Holter monitoring: Are two days better than one? American Journal of Cardiology. 2000; 86(5): 562–4.
27. Safe AF, Maxwell RT. Transtelephonic electrocardiographic monitoring for detection and treatment of cardiac arrhythmia. Postgraduate Medical Journal. 1990; 66(772): 110–2.
28. Assayag P, Chailley O, Lehner JP, Brochet E, Demange J, Rezvani Y et al. [Contribution of sequential voluntary ambulatory monitoring in the diagnosis of arrhythmia: A multicenter study of 1287 symptomatic patients]. Archives des maladies du coeur et des vaisseaux. 1992; 85(3): 281–6. [In French]
29. Shanit D, Cheng A, Greenbaum RA. Telecardiology: Supporting the decision-making process in general practice. Journal of Telemedicine and Telecare. 1996; 2(1): 7–13.

30. Schuchert A, Behrens G, Meinertz T. [Evaluation of infrequent episodes of palpitations with a patient-activated hand-held electrocardiograph]. Zeitschrift für Kardiologie. 2002; 91(1): 62–7. [In German]

31. Brown AP, Dawkins KD, Davies JG. Detection of arrhythmias: Use of a patient-activated ambulatory electrocardiogram device with a solid-state memory loop. British Heart Journal. 1987; 58(3): 251–3.

32. Zimetbaum P, Kim KY, Josephson ME, Goldberger AL, Cohen DJ. Diagnostic yield and optimal duration of continuous-loop event monitoring for the diagnosis of palpitations: A cost-effectiveness analysis. Annals of Internal Medicine. 1998; 128(11): 890–5.

33. Fogel RI, Evans JJ, Prystowsky EN. Utility and cost of event recorders in the diagnosis of palpitations, presyncope, and syncope. American Journal of Cardiology. 1997; 79(2): 207–8.

34. Wu CC, Hsieh MH, Tai CT, Chiang CE, Yu WC, LIn YK et al. Utility of patient-activated cardiac event recorders in the detection of cardiac arrhythmias. Journal of Interventional Cardiac Electrophysiology. 2003; 8(2): 117–20.

35. Grodman RS, Capone RJ, Most AS. Arrhythmia surveillance by transtelephonic monitoring: Comparison with Holter monitoring in symptomatic ambulatory patients. American Heart Journal. 1979; 98(4): 459–64.

36. Klootwijk P, Leenders CM, Roelandt J. Usefulness of transtelephonic documentation of the electrocardiogram during sporadic symptoms suggestive of cardiac arrhythmias. International Journal of Cardiology. 1986; 13(2): 155–61.

37. Visser J, Schuilenburg RM. Trans-telephonic ECG monitoring in the diagnosis of cardiac arrhythmias: A comparison with Holter electrocardiography. Ned Tijdschrift Geneeskund. 1984; 128: 397–401.

38. Kus T, Nadeau R, Costi P, Molin F, Primeau R. Comparison of the diagnostic yield of Holter versus transtelephonic monitoring. Canadian Journal of Cardiology. 1995; 11(10): 891–4.

39. Kinlay S, Leitch JW, Neil A, Chapman BL, Hardy DB, Fletcher PJ. Cardiac event recorders yield more diagnoses and are more cost-effective than 48-hour Holter monitoring in patients with palpitations: A controlled clinical trial. Annals of Internal Medicine. 1996; 124(1Pt 1): 16–20.

40. Scalvini S, Zanelli E, Martinelli G, Baratti D, Giordano A, Glisenti F. Cardiac event recording yields more diagnoses than 24-hour Holter monitoring in patients with palpitations. Journal of Telemedicine and Telecare. 2005; 11(Suppl 1): 14–6.

41. Wu J, Kessler DK, Chakko S, Kessler KM. A cost-effectiveness strategy for transtelephonic arrhythmia monitoring. American Journal of Cardiology. 1995; 75(2): 184–5.

42. Hoefman E, van Weert HCPM, Reitsma JB, Koster RW, Bindels PJE. Diagnostic yield of patient-activated loop recorders for detecting heart rhythm abnormalities in general practice: A randomised clinical trial. Family Practice. 2005; 22(5): 478–84.

43. Roche F, Gaspoz JM, Da Costa A, Isaaz K, Duverney D, Pichot V et al. Frequent and prolonged asymptomatic episodes of paroxysmal atrial fibrillation revealed by

automatic long-term event recorders in patients with a negative 24-hour Holter. Pacing and Clinical Electrophysiology. 2002; 25(11): 1587–93.

44. Balmelli N, Naegeli B, Bertel O. Diagnostic yield of automatic and patient-triggered ambulatory cardiac event recording in the evaluation of patients with palpitations, dizziness, or syncope. Clinical Cardiology. 2003; 26(4): 173–6.

45. Martinez T, Sztajzel J. Utility of event loop recorders for the management of arrhythmias in young ambulatory patients. International Journal of Cardiology. 2004; 97(3): 495–8.

46. Reiffel JA, Schwarzberg R, Murry M. Comparison of autotriggered memory loop recorders versus standard loop recorders versus 24-hour Holter monitors for arrhythmia detection. American Journal of Cardiology. 2005; 95(9): 1055–9.

47. Ng E, Stafford PJ, Ng GA. Arrhythmia detection by patient and auto-activation in implantable loop recorders. Journal of Interventional Cardiac Electrophysiology. 2004; 10(2): 147–52.

48. Giada F, Gulizia M, Francese M, Croci F, Santangelo L, Santomauro M *et al.* Recurrent unexplained palpitations (RUP) study comparison of implantable loop recorder versus conventional diagnostic strategy. Journal ofthe American College of Cardiology. 2007; 49(19): 1951–6.

49. Hoefman E, van Weert HCPM, Boer KR, Reitsma JB, Koster RW, Bindels PJE. Optimal duration of event recording for diagnosis of arrhythmias in patients with palpitations and light-headedness in the general practice. Family Practice. 2006; 24(1): 11–3.

SECTION 4
Infectious Disease

Chapter 25 **Bacterial Meningitis in Children**

> **Highlights**
>
> - All children suspected of having meningitis should undergo a lumbar puncture.
> - The bacterial meningitis score and the Meningitest criteria are simple decision rules that discriminate bacterial meningitis from aseptic meningitis with high sensitivity in children with CSF pleocytosis.

Background

While meningitis in a child may be suspected based on history and physical exam alone, confirmation of the diagnosis requires a lumbar puncture and examination of the cerebrospinal fluid (CSF). There have been many clinical decision rules derived to differentiate children who do not require evaluation with lumbar puncture, but most were published in the pre–*Haemophilus influenzae* type B (HIB) and pneumococcal vaccine eras and have not been internally or externally validated.

Bacterial meningitis can only be ruled out when the CSF analysis is completely normal (CSF WBC count of <5 cells/µL). However, when children have CSF pleocytosis, the disease has not been completely ruled out. CSF pleocytosis is defined as a CSF white blood cell (WBC) count of ≥10 cells/µL, with a correction for the presence of CSF red blood cells (RBC) using a 1:500 ratio of leukocytes to erythrocytes. In children who undergo lumbar puncture (LP), the most common diagnosis is aseptic meningitis (more than 80–90% of cases) in industrialized countries; however, bacterial meningitis is still present in a small proportion of patients. Completely excluding bacterial meningitis requires a negative CSF culture, which is not available for 2–3 days. In order to achieve almost 100% sensitivity, most clinicians admit children

Evidence-Based Emergency Care: Diagnostic Testing and Clinical Decision Rules, Second Edition. Jesse M. Pines, Christopher R. Carpenter, Ali S. Raja and Jeremiah D. Schuur.
© 2013 John Wiley & Sons, Ltd. Published 2013 by John Wiley & Sons, Ltd.

with CSF pleocytosis while treating with broad-spectrum antibiotics and waiting for culture results. The advent of two vaccines, the *Haemophilus influenzae* type B (HIB) and the pneumococcal conjugate vaccine, has significantly reduced the incidence of bacterial meningitis in children in the United States.[1] Because the prevalence of bacterial meningitis in children with CSF pleocytosis is low, a clinical decision rule to identify children who are at very low risk for meningitis at the time of clinical presentation may limit unnecessary hospital admissions and antibiotic use in aseptic meningitis. The bacterial meningitis score (BMS) was recently validated across 20 academic medical centers in the post-HIB and post–pneumococcal vaccine era.

Clinical question

Are clinical decision rules useful in ruling out bacterial meningitis at the time of clinical presentation in children with CSF pleocytosis?

Nigrovic and colleagues developed the BMS to classify patients with CSF pleocytosis who are at very low risk of bacterial meningitis (Table 25.1).[2]

The BMS was derived from 696 children who were hospitalized with CSF pleocytosis at one center. The children ranged in age from 29 days to 19 years. The overall prevalence of bacterial meningitis was 18%. A BMS was calculated by giving two points for a positive CSF Gram stain and one point for each other variable, if present. They found that a BMS equal to 0 identified patients with aseptic meningitis with 100% accuracy and did not misclassify any child with bacterial meningitis in the validation set. The negative predictive value for a score of zero was 100% (CI 97–100%), and a BMS ≥2 predicted the presence of bacterial meningitis with a sensitivity of 87% (CI 72–96%).

The BMS was recently validated using a multicenter retrospective cohort study in 20 US academic medical centers.[3] The authors included all children between the ages of 29 days and 19 years who presented from January 2001 to June 2004 with CSF pleocytosis who had not received any antibiotics before

---

Table 25.1 The original bacterial meningitis score

Patients are at very low risk of bacterial meningitis if they *lack* all of the following criteria:
- Cerebrospinal fluid (CSF) absolute neutrophil count (ANC) of at least 1,000 cells/μL
- CSF protein of at least 80 mg/dL
- Peripheral blood ANC of at least 10,000 cells/μL
- History of seizure before or at the time of presentation

lumbar puncture. In 3,295 patients with CSF pleocytosis, 3.7% (95% CI 3.1–4.4) had bacterial meningitis and the remainder had aseptic meningitis. There were 1,714 children who were categorized as low risk by the BMS (as a score of 0). Of those, two had bacterial meningitis for a sensitivity of 98% (CI 94–100%) and an NPV of 100% (CI 100–100%). Both patients who had bacterial meningitis and had a BMS score of 0 were less than 2 months old. They concluded that the BMS is an accurate clinical decision rule that imparts a very low risk of bacterial meningitis (0.1%) in patients with none of the criteria. An external validation of the BMS has been conducted that has confirmed the sensitivity to be near 100%.[5]

However, because the BMS had a sensitivity of less than 100%, there was further study to refine the rule to include additional criteria to reach 100% sensitivity. Specifically, there was additional work to better define the laboratory cutoff values and also add the serum marker procalcitonin as an additional risk stratifier.[4] With the additional data, the BMS has been refined and named the Meningitest criteria (Table 25.2).

In an external validation of the Meningitest criteria, the sensitivity was 100% (CI 96–100%), and the specificity was 37% (CI 28–47%).[6] The authors concluded that using the rule would make it possible to safely reduce antibiotic treatments and hospitalization in 37% of children with acute meningitis.

Comment

In large multicenter studies, both the BMS and the Meningitest seem to accurately differentiate children with CSF pleocytosis with aseptic meningitis from those with bacterial meningitis with close to 100% sensitivity. Both are simple and easy-to-use scoring systems that involve routinely collected data, although the procalcitonin level required to calculate the Meningitest may not be run frequently by some laboratories. We think that both rules may be very helpful to clinicians in distinguishing children with pleocytosis who may be candidates for outpatient management because they have a very low

Table 25.2 Meningitest criteria

Antibiotic treatment and hospitalization are indicated in children with meningitis and at least one of the following criteria:
Seizure
"Toxic" appearance (irritability, lethargy, or low capillary refill)
Purpura
Positive cerebrospinal fluid (CSF) Gram staining
Procalcitonin >0.5 ng/ml
CSF protein <50 mg/dl

---

likelihood of bacterial meningitis. There have been external validations for both the BMS and the Meningitest.

There are a few considerations that must be taken into account when using either the BMS or the Meningitest to guide clinical management. Because they were both designed to identify patients at low risk for bacterial meningitis only, some patients who may benefit from antimicrobial therapy, such as those with Lyme meningitis and herpes simplex virus (HSV) encephalitis, may not be captured. We therefore recommend that use of both the BMS and Meningitest be used in conjunction with clinical assessment of the patient for other important and treatable infections. In addition, because the two cases of meningitis that were missed by the BMS in the multicenter validation study involved children under 2 months of age, we would recommend exercising caution when applying the BMS to this high-risk population of children.

References

1. Thigpen MC, Whitney CG, Messonnier NE *et al*. Bacterial meningitis in the United States, 1998–2007. New England Journal of Medicine. 2011; 364: 2016–25.
2. Nigrovic LE, Kuppermann N, Malley R. Development and validation of a multivariable predictive model to distinguish bacterial from aseptic meningitis in children in the post–*Haemophilus influenzae* era. Pediatrics 2002; 110: 712–19.
3. Nigrovic LE, Kuppermann N, Macias CG *et al*. Clinical prediction rule for identifying children with cerebrospinal fluid pleocytosis at very low risk of bacterial meningitis. Journal of the American Medical Association. 2007; 297: 52–60.
4. Dubos F, Lamotte B, Bibi-Triki F *et al*. Clinical decision rules to distinguish between bacterial and aseptic meningitis. Archives of Disease in Childhood. 2006; 91: 647–50.
5. Dubos F, Martinot A, Gendrel D *et al*. Clinical decision rules for evaluating meningitis in children. Current Opinion in Neurology. 2009; 22: 288–93.
6. Dubos F, Korczowski B, Aygun DA *et al*. Serum procalcitonin and other biologic markers to distinguish between bacterial and aseptic meningitis in children: A European multicenter case–control study. Archives of Pediatrics & Adolescent Medicine. 2008; 162: 1157–63.

Chapter 26 **Serious Bacterial Infections in Children Aged 1–3 Months**

Highlights

- The main goal of the ED evaluation of the febrile infant 1–3 months of age is to identify patients at risk for serious bacterial infection (SBI).
- Two clinical decision rules, the Philadelphia protocol and Rochester criteria, are highly sensitive and able to identify febrile infants at low risk for SBI.

Background

Children who are 0–28 days of age with fever (defined as a rectal temperature of 38.0°C or higher) have a high prevalence of a serious occult source of infection and should receive a full sepsis workup (labs, urinalysis, lumbar puncture, and blood culture) and empirical antibiotics. For children who are between 29 and 90 days, there are two clinical decision rules designed to identify children who are low risk: the Philadelphia protocol and the Rochester criteria. For children who are not low risk, the recommendations are hospitalization, a full workup, and empiric antibiotic therapy. Those deemed to be low risk can be discharged so long as they can obtain close follow-up and they have reliable parents.

Clinical question

What are the Philadelphia and Rochester criteria, and how do these clinical decision rules differentiate children 1–3 months old with serious bacterial infections (SBI)?

The derivation of the Philadelphia criteria involved a study of 747 consecutive infants who were between 29 and 56 days of age with temperatures of 38.2°C or higher.[1] A total of 460 infants had laboratory or clinical findings worrisome

Evidence-Based Emergency Care: Diagnostic Testing and Clinical Decision Rules, Second Edition. Jesse M. Pines, Christopher R. Carpenter, Ali S. Raja and Jeremiah D. Schuur.
© 2013 John Wiley & Sons, Ltd. Published 2013 by John Wiley & Sons, Ltd.

Table 26.1 The Philadelphia protocol to identify children at low risk for serious bacterial infection

Children are low risk if all criteria are met:
White blood cell (WBC) <15 K with band:neutrophil count <20%
<10 WBC on urinanalysis
<7 WBC on cerebrospinal fluid
Negative chest radiography

Source: Data from [1].

for SBI and were hospitalized and treated empirically with antibiotics. They used a screening criteria for SBI of a WBC >15,000 mm³, a spun urine specimen with more than 10 WBC per high-power field or that was positive on bright-field microscopy, a cerebrospinal fluid (CSF) with a WBC > 8mm³ or a positive CSF Gram stain, or an infiltrate on chest radiography. For the 287 infants with normal physical examination and normal labs, they were assigned to either inpatient observation without antibiotics or outpatient care with a close follow-up. A total of 65 infants (9%) had SBI, and 64 were identified using the screening criteria. The sensitivity was 98% (CI 92–100). Of the 287 who were low risk, only one had SBI. The authors termed these criteria the Philadelphia Protocol (Table 26.1).

These same authors then performed a 3-year prospective cohort study of their protocol.[2] They followed 422 infants who were between 29 and 60 days old and had a fever of >38°C. A total of 101 (24%) were identified as low risk and safe for outpatient management. They reported that, of the 43 children with SBI, none were identified as low risk by the Philadelphia protocol.

The initial derivation of the Rochester criteria involved a 2-year study of 233 infants 3 months or younger.[3] Term infants without perinatal complications or serious underlying diseases, or who had previously received antibiotics, were included. A total of 144 (62%) were considered unlikely to have a SBI, in that they did not have physical exam findings consistent with ear, soft tissue, or skeletal infections; had a WBC of 5–15,000/mm³; had less than 1,500 bands/mm³, and had a normal urinalysis. Of the 144, only one infant had a SBI (0.7%) compared to 22 (25%) in the high-risk group. No patients in the low-risk group had bacteremia compared with 9% of the high-risk group. They termed these low-risk criteria the Rochester criteria (Table 26.2).

The same authors then prospectively examined the criteria in a study published in 1988.[4] They enrolled 237 previously healthy infants 3 months and younger with fever. A total of 149 (63%) were low risk by the following criteria: no findings of soft tissue or skeletal infections, no otitis media, normal urinalysis, <25 WBC per high-power field on stool examination, and WBC

Table 26.2 The Rochester criteria to identify children younger than 2 months of age with serious bacterial infection

Infants are low risk if the following criteria are met:
Full term
Previously healthy
White blood cell (WBC) 5–15 K with less than 1,500 bands
<10 WBC on urinalysis

Source: Data from [3].

5–15,000/mm^3 with less than 1500 band cells/mm^3. No low-risk patients had SBI compared with 24% of high-risk patients and 8% had bacteremia.

A reappraisal of the Philadelphia protocol and the Rochester criteria was recently published.[5] The study involved infants 56 days and younger with a rectal temperature of greater than 38.1°C. As part of the study protocol, the physicians gave their overall impression of sepsis and scored each infant using an Infant Observation Score. They assigned 188 infants to the Philadelphia protocol and 259 to the Rochester criteria. The negative predictive value of the Philadelphia protocol was 97.1% (CI 85.1–99.8%), and the negative predictive value of the Rochester criteria was 97.3% (CI 90.5–99.2%). The authors concluded that the Philadelphia protocol and the Rochester criteria both had high negative predictive values similar to the initial derivation and validation studies.

Clinical question

How well does the Philadelphia protocol work when applied to children younger than 29 days of age?

The Philadelphia protocol was applied retrospectively to a cohort of 254 infants younger than 29 days who were admitted for evaluation of SBI.[6] The overall prevalence of SBI was 12.6%. A total of 109 (43%) infants could have been classified as low risk by the Philadelphia protocol. Five children were found to have a SBI that would have been missed by the Philadelphia protocol. The authors warned that these results demonstrate the unpredictable nature of SBI in infants younger than 29 days of age.

Comment

Any infant younger than 29 days should have a full sepsis workup including a lumbar puncture, be admitted to the hospital, and be treated with empirical antibiotics. Some centers advocate conducting risk stratification using protocols such as the Philadelphia protocol or Rochester criteria in children who are nontoxic appearing and between 29 and 90 days old. Through analyses of laboratory, urine, and/or CSF findings, can identify low-risk infants with reliable parents who can be sent home with close follow-up and without antibiotics.[7,8] However, many of the studies that used the Philadelphia and Rochester criteria are small single-center studies and have not been validated in large cohorts of children.

References

1. Baker MD, Bell LM, Avner JR. Outpatient management without antibiotics of fever in selected infants. New England Journal of Medicine. 1993; 329(20): 1437–41.
2. Baker MD, Bell LM, Avner JR. The efficacy of routine outpatient management without antibiotics of fever in selected infants. Pediatrics. 1999; 103(3): 627–31.
3. Dagan R, Powell KR, Hall CB, Menegus MA. Identification of infants unlikely to have serious bacterial infection although hospitalized for suspected sepsis. Journal of Pediatrics. 1985; 107(6): 855–60.
4. Dagan R, Sofer S, Phillip M, Shachak E. Ambulatory care of febrile infants younger than 2 months of age classified as being at low risk for having serious bacterial infections. Journal of Pediatrics. 1988; 112(3): 355–60.
5. Garra G, Cunningham SJ, Crain EF. Reappraisal of criteria used to predict serious bacterial illness in febrile infants less than 8 weeks of age. Academic Emergency Medicine. 2005; 12(10): 921–5.
6. Baker MD, Bell LM. Unpredictability of serious bacterial infections in febrile infants from birth to 1 month of age. Archives of Pediatrics & Adolescence Medicine. 1999; 153: 508–11.
7. Available from: www.cincinnatichildrens.org
8. Available from: http://pediatrics.uchicago.edu/chiefs/inpatient/documents/FebrileInfant.pdf

Chapter 27 **Necrotizing Fasciitis**

Highlights

- Necrotizing fasciitis is a rare but potentially lethal condition that requires early recognition and aggressive surgical treatment.
- The Laboratory Risk Indicator for Necrotizing Fasciitis (LRINEC) criteria use routine blood test results that can discriminate between necrotizing fasciitis and severe cellulitis or abscess. The LRINEC criteria still need to be validated in a larger trial in an external setting before widespread use can be recommended.
- In a small single-center retrospective study, CT scanning was found to be 100% sensitive with a 100% negative predictive value for necrotizing soft tissue infections, indicating that CT may be helpful in ruling out necrotizing fasciitis in the ED.

Background

Necrotizing fasciitis is a rapidly progressive infection involving the fascia and subcutaneous tissue. Differentiating necrotizing fasciitis from other skin and soft tissue infections (Figure 27.1) is important in the emergency department (ED), because while necrotizing fasciitis is a rare disease, it results in considerable morbidity and mortality. By some reports, mortality from necrotizing fasciitis can approach 34%. Necrotizing fasciitis is a surgically treated disease, and early recognition and debridement of necrotic fascia and other involved areas are major determinants of overall outcome (Figure 27.2). A delay in debridement has been associated with poorer survival.

Early on, necrotizing fasciitis can be difficult to distinguish from other forms of soft tissue infections, such as cellulitis and abscess. While computed tomography (CT), magnetic resonance imaging (MRI), and ultrasound have been shown to be useful in distinguishing necrotizing fasciitis from other clinical entities, choice of which patients to perform imaging studies on has been a source of controversy.

Evidence-Based Emergency Care: Diagnostic Testing and Clinical Decision Rules, Second Edition.
Jesse M. Pines, Christopher R. Carpenter, Ali S. Raja and Jeremiah D. Schuur.
© 2013 John Wiley & Sons, Ltd. Published 2013 by John Wiley & Sons, Ltd.

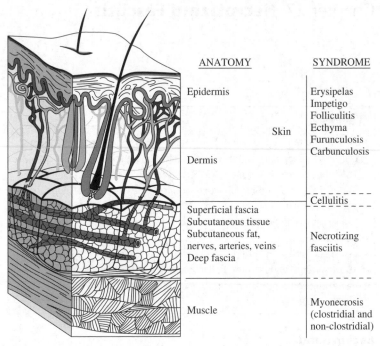

ANATOMY		SYNDROME
Epidermis		Erysipelas
		Impetigo
		Folliculitis
	Skin	Ecthyma
		Furunculosis
		Carbunculosis
Dermis		
		Cellulitis
Superficial fascia		
Subcutaneous tissue		
Subcutaneous fat,		Necrotizing
nerves, arteries, veins		fasciitis
Deep fascia		
Muscle		Myonecrosis (clostridial and non-clostridial)

Figure 27.1 Schematic of the different layers of the skin and the corresponding infections associated with each layer.

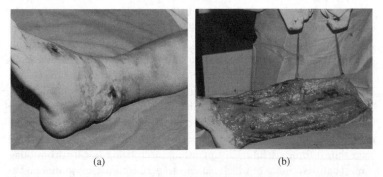

(a)   (b)

Figure 27.2 (a) A suspected case of necrotizing fasciitis. Left foot shown with oozing wound, dusky skin, and bullae formation. (b) Surgical exploration resulted in extensive debridement. (Reproduced from [5], Hall et al Principles of Critical Care 3rd edition, Copyright 2005, with permission of The McGraw-Hill Companies).

Clinical question

Can laboratory tests be reliably used in the ED to distinguish necrotizing fasciitis from other skin and soft tissue infections?

The Laboratory Risk Indicator for Necrotizing Fasciitis (LRINEC) investigators developed a scoring system to differentiate necrotizing fasciitis from other skin and soft tissue infections.[1] They derived the LRINEC scoring system in a retrospective cohort of 314 patients and validated it in 140 patients in two teaching hospitals in Singapore. They included 140 patients who had necrotizing fasciitis and 309 patients with severe cellulitis or abscesses. They found that WBC, hemoglobin, sodium, glucose, creatinine, and C-reactive protein were associated with a diagnosis of necrotizing fasciitis. They constructed the LRINEC score through conversion of the independent predictors of necrotizing fasciitis into an integer scoring system. This scoring system is detailed in Table 27.1.

Using a cutoff of 6 points or higher, there was a positive predictive value of 92% and a negative predictive value of 96%. The authors did not report sensitivities and specificities in their results section. The area under the ROC curve was 0.98 in the derivation set and 0.976 in the validation cohort, showing a high degree of accuracy in differentiating necrotizing fasciitis from cellulitis or abscess.

In 2009, a single-center retrospective study was published from Australia that aimed to externally validate the LRINEC.[2] The authors calculated the performance of a LRINEC score of ≥ 6 compared with the findings of a surgical biopsy. In 28 patients who were identified with an admission

Table 27.1 The LRINEC score to differentiate necrotizing fasciitis from severe cellulitis

Variable, units		Score
C-reactive protein, mg/L $\geq$150		4
WBC (per mm3)	15–25	1
WBC (per mm3)	>25	2
Hemoglobin	11–13.5	1
Hemoglobin	<11	2
Sodium, mmol/L	<135	2
Creatinine, mg/dL	>1.6	2
Glucose, mg/dL	<180	1

Source: A score $\geq$6 is a positive test.
WBC = white blood cell.

diagnosis of necrotizing fasciitis, 10 had biopsy-proven necrotizing fasciitis. In this small group of patients using a score ≥6, the LRINEC score had a sensitivity of 80%, a specificity of 67%, a positive predictive value of 57%, and a negative predictive value of 86% in distinguishing the patients with proven necrotizing fasciitis from those with severe soft tissue infections. The author concluded that at this cutoff level, the LRINEC score would have only minimal effect on posttest probability for having necrotizing fasciitis.

In another 2010 study in France, a LRINEC ≥6 was retrospectively applied to risk-stratify patients for the diagnosis of necrotizing fasciitis.[3] Three criteria were used: time from initiation of antibiotics to regression of erythema, duration of fever, and occurrence of complications (abscess, surgery, septic shock, necrotizing fasciitis, death, and transfer to intensive care). There were several potential predictor variables, including a LRINEC score ≥6 at admission. In 50 patients, the authors reported that the complication rate was higher for patients with a LRINEC score ≥6 (54%) than for patients with a score <6 (12%, P = 0.008). However, a LRINEC score ≥6 did not appear to be related to an increased duration of erythema or fever.

Clinical question

What are the sensitivity and specificity of CT to rule out necrotizing fasciitis?
A recent study investigated the sensitivity of CT to detect necrotizing fasciitis in a single academic medical center from January 2003 to April 2009 (all patients were scanned with either 16- or 64-section helical CT).[4] They considered a CT result positive if inflamed and necrotic tissue was detected with or without gas or fluid collections. The criterion standard for necrotizing fasciitis was a necrotizing soft tissue infection found on surgical exploration and pathological analysis, while the diagnosis was excluded if surgical exploration or pathological analysis did not find either, or if the patient improved without surgical exploration. In the 67 patients meeting inclusion criteria, 58 had a surgical exploration, and necrotizing infections were found in 25 (43% of the sample). The remainder either had non-necrotizing infections on exploration (33) or were treated non-operatively and their symptoms resolved. The authors reported that the sensitivity of CT was 100%, the specificity was 81%, the positive predictive value was 76%, and the negative predictive value was 100%. The authors concluded that a negative CT reliably excludes the diagnosis of necrotizing soft tissue infections.

Comment

The LRINEC score had good discrimination in detecting clinically early cases of necrotizing fasciitis in the derivation and validation cohorts in two academic medical centers in Singapore. However, it was not shown to be particularly helpful in the small Australian study, while it was found to be a predictor of complications in a somewhat larger French study (50 patients). Given the high specificity of the LRINEC to differentiate necrotizing fasciitis from other less severe infections, ED physicians may consider using the LRINEC scoring system or the laboratory abnormalities detailed in the scoring system along with their clinical evaluation in identifying high-risk patients in whom to obtain surgical consultation or further diagnostic studies to rule out necrotizing fasciitis. We would not recommend using the LRINEC to rule out necrotizing fasciitis.

In a single-center study, multidetector CTs were able to reliably distinguish patients who had necrotizing soft tissue infections. Although it was a small sample (67 patients), CT showed a perfect ability to rule out necrotizing fasciitis. While we believe that additional studies should be done to confirm these study findings, at this time, we recommend CT as the initial test of choice to rule out necrotizing fasciitis in the ED.

References

1. Wong CH, Khin LW, Heng KS *et al*. The LRINEC (Laboratory Risk Indicator for Necrotizing Fasciitis) score: A tool for distinguishing necrotizing fasciitis from other soft tissue infections based on routine laboratory testing. Critical Care Medicine. 2004; 32(7): 1535–41.
2. Holland MJ. Application of the Laboratory Risk Indicator in Necrotising Fasciitis (LRINEC) score to patients in a tropical tertiary referral centre. Anaesthesia and Intensive Care. 2009; 37: 588–92.
3. Corbin V, Vidal M, Beytout J *et al*. [Prognostic value of the LRINEC score (Laboratory Risk Indicator for Necrotizing Fasciitis) in soft tissue infections: A prospective study at Clermont-Ferrand University hospital]. Annales de Dermatologie et de Vénéréologie. 2010 Jan; 137(1): 5–11. [Article in French]
4. Zacharias N, Velmahos GC, Salama A *et al*. Diagnosis of necrotizing soft tissue infections by computed tomography. Archives of Surgery. 2010; 145: 452–5.
5. Hall JB, Schmidt GA, Wood L. Principles of critical care. 3rd ed. New York: McGraw-Hill Companies; 2005.

Chapter 28 **Infective Endocarditis**

Highlights

- Infective endocarditis is a challenging diagnosis in the ED.
- The Duke major criteria rely heavily on blood culture and echocardiography results.
- The Duke minor criteria provide risk factors that emergency physicians can use to stratify a patient's risk of endocarditis.
- Transesophageal echocardiography is currently the best method of evaluation for endocarditis because it is more sensitive in both native and prosthetic heart valves.

Background

Infective endocarditis is a microbial infection of the endocardial surface of the heart and has an incidence of between 1.8 and 7.0 per 100,000 patients per year. It is challenging to diagnose, primarily because of the presence of nonspecific clinical features at emergency department (ED) presentation. Because a missed diagnosis of endocarditis can lead to poor outcomes, emergency physicians must have a low threshold for the consideration of this potentially lethal disease. Fever is the most common symptom of endocarditis, leading some sources to state that relapsing fevers for a week or more should prompt consideration of the diagnosis. The second most common clinical feature is the presence of a murmur or other evidence of valvular heart disease. Other common signs include splenomegaly, microscopic hematuria, anemia, and leukocytosis.

Over the past 30 years, a shift in the epidemiology of endocarditis has decreased the prevalence of common classic cutaneous and ophthalmologic manifestations of endocarditis, including Osler's nodes, Roth's spots, Janeway lesions (Figure 28.1), splinter hemorrhages, and oral petichiae.[1] These

---

Evidence-Based Emergency Care: Diagnostic Testing and Clinical Decision Rules, Second Edition.
Jesse M. Pines, Christopher R. Carpenter, Ali S. Raja and Jeremiah D. Schuur.
© 2013 John Wiley & Sons, Ltd. Published 2013 by John Wiley & Sons, Ltd.

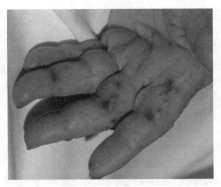

Figure 28.1 Janeway lesions from bacterial endocarditis. (Reproduced from [9], Fitzpatrick T, Johnson RA, Wolff K, and Suurmond D . Color Atlas and Synopsis of Clinical Dermatology 4th Edition ©2001 with permission of The McGraw-Hill Companies).

changes are primarily attributable to the increase in incidence of endocarditis in prosthetic valve recipients, intravenous drug users (IVDU), and geriatric patients.[2] There has also been a shift in the microbiology of endocarditis from primarily streptococcal species to coagulase-positive and coagulase-negative staphylococcus. This has led to a change in the classic presentation of infective endocarditis, where most commonly a patient with IVDU may present acutely with right-sided valvular infection caused by *Staphylococcus aureus* and without the classic peripheral stigmata of endocarditis listed in this section.

Clinical question

What is the most accurate method to diagnose suspected infective endocarditis in the ED?

The best criteria for the diagnosis of endocarditis are the Duke criteria, which were initially suggested in 1994 by Dureck et al.[3] The Duke criteria were derived using 405 consecutive cases of suspected infective endocarditis in 353 patients between 1985 and 1992. The authors defined two "major criteria" (positive blood culture and positive echocardiogram; Figure 28.2) and six "minor criteria" (predisposition, fever, vascular phenomena, immunologic phenomena, suggestive echocardiogram, and suggestive microbiologic findings). They also defined three distinct diagnostic categories: *definite* by pathologic or clinical criteria, *possible*, and *rejected*. A definite case was defined as direct evidence of infectious endocarditis based on histology or bacteriology of a vegetation or peripheral embolus. There were a total of 69 pathologically confirmed cases of definite endocarditis; 55 (80%)

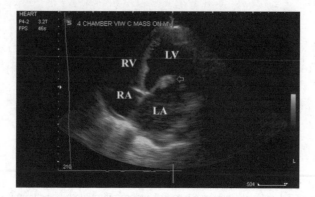

Figure 28.2 Apical four-chamber view demonstrating a large mitral valve vegetation (*arrow*). (Courtesy of Anthony J. Dean, MD Pennsylvania).
Note: RA = right atrium; LA = left atrium; LV = left ventricle; and RV = right ventricle.

pathologically confirmed cases were classified as clinically definite endocarditis. Table 28.1 provides a list of the Duke criteria.

Other studies have investigated how well the Duke criteria work in excluding a diagnosis of infective endocarditis. Dodd et al investigated the long-term follow-up of 49 episodes of suspected endocarditis in which the diagnosis of endocarditis was rejected by the Duke criteria.[4] Of those, 63% had a firm alternative diagnosis established at the time of initial evaluation. Thirty-five percent had syndromes that resolved spontaneously following 4 or fewer days of antibiotics, and one patient had endocarditis ruled out at the time of heart surgery. There was follow-up information on all patients at 3 months post hospitalization, and only one patient eventually had a diagnosis of prosthetic-valve endocarditis, with another who died and had a diagnosis of possible endocarditis on autopsy.

The Duke criteria have also been applied to a group of 100 patients with fever of unknown origin who had multiple blood cultures and underwent echocardiography, in order to calculate the specificity of the criteria.[5] Similar to the Dodd study, 65% had an alternative diagnosis and 35% had a clinical syndrome that resolved after either short-term or no antibiotic therapy. There was only one patient who was misclassified as negative by the Duke criteria, making the criteria 99% specific.

Recent proposals have advocated revisions of the Duke criteria, including the elimination of the minor criterion *echocardiogram consistent with infective endocarditis* (given the use of transesophageal echocardiography as a more definitive test) and the addition of new minor criteria, such as splenomegaly and an elevated C-reactive protein (CRP) of >100 mg/L.[6]

Table 28.1 The Duke criteria for infective endocarditis

Definite infective endocarditis
Pathologic criteria
- Microorganisms: demonstrated by culture or histology in a vegetation, in a vegetation that has embolized, or in an intracardiac abscess; or
- Pathologic lesions: vegetation or intracardiac abscess present, confirmed by histology showing active endocarditis.

Clinical criteria
- 2 major criteria, 1 major and 3 minor criteria, or 5 minor criteria (defined in this table)

Possible infective endocarditis
- Findings of endocarditis that fall short of definite, but not rejected

Rejected (i.e., not endocarditis)
- Firm alternate diagnosis explaining evidence of infective endocarditis; or
- Resolution of endocarditis syndrome, with antibiotic therapy for 4 days or less; or
- No pathologic evidence of infective endocarditis at surgery or autopsy, after antibiotic therapy of 4 days or less.

Major criteria
Positive blood culture for infectious endocarditis
- Typical microorganism for infective endocarditis from 2 separate blood cultures.
- Viridans streptococci, *Streptococcus bovis*, HACEK group; or
- Community-acquired *Streptococcus aureus* or enterococci, in the absence of a primary focus or
- Persistently positive blood culture, defined as recovery of a microorganism consistent with infective endocarditis from.
- Blood cultures drawn more than 12 hours apart; or
- All or 3, or majority of 4 or more separate blood cultures, with first and last drawn at least 1 hour apart.

Evidence of endocardial involvement on echocardiogram
- Oscillating intracardiac mass, on valve or supporting structures, or in the path of regurgitant jets, or on implanted material, in the absence of an alternative anatomic explanation; or
- Abscess; or
- New partial dehiscence of a prosthetic valve; or
- New valvular regurgitation (increase or change in preexisting murmur not sufficient).

Minor criteria
- Predisposition: predisposing heart condition or intravenous drug use
- Fever $\geq$38.0°C (100.4°F)
- Vascular phenomena: major arterial emboli, septic pulmonary infarcts, mycotic aneurysm, intracranial hemorrhage, conjunctival hemorrhages, Janeway lesions
- Immunologic phenomenon: glomerulonephritis, Osler's nodes, Roth's spots, rheumatoid factor
- Echocardiogram consistent with infective endocarditis but not meeting major criteria above
- Microbiological evidence: positive blood culture but not meeting major criteria.

Note: HACEK = grouping of Gram-negative bacilli; *Haemophilus* species (*H. parainfluenzae, H. aphrophilus,* and *H. paraphrophilus*), *Actinobacillus actinomycetemcomitans, Cardiobacterium hominis, Eikenella corrodens,* and *Kingella* species.

In addition, other adjunctive tests, including procalcitonin levels, have been suggested as potential aids for the diagnosis of infective endocarditis. Mueller et al performed a prospective cohort study in 67 patients admitted with the suspicion of infective endocarditis and inpatients with suspected endocarditis.[7] Infective endocarditis was diagnosed by the Duke criteria and confirmed in 21 patients. Procalcitonin levels were higher in patients with endocarditis (median 6.56 ng/mL) than in those without endocarditis (median 0.44 ng/mL, P < 0.001). The optimal concentration of procalcitonin to calculate positive and negative predictive values was 2.3 ng/mL. With this cutoff, test characteristics of procalcitonin were: sensitivity 81%, specificity 85%, negative predictive value 92%, and positive predictive value 72%.

The choice of echocardiographic imaging technique has also shifted, with the transesophageal (TEE) approach replacing the transthoracic (TTE) approach. Since the TEE allows closer proximity to the heart, there is an improved ability to visualize smaller structures, including small vegetations, leaflet perforations, and small (<5 mm) abscesses. TEE is currently the superior method of evaluation for endocarditis as it is more sensitive in both native and prosthetic heart valves.

Comment

In the context of the diagnosis of endocarditis in the ED, the major microbiological Duke criteria cannot be met on initial evaluation unless blood cultures are drawn in advance. Echocardiogram, specifically TEE, is the currently recommended test to rule out endocarditis, particularly for patients with suspected complicated infective endocarditis and patients with suspected prosthetic valve endocarditis.[8] However, a TEE is technically challenging in the ED because it requires sedation. Echocardiograms are also not a commonly ordered ED test unless patients are unstable or the emergent echocardiogram will alter ED management. Even in emergency cases, some hospital EDs may have limited access to echocardiography.

However, an emergency echocardiogram can change ED management of a patient, particularly in the presence of an intracardiac abscess. The most common life-threatening complication of infective endocarditis is congestive heart failure, with the most common cause being infection-induced valvular damage. Because heart failure is a common ED presentation, infective endocarditis should be considered in patients with new murmurs and acute congestive heart failure in the appropriate clinical setting (e.g., other risk factors such as IVDU).

In lieu of TEE, procalcitonin levels (if available) may be helpful in diagnosing endocarditis in the ED. If procalcitonin testing is not available, C-reactive protein levels, while relatively nonspecific, may be easier to order on an emergent basis.

The Duke minor criteria provide risk factors by which an emergency physician may stratify a patient's risk of endocarditis. The presence of a predisposing heart condition such as rheumatic heart disease, valvular heart disease or other abnormalities, or IVDU should raise suspicion for endocarditis in the context of a fever or other symptoms of infection. Other risk factors include indwelling catheters, long-term hemodialysis, and the presence of a previously undocumented heart murmur. Vascular phenomena and immunologic phenomena should be evaluated on physical examination in these patients as these are minor criteria; however, given the change in the microbiology and epidemiology of endocarditis over the past 30 years, these types of lesions are less frequently seen. Consideration should also be given to include the presence of leukocytosis, microscopic hematuria, and anemia in the evaluation of suspected endocarditis, as these are commonly ordered tests and may be present in endocarditis.

Blood cultures remain the most important laboratory test in patients with suspected endocarditis. In addition to their diagnostic utility, blood cultures provide antibiotic susceptibility results that guide long-term treatment, which has resulted in the current recommendation to draw three sets of blood cultures in these patients.

References

1. Bayer AS. Diagnosis and management of infectious endocarditis. Cardiology Clinics. 1996; 345–51.
2. Bayer AS. Infectious endocarditis: State-of-the-art. Clinical Infections Diseases. 1993; 17: 313–22.
3. Dureck DT, Lukes AS, Bright DK. New criteria for diagnosis of infective endocarditis: Utilization of specific echocardiographic findings. Duke Endocarditis Service. American Journal of Medicine. 1994; 96(3): 200–9.
4. Dodds GA III, Sexton DJ, Durack DT *et al.* and the Duke Endocarditis Service. Negative predictive value of the Duke criteria for infective endocarditis. American Journal of Cardiology. 1996; 77: 403–7.
5. Hoen B, Beguinot I, Maignan M *et al.* The Duke criteria for the diagnosis of infective ednocarditis are specific: An analysis of 100 patients with acute fever or fever of unknown origin. Clinical Infections Diseases. 1996; 23(2): 298–302.
6. Li JS, Sexton DJ, Mick N, et al. Proposed Modifications to the Duke Criteria for the Diagnosis of Infective Endocarditis. Clin Inf Dis. 2000; 3(4): 633–638.
7. Mueller C, Huber P, Laifer G *et al.* Procalcitonin and the early diagnosis of endocarditis. Circulation 2004; 109: 1707–10.
8. Horstkotte D, Follath F, Gutschik E *et al.* Guidelines on prevention, diagnosis and treatment of infective endocarditis – executive summary. European Heart Journal. 2004; 25: 267–76.
9. Fitzpatrick T, Johnson RA, Wolff K, and Suurmond D. Color Atlas and Synopsis of Clinical Dermatology: McGraw-Hill Companies; 2001.

Chapter 29 **Pharyngitis**

> **Highlights**
>
> - Differentiating bacterial pharyngitis (group A streptococci) from other causes of sore throat can be challenging.
> - The Centor criteria with the McIssac classification can predict the probability of GAS infection based on clinical criteria.
> - Patients with intermediate scores may benefit from confirmatory rapid strep testing or cultures before starting therapy to avoid overtreatment of viral infections.

Background

The complaint of sore throat is common in emergency medicine. In 2006, there were more than 650,000 visits to US emergency departments (EDs) for acute pharyngitis.[1] The most common bacterial cause for sore throat is group A streptococci (GAS). The value of using antibiotics has been debated in this disease because it usually resolves spontaneously without complications. In fact, in adults without a previous history of rheumatic heart disease the number needed to treat to prevent one case of rheumatic heart disease is 3 million.[2] However, antibiotics are recommended for patients in cases where there is a high likelihood of, or culture-confirmed, streptococcal infection in the throat.[3]

The reasons to treat patients with antibiotics are to prevent complications, reduce symptoms, and prevent transmission of the disease to others. A Cochrane review found that at 3 days, antibiotics reduced symptoms of sore throat, headache, and fever.[4] Complications following GAS pharyngitis include suppurative (acute otitis media and acute sinusitis) and nonsuppurative complications (acute glomerulonephritis and acute rheumatic fever). In general, antibiotics tend to reduce the incidence of suppurative complications considerably, by about one-quarter in acute otitis media and by about

Evidence-Based Emergency Care: Diagnostic Testing and Clinical Decision Rules, Second Edition.
Jesse M. Pines, Christopher R. Carpenter, Ali S. Raja and Jeremiah D. Schuur.
© 2013 John Wiley & Sons, Ltd. Published 2013 by John Wiley & Sons, Ltd.

one-half in acute sinusitis. Antibiotics reduce the likelihood of rheumatic fever by about one-third.

There is no standardized diagnostic testing guideline for which ED patients with sore throat require antibiotics. However, clinical decision rules such as the Centor criteria can be very helpful in risk-stratifying patients who require testing and treatment. In fact, according to the American Academy of Family Practice, the statement, "Use of clinical decision rules for diagnosing GABHS pharyngitis improves quality of care while reducing unwarranted treatment and overall cost" was given an evidence grade A.[5] However, many guidelines base their strategy on a clinical scoring system to not treat, further test (with either rapid strep testing or throat culture), or empirically treat pharyngitis with antibiotics.

Clinical question

Which physical examination findings significantly alter the likelihood of a positive GAS culture in patients with sore throat?

A diagnostic systematic review compiled data and calculated likelihood ratios (LR+ and LR−) for clinical findings and the chance of a positive GAS culture.[6] All data are reported here with either the 95% CI or the ranges provided by the studies. The most predictive elements included pharyngeal exudates LR+ 2.1(CI 1.4−3.1), LR− 0.90 (CI 0.75−1.1); tonsillar swelling or enlargement LR+ 1.8 (CI 1.5−2.3), LR− 0.63 (CI 0.56−0.72); tender anterior cervical nodes LR+ 1.2−1.9, LR− 0.60 (CI 0.49−0.71); tonsillar exudates LR+ 3.4 (1.8−6.0), LR− 0.72 (0.60−0.88); no cough LR+ 1.1−1.7, LR− 0.53−0.89; and strep exposure within the previous 2 weeks, LR+ 1.9 (1.3−2.8), LR− 0.92 (0.86−0.99). Notably, no single clinical finding showed a sufficient accuracy to discriminate through its presence or absence between GAS-positive and GAS-negative patients with sore throat.

Clinical question

What are the clinical prediction rules for GAS pharyngitis, and how can they guide therapy for ED patients with sore throat?

The Centor criteria is a prediction rule based on selected signs and symptoms in patients with pharyngitis and can identify patients at low risk for GAS pharyngitis.[7] The Centor criteria include (i) history of fever, (ii) anterior cervical adenopathy, (iii) tonsillar exudates, and (iv) absence of cough. Using a positive culture for GAS as a criterion standard, in the initial derivation study of the Centor criteria, probabilities assigned to each score include: a 56% probability of positive culture in patients with four criteria, a 32%

Table 29.1 The Centor Strep Score with the McIssac modification, likelihood ratio (LR), and probability of strep infection

Points	Likelihood ratio	Probability of infection
−1 or 0	0.05	1%
1	0.52	10%
2	0.95	17%
3	2.5	35%
4 or 5	4.9	51%

Source: Data from [5].

probability with three criteria, a 15% probability with two, 6.5% with one, and 2.5% with zero.[8] Since the probability of a strep infection is higher in children than adults, McIssac et al suggested an age-based revision to the Centor criteria.[9] In the McIssac revision to the Centor criteria, patients who are <5 years old receive an additional point, whereas if they are >45 years old they have a point subtracted. Using the McIssac modification, the risk of streptococcal infection is listed in Table 29.1.

Comment

Specific signs and symptoms can increase or reduce the likelihood of patients with sore throat having positive throat cultures for GAS. The Centor criteria with the McIssac modification have been validated in both adults and children for use in predicting the probability of GAS pharyngitis.[9] Using these criteria will guide effective testing and antimicrobial treatment decisions in the ED.

There is, however, considerable controversy over how these rules should be applied in clinical practice. Multiple management strategies have been suggested. Using two separate criteria as an example, the Infectious Disease Society of America (IDSA) and the American College of Physicians–American Society of Internal Medicine (ACP-ASIM) have proposed different management strategies for adults with pharyngitis (see Table 29.2).[10]

The clinical balancing act centers on overtreatment (which may result in inappropriate use of antibiotics for cases that are not GAS) versus undertreatment, which may result in missed cases and potentially lead to complications such as longer times to clinical improvement and higher rates of both suppurative and nonsuppurative complications of GAS.[4] Given that the prevalence of GAS is higher among children as compared to adults, a more liberal approach to testing makes more sense to conform with IDSA

Table 29.2 Adult pharyngitis guidelines for diagnostic testing and treatment with antibiotics (abx) based on the Centor Score

Centor Score		IDSA	ACP-ASIM
0	Test	No	No
	Treat	No	No
1	Test	No	No
	Treat	No	No
2	Test	Rapid strep	Rapid strep
	Treat	Abx if rapid strep +	Abx if rapid strep +
3	Test	Rapid strep	No test/rapid strep
	Treat	Abx if rapid strep +	Empirical abx/abx if strep +
4	Test	Rapid strep	No test
	Treat	Abx if rapid strep +	Empiric abx

Note: IDSA = Infectious Disease Society of America; and ACP-ASIM = American College of Physicians–American Society of Internal Medicine. Reproduced from [10] Centor R, Allison JJ, Cohen SJ. Pharyngitis Management: Defining the Controvery. J Gen Intern Med 2007; 22: 127–130 With kind permission from Springer Science and Business Media.

guidelines. However, rapid strep tests have different test sensitivities at different Centor scores (likelihoods of GAS pharyngitis).[11] According to this study, the Centor score corresponded to the following probabilities of the rapid strep test being positive: Centor 0 or 1: 61%; Centor 2: 76%; Centor 3: 90%; and Centor 4: 97%. Given that rapid strep testing is not 100% sensitive, the recommendation of the American Academy of Pediatrics (AAP) is to culture all negative rapid strep tests.[12]

References

1. Pitts SR, Niska RW, Xu J, Burt CW. National Hospital Ambulatory Medical Care Survey: 2006 Emergency department summary. National Health Statistics Reports. 2008; 7: 1–38.

2. Newman D. Hippocrates' shadow. New York: Simon & Schuster; 2009.

3. Infectious Diseases Society of America (IDSA). Practice guidelines for the diagnosis and management of group A streptococcal pharyngitis. Clinical Infectious Diseases. 2002; 35: 113–25.

4. Spinks A, Glasziou PP, Del Mar CB. Antibiotics for sore throat (Cochrane Methodology Review). In: The Cochrane Library, Issue 9. Chichester, UK: John Wiley & Sons, Ltd, 2011.

5. Choby BA. Diagnosis and treatment of streptococcal pharyngitis. American Family Physician. 2009; 79: 383–90.

6. Ebell MH, Smith MA, Barry HC *et al*. The rational clinical examination: Does this patient have strep throat? Journal of the American Medical Association. 2000; 284: 2912–18.

7. Centor R, Witherspoon J, Dalton H, Brody C, Link K. The diagnosis of strep throat in adults in the emergency room. Medical Decision Making. 1981; 1(3): 239–46.

8. McIsaac WJ, Goel V, To T *et al*. The validity of a sore throat score in family practice. Canadian Medical Association Journal. 2000; 168: 811–15.

9. McIsaac WJ, Kellner JD, Aufricht P, Vanjaka A, Low DE. Empirical validation of guidelines for the management of pharyngitis in children and adults. Journal of the American Medical Association. 2004; 291: 1587–95.

10. Centor R, Allison JJ, Cohen SJ. Pharyngitis management: Defining the controversy. Journal of General Internal Medicine. 2007; 22: 127–30.

11. DiMatteo LA, Lowenstein SR, Brimhall B *et al*. The relationship between the clinical features of pharyngitis and the sensitivity of a rapid antigen test: Evidence of spectrum bias. Annals of Emergency Medicine. 2001; 38: 648–52.

12. American Academy of Pediatrics. Red book: 2003 report of the Committee on Infectious Diseases. 26th ed. Elk Grove Village (IL): American Academy of Pediatrics; 2003: 576–8.

Chapter 30 **Rhinosinusitis**

Highlights

- The vast majority of patients with symptoms of nasal and sinus congestion in the ED have viral infections.
- Certain clinical symptoms and signs are suggestive of acute bacterial rhinosinusitis including a "double sickening," length of symptoms >10 days, unilateral facial pain, mucopurulent nasal discharge, unilateral maxillary tenderness, and maxillary toothache.
- The criterion standard for the diagnosis of bacterial rhinosinusitis is sinus puncture, which is not practical in the ED.
- Sinus imaging has been used as a criterion standard in some studies, but sinus imaging is not currently recommended in the ED unless invasive disease is suspected.

Background

The complaint of nasal and sinus congestion is very common in emergency care. The majority of patients with these complaints have viral infections, while a small subset will have acute bacterial rhinosinusitis – requiring treatment with antibiotics. Acute bacterial rhinosinusitis is typically preceded by a viral upper respiratory tract infection and, less commonly, allergic rhinitis. Approximately 0.5–2.0% of adult cases of acute viral upper respiratory tract infections will be complicated by acute bacterial rhinosinusitis, while in children the proportion is considerably higher: 6–13%. Therefore, differentiating patients who present with symptoms of sinus inflammation caused by viral or allergic causes compared with bacterial causes is a clinical challenge for emergency and primary care physicians. The criterion standard diagnosis for acute bacterial rhinosinusitis is sinus puncture and culture, both of which are impractical in the emergency department (ED) setting. Sinus imaging has

Evidence-Based Emergency Care: Diagnostic Testing and Clinical Decision Rules, Second Edition. Jesse M. Pines, Christopher R. Carpenter, Ali S. Raja and Jeremiah D. Schuur.
© 2013 John Wiley & Sons, Ltd. Published 2013 by John Wiley & Sons, Ltd.

been used in some studies as a criterion standard. However, imaging is not 100% accurate. In many cases, sinus imaging is interpreted to show bacterial disease, but if cultured the sinusitis is of viral etiology. Sinus imaging is not currently recommended for patients unless more invasive (i.e., orbital) disease is suspected.

Clinical question

Which clinical features are associated with acute bacterial rhinosinusitis in ambulatory ED patients?

Given the limitations of imaging and cultures, the diagnosis of acute bacterial sinusitis and the treatment with antibiotics are often made on clinical grounds based on the history and physical examination. A strong factor in distinguishing patients with acute bacterial rhinosinusitis is duration of symptoms. One trial studied the natural course of rhinosinusitis and found that 60% of patients whose symptoms persisted for 10 days or longer had a positive bacterial culture from a sinus aspirate. On that basis, consensus groups have recommended different time intervals for making a diagnosis of acute bacterial rhinosinusitis and subsequently treating with antibiotics. Some groups recommend 7 days of symptoms as an appropriate time at which to use antibiotics; others have recommended antibiotics should be withheld for up to 10 days in children. This recommendation was based on a study of 2,013 children that found that of those screened at 10 days with Waters view radiography, 92% had a confirmed radiographic diagnosis of rhinosinusitis.[1] Others recommend treatment based on a worsening clinical status after 5–6 days, regardless of overall duration of illness.[2]

Studies on the signs and symptoms of rhinosinusitis are limited by the choice of a criterion standard. No studies have used a criterion standard as reliable as bacterial growth of 10^5 CFU/mL or greater from a sinus aspirate. Studies have varied considerably in their use of a criterion standard from purulent sinus aspirates to sinus radiography. One early study (from 1988) evaluated 155 patients with acute sinusitis and found that predominantly unilateral purulent nasal discharge, unilateral facial pain, physical examination findings of purulent nasal discharge, and pus in the nasal cavity were highly associated with positive radiography for rhinosinusitis. They calculated a sensitivity of 81% and a specificity of 88% in patients with three or four of these signs or symptoms.[3]

A study of 247 men in the Veterans Administration system with rhinorrhea, facial pain, or self-suspected sinusitis used plain radiography as the criterion standard and found five independent predictors of rhinosinusitis: (i) maxillary toothache (OR 2.9), (ii) lack of transillumination (OR 2.7), (iii) poor response to nasal decongestants or antihistamines (OR 2.4), (iv) report of colored nasal discharge (OR 2.2), and (v) purulent mucus found on physical examination (OR 2.9).[4]

Another study of 201 patients with clinically diagnosed acute rhinosinusitis used CT findings as the criterion standard.[5] More than half met the CT criteria for acute bacterial rhinosinusitis (an air-fluid level or total opacification of any sinus). Four signs or symptoms were independently (and significantly) associated with a CT diagnosis of bacterial rhinosinusitis: (i) purulent secretion from the nose, (ii) purulent rhinorrhea, (iii) "double sickening" (defined as a presence of two phases of illness history), and (iv) an erythrocyte sedimentation rate of > 10 mm. The presence of three or more of these yielded a sensitivity of 66% and a specificity of 81%. The authors felt that "double sickening," which had an OR of 2.8, was particularly relevant given the association with the natural history of a viral upper respiratory infection followed by a secondary bacterial infection. CT-confirmed rhinosinusitis was present in only 20% with symptoms of less than 7 days' duration.

A more recent study used three separate criterion standards in 174 adult patients with suspected rhinosinusitis: CT, sinus aspiration, and culture.[6] Of the 70% with abnormal CT findings, only half met the diagnostic criteria for acute bacterial rhinosinusitis (i.e., the presence of purulent or mucopurulent sinus aspirate). Signs and symptoms associated with a positive culture included unilateral facial pain (OR 1.9), maxillary toothache (OR 1.9), unilateral maxillary tenderness (OR 2.5), and mucopurulent nasal discharge (OR 1.6) (Figure 30.1).

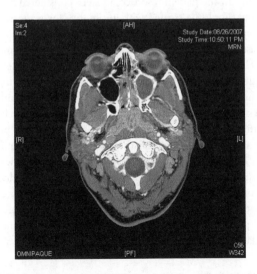

Figure 30.1 Computed tomography (CT) showing left maxillary sinusitis.

Taken together, these results suggest that acute bacterial rhinosinusitis may be characterized by the clinical signs and symptoms of (i) unilateral facial pain, (ii) mucopurulent nasal discharge, (iii) unilateral maxillary tenderness, and (iv) maxillary toothache. No single clinical finding is sensitive and specific to diagnose acute bacterial rhinosinusitis. In 2000, the Task Force on Rhinosinusitis of the American Academy of Otolaryngology – Head and Neck Surgery has provided guidance by stratifying specific diagnostic factors into major and minor categories.[7] They stratified the diagnosis of acute bacterial rhinosinusitis on the basis of at least two major factors (facial pain or pressure, facial congestion or fullness, nasal obstruction, nasal purulence or discolored postnasal discharge, hyposmia or anosmia, or fever) or one major and two minor factors (headache, halitosis, fatigue, dental pain, cough, ear pain, pressure, fullness, or fever). The validity of this classification system is based not on culture results of sinus aspirates but on sinus imaging, which is not a validated criterion standard.

Comment

The diagnosis of acute bacterial rhinosinusitis in the ED setting is a challenge due to the absence of an empirically validated decision rule to identify which patients to treat with antibiotics. As most patients (>90%) have a viral cause of their sinus symptoms, clinicians should not routinely prescribe antibiotics to all patients with rhinosinusitis. Clinical signs and symptoms, duration of illness, and patient resources must be considered in determining which patients should be treated with antibiotics for acute rhinosinusitis. Guidelines regarding treatment of acute bacterial rhinosinusitis have been primarily based on the literature discussed in this chapter and on expert consensus. However, in comparison to the primary care setting, in the ED, we frequently cannot rely on patient follow-up as part of the diagnostic algorithm, and have to make a decision about whether to treat with antibiotics on the first visit. We recommend the following strategy. Obtain imaging only in cases with suspected invasive disease. In well-appearing patients with low clinical suspicion for bacterial rhinosinusitis, recommend outpatient follow-up in 7 days. In patients with equivocal findings or in whom follow-up is not assured, write a prescription for patients with clinical signs and symptoms suspicious for rhinosinusitis with explicit recommendations to fill the prescription if symptoms do not remit within 7 days. Finally, we recommend prescribing antibiotics for patients with signs and symptoms highly associated with bacterial rhinosinusitis.

References

1. Ueda D, Yoto Y. The ten-day mark as a practical diagnostic approach for acute paranasal sinusitis in children. Pediatric Infectious Disease Journal. 1996; 15: 576–9.
2. Scheid DC, Hamm RM. Acute bacterial rhinosinusitis in adults: Part II. Treatment. American Family Physician. 2004; 70: 1697–704.
3. Berg O, Carenfelt C. Analysis of symptoms and clinical signs in the maxillary sinus empyema. Acta Oto-Laryngologica. 1988; 105: 343–9.
4. Williams JW Jr, Simel DL, Roberts L *et al*. Clinical evaluation for sinusitis: Making the diagnosis by history and physical examination. Annals of Internal Medicine. 1992; 117: 705–10.
5. Lindbaek M, Hjortdahl P, Johnsen UL. Use of symptoms, signs, and blood tests to diagnose acute sinus infections in primary care: Comparison with computed tomography. Family Medicine. 1996; 28: 183–8.
6. Hansen JG, Schmidt H, Rosborg J *et al*. Predicting acute maxillary sinusitis in a general practice population. British Medical Journal. 1995; 311: 233–6.
7. Brooks I, Gooch WM III, Jenkins SG *et al*. Medical management of acute bacterial sinusitis: Recommendations of a clinical advisory committee on pediatric and adult sinusitis. Annals of Otology, Rhinology and Laryngology. 2000; 182(Suppl): 2–20.

Chapter 31 **Pneumonia**

Highlights

- The presence or absence of several elements of the history, physical examination, and laboratory testing can raise or lower the likelihood of a radiographic diagnosis of pneumonia.
- The Pneumonia Severity Index accurately determines which patients are at low risk for 30-day mortality.
- The CURB-65 rule accurately stratifies patients at high risk for 30-day mortality.
- Risk stratification tools can improve clinical decision making and help identify a group of patients who can be safely managed as outpatients.

Background

Community-acquired pneumonia (CAP) is an acute infection of the lung's parenchyma accompanied by symptoms of acute illness (Figure 31.1). There are several challenges in the ED evaluation of patients with CAP. The question whether a patient has pneumonia informs whether patients should be treated with antimicrobials, and several elements of the history and physical examination may increase or decrease the likelihood of having CAP. In addition, illness severity in CAP often guides decisions about admission, further diagnostic testing in the ED, and the choice of antibiotics. Several scoring systems have been developed to aid in ED decision making regarding patients with CAP.

Probably the most widely used scoring system is the Pneumonia Severity Index (PSI) which was developed by Fine et al.[1] Table 31.1 details the elements of the PSI and its association with risk of death at 30 days. The primary purpose of the PSI was to identify patients who were at low-risk

---

Evidence-Based Emergency Care: Diagnostic Testing and Clinical Decision Rules, Second Edition. Jesse M. Pines, Christopher R. Carpenter, Ali S. Raja and Jeremiah D. Schuur.
© 2013 John Wiley & Sons, Ltd. Published 2013 by John Wiley & Sons, Ltd.

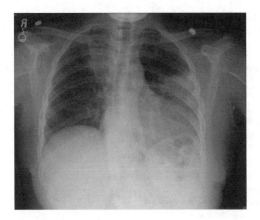

Figure 31.1 Left lower lobe pneumonia.

for mortality and could be managed on an outpatient basis (i.e., at home). The authors have suggested that groups I, II, and III have mortality rates sufficiently low for these patients to be treated as outpatients.

Another risk score, the CURB-65, was developed by the British Thoracic Society. The purpose of the CURB-65 is to identify patients who are at high risk of mortality from pneumonia. The elements of the CURB-65 are detailed in Table 31.2. In the CURB-65, similar to the PSI, higher numbers of points correlated with higher 30-day mortality rates. In an international derivation and validation study, the 30-day mortality rates for the CURB-65 were 0.7% for score 0, 3.2% for score 1, 3% for score 2, 17% for score 3, 41.5% for score 4, and 57% for score 5. The authors of the CURB-65 criteria have suggested that patients who score 0 or 1 are at low risk for mortality and can be managed as outpatients, while those who have a score of 2 are at intermediate risk, and those with scores >2 have severe CAP and are at high risk and should be managed in an intensive care unit.

Clinical question

Which elements of the history and physical examination findings are associated with a diagnosis of pneumonia?
Metlay et al addressed this question in a systematic review evaluating history and physical findings against the criterion standard of findings on chest radiography.[2] They reported likelihood ratios based on history and physical examination findings where there were two or more studies; however, an important limitation of this approach is that chest radiography is neither

Table 31.1 The Pneumonia Severity Index

Characteristic	Points assigned	
Demographic factor		
Men	Age (years)	
Women	Age (years)−10	
Nursing home resident	+10	
Coexisting illnesses		
Neoplastic disease	+30	
Liver disease	+20	
Congestive heart failure	+10	
Cerebrovascular disease	+10	
Renal disease	+10	
Physical examination findings		
Altered mental status	+20	
Respiratory rate 30 breaths/min	+20	
Systolic blood pressure <90 mm Hg	+20	
Temperature <35°C (95°F) or	+15	
40°C (104°F) Pulse 125 beats/min	+10	
Laboratory and radiographic findings (if study performed)		
Arterial blood pH < 7.35	+30	
Blood urea nitrogen level 30 mg/dL	+20	
Sodium level < 130 mmol/L	+20	
Glucose level 250 mg/dL	+10	
Hematocrit < 30%	+10	
Partial pressure of arterial	+10	
02 < 60 mm Hg or 02 Sat <90%	+10	
Pleural effusion	+10	
Class	Points	Mortality
I	<51	0.1%
II	51–70	0.6%
III	71–90	0.9%
IV	91–130	9.5%
V	>130	26.7%

Source: Data from [1].

100% sensitive nor specific for the diagnosis of pneumonia. These likelihood ratios are listed in Table 31.3.

Clinical question

Can procalcitonin be used to predict a bacterial etiology of infection and survival in pneumonia?

One study followed 185 patients who had procalcitonin levels measured within 24 hours of admission for CAP.[3] They found that higher procalcitonin

Table 31.2 The CURB-65 scoring system*

Confusion
Elevated blood urea nitrogen (BUN) (>7 mmol/L)
Respiratory rate (≥30/min)
Blood pressure (systolic <90 mmHg or diastolic ≤60 mmHg)
Age ≥65 years

*Each element, when positive, is assigned one point.

Table 31.3 Positive and negative likelihood ratios for history, examination, and laboratory findings in diagnosing pneumonia

Finding	Likelihood ratio positive (LR+)	Likelihood ratio negative (LR−)
Patient history		
Fever	1.7–2.1	0.6–0.7
Chills	1.3–1.7	0.7–0.9
Vital signs		
Tachypnea	1.5–3.4	0.8
Tachycardia	1.6–2.3	0.5–0.7
Hyperthermia	1.4–4.4	0.6–0.8
Chest examination		
Dullness to percussion	2.2–4.3	0.8–0.9
Decreased breath sounds	2.3–2.5	0.8–0.9
Crackles	1.6–2.7	0.6–0.9
Rhonchi	1.4–1.5	0.8–0.9
Egophony	2.0–8.6	0.8–1.0
Laboratory findings		
Leukocytosis	1.9–3.7	0.3–0.6

Note: The intervals represent ranges in published studies.
Source: Data from [2].

levels correlated with PSI score and also predicted complications including the development of empyema, need for mechanical ventilation, septic shock, and mortality. An interesting finding of this study was that procalcitonin predicted a bacterial etiology for pneumonia in patients with low PSI scores, but these findings did not apply to those with more severe CAP.

Another large trial studied 1,641 ED patients with dyspnea and measured procalcitonin levels, as well as several other biomarkers.[4] The diagnosis of pneumonia was made based on strict, validated guidelines. They found that a model that used procalcitonin was more accurate with an area under the curve of 72%, than any other clinical variable for a strict diagnosis of pneumonia. They reported that combining physician estimates of the probability of pneumonia along with procalcitonin levels increased the accuracy of diagnosis to greater than 86%. They found that patients with a diagnosis of acute heart failure and an elevated procalcitonin level (>0.21 ng/mL) had a worse outcome if they were not treated with antibiotics (p < 0.05). Patients with lower procalcitonin levels (<0.05 ng/mL) had better outcomes if they did not receive any antibiotic therapy (p < 0.05).

Clinical question

Which severity adjustment tool provides the best discriminatory power in predicting survival in patients with pneumonia in the emergency department?
A recent retrospective study compared PSI to CURB-65 in 3,181 ED patients.[5] Both PSI and CURB-65 were good predictors of 30-day mortality and for identifying patients at low risk for mortality. However, PSI appeared to discriminate better in identifying patients at lower risk of mortality. Using PSI, 68% were identified as low risk (class I–III) with a mortality rate of 1.4% while CURB-65 identified 61% as low risk (score of 0 or 1) with a mortality rate of 1.7%. In more severe CAP (score of 2 or higher), CURB-65 seemed to be somewhat more valuable because each score (2, 3, 4, or 5) was associated with a progressive increase in mortality while PSI only discriminated a high-risk versus a low-risk group. Another study used PSI and CURB-65 in a large group of both inpatients and outpatients with CAP in Spain.[6] They found that the CURB-65 and CRB-65 (which is a simpler version that excludes the BUN measurement) accurately predicted 30-day mortality rate, mechanical ventilation, and to some degree, hospitalization. CURB-65 also correlated with time to clinical stability and was predictive of a longer duration of intravenous antibiotics. Higher PSI numbers also predicted increased mortality, similarly to previous studies.

Comment

Several findings in the history, physical examination, and laboratory results are associated with a diagnosis of pneumonia on chest radiography. The presence of a single finding does not have a major impact on the overall probability of disease, reflecting the fact that combinations of findings are typically more important in predicting a radiographic diagnosis. Several studies have demonstrated that a combination of findings together are associated with considerably higher likelihoods of disease.[8,9]

Procalcitonin may be a promising tool for predicting which patients with pneumonia (particularly equivocal diagnoses) may benefit from empiric antibiotic therapy. As there has only been one randomized prospective trial, additional studies are needed to confirm this finding.

PSI and CURB-65 are the two major widely studied scoring systems for severity of illness in CAP. PSI better identifies patients who are at low risk of mortality. There is a tendency with PSI, however, to underestimate severity of illness in younger patients with comorbid illness because it places heavy weights on age and comorbidities. CURB-65 seems somewhat better at identifying patients at higher risk for mortality and discriminates better among more severely ill patients. One problem with CURB-65 is that it does not account as well for comorbidities. It also may be difficult to use in older patients with other chronic conditions who are at high risk for mortality, even though they may have a lower CURB-65 score.

While both scoring systems predict 30-day survival in large populations, neither can perfectly predict which patients with CAP can be safely admitted or discharged from ED. Additionally, clinical variables, social circumstances, and adequate access to follow-up care, among other factors, must be considered in the disposition plan. A recent commentary has suggested that PSI and CURB-65 be combined, recognizing that each system has its own limitations.[5] The authors suggested that low-risk patients (PSI classes I to III or CURB-65 scores of 0–1) could be managed at home if there are no vital sign abnormalities or significant comorbidities, as measured by both scoring systems, and if no other factors (such as social situation) necessitate hospital admission.

References

1. Fine MJ, Auble TE, Yealy DM *et al.* A prediction rule to identify low-risk patients with community-acquired pneumonia. N Engl J Med 1997; 336: 243–50.
2. Metlay JP, Fine MJ. Testing strategies in the initial management of patients with community-acquired pneumonia. Ann Intern Med. 2003; 138: 109–18.
3. Masia M, Gutierrez F, Shum C *et al.* Usefulness of procalcitonin levels in community-acquired pneumonia according to the patients outcome research team pneumonia severity index. Chest 2005; 128: 2223–9.
4. Maisel A, Neath SX, Landsberg J *et al.* Use of procalcitonin for the diagnosis of pneumonia in patients presenting with a chief complaint of dyspnoea: results from the BACH (Biomarkers in Acute Heart Failure) trial. Eur J Heart Fail. 2012 Feb 2:epub ahead of print.
5. Aujesky D, Auble TE, Yealy DM *et al.* Prospective comparison of three validated prediction rules for prognosis in community-acquired pneumonia. Am J Med 2005; 118: 384–92.
6. Capelastegui A, Espana PP, Quintana JM *et al.* Validation of a predictive rule for the management of community-acquired pneumonia. Eur Respir J 2006; 27: 151–7.

7. Niederman MS, Feldman C, Richards GA. Combining information from prognostic scoring tools for CAP: an American view on how to get the best of all worlds. Eur Respir J 2006; 27: 9–11.
8. Macfarlane J, Holmes W, Gard P, Macfarlane R, Rose D, Weston V *et al.* Prospective study of the incidence, aetiology and outcome of adult lower respiratory tract illness in the community. Thorax. 2001; 56: 109–14.
9. Diehr P, Wood RW, Bushyhead J, Krueger L, Wolcott B, Tompkins RK. Prediction of pneumonia in outpatients with acute cough – a statistical approach. J Chronic Dis. 1984; 37: 215–25.

Chapter 32 **Urinary Tract Infection**

Highlights

- Urinary tract infections (UTIs) commonly affect women and older men with disorders of the prostate.
- Urine culture is the criterion standard for UTIs, but its results are not available at the time of ED care.
- Urine dipsticks are not highly sensitive indicators of positive urine cultures; however, information from the urine dipstick can be combined with clinical pretest probability to improve accuracy.
- Because UTI symptoms and dipstick testing are not highly sensitive and specific, patients should receive a full examination (including pelvic examinations), especially if vaginal symptoms are present.

Background

Urinary tract infections (UTIs) are common complaints in emergency medicine practice. In 2005, 1.8 million patients in US emergency departments (EDs) were diagnosed with a UTI, and almost 5% of patients had a genitourinary complaint.[1] UTIs are relatively uncommon in young men but do affect older men and are often associated with disorders of the prostate. The most common way to diagnose UTI in the emergency department (ED) is either a urine dip or laboratory urinalysis. The dipstick urine test measures leukocytes, nitrite, blood, protein, and pH, while a urinalysis quantifies cell counts such as white blood cells, red blood cells, and squamous cells. The diagnosis of UTI can be difficult in the ED because of the inconsistent relationship between the clinical symptoms, bacteriuria, and pyuria. In addition, because the criterion standard test (a clean-catch or catheterized specimen urine culture) cannot be completed in the ED because it can take 2–3 days to grow, emergency physicians must diagnose and treat UTIs without criterion standard testing. Distinguishing sexually transmitted diseases (STDs),

Evidence-Based Emergency Care: Diagnostic Testing and Clinical Decision Rules, Second Edition. Jesse M. Pines, Christopher R. Carpenter, Ali S. Raja and Jeremiah D. Schuur. © 2013 John Wiley & Sons, Ltd. Published 2013 by John Wiley & Sons, Ltd.

other vaginal infections, and UTIs can be a challenge because of overlapping symptoms and signs.[2]

Clinical question

What is the diagnostic accuracy of clinical symptoms for UTI?

A 2002 diagnostic systematic review addressed this question and reported LR+s and LR−s for several symptoms and signs and combinations using data from published literature, although only one of the nine included studies was based in the ED.[3] These are listed in Table 32.1 ("Symptoms and Signs") and Table 32.2 ("Combination of Symptoms and Signs"). In isolation, signs and symptoms do not demonstrate large positive or negative LRs to predict the presence of UTI, except for the presence of vaginal discharge, which considerably lowers the likelihood of UTI and the absence of which considerably raises the likelihood of UTI. Combinations of signs and symptoms seem to dramatically impact the likelihood of UTI.

Clinical question

What is the best way to interpret positive urine dipsticks in the ED?

In the early 1990s, one paper aggregated 51 previous studies published to date that had reported 2 × 2 tables regarding the accuracy of urine dipsticks to diagnose UTIs, using urine culture as the criterion standard.[4] The study assessed four separate categories: nitrite only, leukocyte esterase only, and two pairings (dipstick positive if nitrite, leukocyte esterase, or both were positive, and dipstick positive only if both nitrite and leukocyte esterase were positive). When the authors plotted true-positive rates versus false-positive rates, the scatterplots demonstrated wide heterogeneity. They concluded that of the four ways to interpret urine dipsticks, defining a "positive" as "nitrite,

Table 32.1 Symptoms and signs predicting urinary tract infections (UTIs)

	LR+ (95% CI)	LR− (95% CI)
Dysuria	1.5 (CI 1.2–2.0)	0.5 (CI 0.3–0.7)
Frequency	1.8 (1.1–3.0)	0.6 (0.4–1.0)
Hematuria	2.0 (1.3–2.9)	0.9 (0.9–1.0)
Fever	1.6 (1.0–2.6)	0.9 (0.9–1.0)
Flank pain	1.1 (0.9–1.4)	0.9 (0.8–1.1)
Lower abdominal pain	1.1 (0.9–1.4)	0.9 (0.8–1.1)
Vaginal discharge	0.3 (0.1–0.9)	3.1 (1.0–9.3)

Source: Data from [3].

Table 32.2 Combination of symptoms and signs

	Posttest probability of urinary tract infection (%)	Summary likelihood ratio
Dysuria and frequency present, and vaginal discharge and vaginal irritation absent	77%	24.6
Dysuria absent and vaginal discharge or irritation present	4%	0.3
Dysuria or frequency present and vaginal discharge or irritation present	9%	0.7

Source: Data from [3].

leukocyte esterase, or both being positive" had the greatest accuracy. They also concluded that a negative urine dipstick does not exclude the diagnosis of UTI in patients with high pretest probabilities.

One ED-specific study compared urine dipsticks with urinalysis.[5] This was a prospective observational study investigating test characteristics of both urine dipstick and urinalysis using multiple test cutoff points in females seen in the ED with symptoms of UTI (dysuria, urgency, or urinary frequency on history OR suprapubic or costovertebral angle tenderness on exam). The authors excluded patients who had taken antibiotics within 72 hours or had indwelling Foley catheters, symptomatic vaginal discharge, diabetes, or HIV. A positive urine culture in this study was treated as the criterion standard and defined as more than 10^5 CFU/mL of one or two uropathogenic bacteria at 48 hours from collection. In 349 patients, a little fewer than half had positive cultures. Urine dipstick results were defined as positive when either nitrite was positive *or* leukocyte esterase was positive or blood was more than trace. Using this definition of positive, the overtreatment rate was 47% (defined as one minus the positive predictive value) and the undertreatment rate was 13%. By defining a positive urinalysis as >3 WBC per high-power field or when RBC are more than 5 per high power field, the overtreatment rate was 44% and the undertreatment rate was 11%. The authors concluded that there were similar overtreatment and undertreatment rates identified for various test cutoff points for urine dipstick tests and urinalysis.

Comment

This chapter highlights the continued difficulty in identifying ED patients with UTIs without criterion standard testing. In the context of clinical

ED practice, this review identifies a number of conclusions and observations from the literature describing the care of females with suspected UTI. Clinical symptoms alone are not particularly helpful in diagnosing UTI; however, the presence of vaginal symptoms should prompt further investigation into other causes because of the low positive likelihood ratio (0.3). Combinations of symptoms appear to be highly predictive of urinary tract infections, while similarly the presence of vaginal symptoms along with other urinary symptoms further demonstrates that any vaginal symptom should be thoroughly evaluated, even in women with symptoms suggestive of UTI. The test performance of urinary dipstick is highly variable across studies, and the most accurate way to define a positive is either positive leukocyte esterase or positive nitrite or both being positive. One paper found that urine dipsticks and urinalysis are similarly predictive of positive urine cultures in ED patients. While one paper should not necessarily change practice, a point-of-care urine dipstick may be a reasonable diagnostic endpoint in a classic presentation of UTI (i.e., a high pretest probability). However, the absence of leukocyte esterase, nitrite, and blood does not fully exclude UTI.

References

1. Nawar EW, Niska RW, Xu J. National Hospital Ambulatory Medical Care Survey: 2005 Emergency department summary. Advance Data. 2007; 386: 1–32.
2. Komaroff AL. Acute dysuria in women. New England Journal of Medicine. 1984; 310: 368–75.
3. Bent S, Nallamothu BK, Simel DL *et al*. Does this woman have an acute uncomplicated urinary tract infection? Journal of the American Medical Association. 2002; 287: 2701–10.
4. Hurlbut TA 3rd, Littenberg B. The diagnostic accuracy of rapid dipstick tests to predict urinary tract infection. American Journal of Clinical Pathology. 1991; 96: 582–8.
5. Lammers RL, Gibson S, Kovacs D *et al*. Comparison of test characteristics of urine dipstick and urinalysis at various test cutoff points. Annals of Emergency Medicine. 2001; 38: 505–12.

Chapter 33 **Sepsis**

Highlights

- Sepsis is a clinical syndrome of systemic inflammatory response due to acute infection; early detection difficult solely based on clinical parameters.
- Approximately 500,000 patients with severe sepsis are treated in emergency departments and admitted to hospital in the United States each year.
- Mortality from sepsis increases along the continuum from approximately 7% for SIRS to over 40% for septic shock.
- Elevated serum lactate is an independent predictor of mortality in patients with sepsis.
- The Mortality in Emergency Department Sepsis (MEDS) score can accurately predict in-hospital death among ED patients admitted for infectious conditions.

Background

Sepsis is a clinical syndrome of systemic inflammatory response that is a sequela of acute infection. Four conditions along the sepsis continuum have been defined from least severe to most: systemic inflammatory response syndrome (SIRS), sepsis, severe sepsis, and septic shock.[1] Table 33.1 defines SIRS. *Sepsis* exists if infection causes two or more abnormalities in temperature, heart rate, respiration, or white blood cell (WBC) count; *severe sepsis* refers to sepsis and at least one sign of hypoperfusion or organ dysfunction; finally, *septic shock* refers to severe sepsis with either hypotension or the requirement for a vasopressor. Estimates indicate that annually in the United States, 500,000 patients with severe sepsis are initially treated in emergency departments (EDs) and at least 750,000 people are admitted to hospital.[2,3]

The mortality rate from sepsis ranges from 20% to 50%, although it has decreased over the last 30 years.[4] Mortality rates increase across the spectrum of disease severity, from SIRS (7%), to sepsis (16%), severe sepsis (20%),

Evidence-Based Emergency Care: Diagnostic Testing and Clinical Decision Rules, Second Edition. Jesse M. Pines, Christopher R. Carpenter, Ali S. Raja and Jeremiah D. Schuur.
© 2013 John Wiley & Sons, Ltd. Published 2013 by John Wiley & Sons, Ltd.

Table 33.1 Systemic inflammatory response syndrome (SIRS)

SIRS is defined as the presence of two or more of the following:
- Heart rate >90 beats/min
- Respiratory rate >20 breaths/min or oxygen saturation <90% or need for >0.4 FiO_2 to maintain saturation
- Temperature >38°C or <35.5°C
- White blood cell count >15,000 cells/mm^3 or bands >10%

Source: Data from [1].

and septic shock (46%).[5] In the ED, clinicians are challenged to identify sepsis early in its course and to identify those patients at risk of adverse events. Early identification is required to initiate early goal-directed therapy, a bundle of hemodynamically based interventions that has been associated with improved outcomes.[6]

Early diagnosis of sepsis can be difficult because it is largely a clinical diagnosis which can be mistaken for other causes of shock. Heffner et al prospectively evaluated the cause of illness in 211 adult patients initially determined to have sepsis and admitted to the hospital from the ED after initial management with a sepsis protocol.[7] Three-quarters of the patients were diagnosed with infectious etiologies: 45% had positive cultures, 24% were diagnosed with culture-negative clinical infections, and 4% had atypical infections. A noninfectious mimic was diagnosed in 18% of patients, including inflammatory colitis, hypovolemia, medication effect, adrenal insufficiency, acute myocardial infarction, and pulmonary embolism. In 9% of the patients, the final diagnosis was indeterminate. Early indicators of infection did not differ between infectious and non-infectious causes including temperature, WBC count, vital signs in the ED, median lactate levels, or illness severity scores. Patients with infections had higher mortality rates than those with non-infectious diagnoses (15% vs. 9%). The authors concluded that about one in five patients with an early diagnosis of sepsis in the ED was ultimately diagnosed with a noninfectious illness, and may have benefited from alternative management.

Clinical question

Which laboratory tests are useful in risk stratifying ED patients with sepsis?
Lactic acid, procalcitonin, and central venous oxygen saturation ($ScvO_2$) have been prospectively studied as prognostic tests in sepsis. During sepsis, lactate production exceeds the rate of lactate removal, which leads to accumulation in venous blood. Multiple studies have identified an association between elevated serum lactate levels and mortality in critically ill ED patients, including those with sepsis, burns, and traumatic injuries. This could indicate

that the severity of sepsis is independently associated with lactate elevations, or elevated lactate could be reflective of organ dysfunction due to patient factors such as age and comorbidity.

Mikkelsen et al evaluated the association of elevated serum lactate in severe sepsis with 28-day mortality in 830 adult patients admitted with sepsis from an urban, academic ED.[8] They collected and evaluated other potential causes of sepsis in order to test whether the association between initial serum lactate level and mortality was independent of organ dysfunction and shock. They classified initial venous lactate (mmol/L) as low (<2), intermediate (2.0–3.9), or high (≥ 4) and evaluated other variables including age, sex, race, acute and chronic organ dysfunction, severity of illness, and initiation of early goal-directed therapy using multivariable logistic regression. Mortality at 28 days was 23%, and median serum lactate was 2.9 mmol/L. Intermediate (odds ratio (OR) = 2.1) and high serum lactate levels (OR = 4.9) were associated with mortality in the subgroup without shock. In patients with shock, intermediate (OR = 3.3) and high serum lactate levels (OR = 4.9) were also associated with mortality. After adjusting for potential confounders, intermediate and high serum lactate levels remained significantly associated with mortality among patients with and without shock.

As lactate analysis performed in a central laboratory can require 30–90 minutes including transport to generate results for ED clinicians, point-of-care (POC) lactate tests have been developed. Shapiro et al conducted a prospective study of 699 ED patients with suspected sepsis to evaluate the diagnostic utility of POC lactate to predict mortality.[9] The study, funded by the POC test manufacturer, evaluated POC lactate measurement, base excess, and pH, compared to lab measurement of lactate. The mortality rate in these patients was 4.9%. POC lactate levels were 0.3 lower than central lab values on average (range −1.1 to 0.5). The average POC lactate was 3.2 mmol/L in patients who died versus 1.7 mmol/L in survivors, and the corresponding mean lab lactate levels were 3.8 mmol/L versus 2.0 mmol/L, respectively. Lactate levels, both POC and laboratory, were correlated with mortality (area under the curve (AUC) 0.72 for the POC lactate and 0.70 for lactate levels measured in the laboratory), and both were more useful predictors than the pH and/or base excess (AUC 0.60 each). The authors conclude that POC lactate testing in the ED is useful to identify at-risk patients, in whom early goal-directed therapy may be beneficial.

Some studies, in particular the Rivers study of early goal-directed therapy, have recommended use of $ScvO_2$ as a prognostic and diagnostic tool to judge adequacy of resuscitation.[6] As $ScvO_2$ requires invasive monitoring via a central line with a special probe or repeated analysis from central blood specimens, it is important to know if it adds value above routine lactate testing. Jones et al conducted a multicenter, randomized, non-inferiority trial to test the hypothesis that lactate clearance and $ScvO_2$ are non-inferior as goals of early sepsis resuscitation for the outcome of in-hospital mortality.[10] They included patients with severe sepsis and evidence of hypoperfusion or septic shock who were admitted from the ED at one of three urban hospitals in the United States. They randomly assigned patients to one of two resuscitation protocols: $ScvO_2$ or lactate clearance. All patients were resuscitated to normalize central venous pressure and mean arterial pressure. Additionally, the $ScvO_2$ group was resuscitated to $ScvO_2$ of at least 70%, while the lactate clearance group was resuscitated to lactate clearance of at least 10%. The study protocol was continued until all goals were achieved or for up to 6 hours, and clinicians who cared for the patients after the protocol was completed were blinded to the treatment assignment. They enrolled 300 patients (150 in each group), and randomization produced well-matched groups including no differences in initial treatments (first 72 hours). In-hospital mortality was 23% (CI 17–30%) in the $ScvO_2$ group compared with 17% (CI 11–24%) in the lactate clearance group, not meeting the predefined 10% threshold for non-inferiority. There were no differences in treatment-related adverse events between the groups. The authors concluded that among patients with septic shock who were treated to normalize central venous and mean arterial pressure, additional management to normalize $ScvO_2$ compared with management to normalize lactate clearance did not alter in-hospital mortality.

Procalcitonin (PCT) is a peptide precursor of the hormone calcitonin, which is involved with calcium homeostasis. In healthy individuals the level of procalcitonin is below the limit of detection of clinical assays (10 pg/mL), but it rises in response to proinflammatory stimuli, for example bacterial infection. Some studies have reported that procalcitonin levels are a reliable method of diagnosing severe bacterial infection and sepsis. Two systematic reviews of procalcitonin were published in 2007. Tang et al performed a systematic review and meta-analysis to assess accuracy of procalcitonin for sepsis diagnosis in critically ill patients, and included 18 studies.[11] Pooled sensitivity and specificity were both 71% (CI 67–76%) with an AUC of 0.78 (CI 0.73–0.83). Jones et al conducted a systematic review and meta-analysis to evaluate the diagnostic performance of procalcitonin for the diagnosis of bacteremia in the ED population.[12] They identified prospective studies that assessed the diagnostic accuracy of procalcitonin for bacteremia, with blood culture as the criterion standard, and included investigations of adults and children with suspected infection studied in the ED or at admission. They calculated unweighted summary AUC and random-effects pooled sensitivity and specificity. Seventeen studies including 2,008 patients met the inclusion criteria. There was a substantial degree of inconsistency between studies.

As different studies used different test thresholds, they analyzed the subgroup of studies that used a test threshold of 0.5 or 0.4 ng/mL and calculated pooled estimates for sensitivity of 76% (CI 66–84%) and specificity of 70% (CI 60–79%). The unweighted summary AUC was 0.84 (CI 0.75–0.90). The authors of both studies concluded that procalcitonin cannot reliably differentiate sepsis from other non-infectious causes of SIRS in critically ill adult patients, and suggest further testing in ambulatory populations.

Several recent studies have examined procalcitonin as a diagnostic test for infection in the ED. Riedel et al studied procalcitonin as a marker for the detection of bacteremia and sepsis in adults admitted to a single urban ED with symptoms of systemic infection.[13] They enrolled 367 patients and analyzed data on the 295 patients in whom a serum sample was obtained at the same time as blood cultures, allowing analysis of procalcitonin. Procalcitonin levels were compared with blood culture results and other clinical data obtained during the ED visit – positive cultures were classified as representing real disease or contaminants according to accepted protocols. Using a predefined procalcitonin test threshold of 0.1 ng/mL led to a sensitivity of 75% and a specificity of 71% for clinically significant bacteremia. Lai et al prospectively examined 370 adult ED patients with fever and suspected bacterial infection in one urban ED.[14] Bacterial infection was confirmed in 72% of patients; pneumonia was the most common infection (31%) followed by bacteremia (26%), urinary tract infection (27%), intra-abdominal infection (19%), skin and soft tissue infection (15%), and others (2%). The AUC for identification of bacteremia by procalcitonin was 0.76 (CI 0.70–0.81). Using a retrospectively derived cutoff level of 0.47 ng/mL, the sensitivity and specificity of procalcitonin for diagnosing bacteremia in patients with fever at admission to the ED were 75% and 70%, respectively. While the authors of both studies concluded that procalcitonin is useful in the diagnosis of bacterial infection in ED patients with symptoms of systemic infection, we think this oversimplifies the issue. As the sensitivity and specificity of procalcitonin are below 80%, it is not accurate enough to either rule in or rule out bacterial infection. It may be reasonable for clinicians to use procalcitonin to identify patients at higher risk and prioritize such patients for interventions, such as early, broad-spectrum antibiotics, but such algorithms need to be studied independently.

Clinical question

Can clinical scoring systems accurately risk-stratify septic patients from the ED?
Many scoring systems for severity of illness and organ dysfunction have been developed and are used to predict the risk of mortality in intensive

care unit (ICU) patients, but their usefulness in patients with suspected infection in the ED is less well studied. The SIRS criteria are neither sensitive nor specific enough to be of use in an undifferentiated ED population. Calle et al conducted a systematic review of severity scores in ED patients with suspected infection published in 2011.[15] They conducted a systematic review, and included 21 studies that compared different severity scores, 19 of which were ED based. They found that the operating characteristics to evaluate the accuracy (calibration and discrimination) of the different scores were insufficiently assessed in most studies. Only two studies evaluated the calibration, and less than half of the studies evaluated the discrimination, using the AUC. They concluded that the literature did not provide enough information to assess the comparative accuracy of the prognostic models in patients with suspected infection admitted from the ED and hospital ward.

Only one score, the Mortality in Emergency Department Sepsis (MEDS) score, was developed in the ED setting. The MEDS score was derived by Shapiro et al in a single-center study at a tertiary, academic ED in the United States to identify risk factors for mortality in ED patients with suspected infection.[16] All adults older than 18 years for whom a blood culture was sent were eligible. Over 1 year, 3,179 patient visits were included, 2,070 were randomly assigned to the derivation group, and the other 1,109 were assigned to the validation group. Patient characteristics including clinical and laboratory data, demographics, and terminal illness (defined as $>50\%$ likelihood of death within 30 days) were assessed retrospectively by medical record review. The outcome was 28-day in-hospital mortality. The association of predictive variables with mortality was assessed using multivariate logistic regression. In-hospital mortality was 5.3% in the derivation group and 5.7% in the validation group. Nine variables were independently associated with mortality and make up the MEDS score (Table 33.2). The AUC for the derivation set was 0.82, and 0.76 in the validation set. Mortality increased with higher MEDS scores in the validation group.

Several studies have subsequently studied the MEDS score. Chen et al retrospectively studied 1,696 adult patients admitted to nonsurgical ICUs in an academic teaching hospital in Taiwan.[17] Eligible patients were identified from an electronic database and data were collected by record review, and included only patients with severe sepsis. MEDS scores for each patient were retrospectively calculated, and subjects were stratified into high-risk (MEDS 12–27; 52%) or low-risk (MEDS <12; 48%) subsets. High-risk patients had higher 28-day mortality than those in the low-risk group (49% vs. 18%, $p < 0.01$). The MEDS score also had a significantly better discriminatory performance than the APACHE II score (ROC area 0.75 vs. 0.26, $p < 0.01$).

Table 33.2 Mortality in Emergency Department
Sepsis (MEDS) score

	Points
Rapidly terminal comorbid illness	6
Age >65 years	3
Bands >5%	3
Tachypnea or hypoxemia	3
Shock	3
Platelet count <150,000 mm^3	3
Altered mental status	2
Nursing home resident	2
Lower respiratory infection	2

Source: Data from [16].

Howell et al studied several severity scores including the MEDS in 2,132 ED patients in whom clinicians had a concern for infection.[18] This was a secondary analysis of a prospective observational cohort including patients identified by daily review of ED census logs. Physicians' medical decision-making documentation was analyzed to determine clinicians' concern for infection. The primary outcome was 28-day mortality, which occurred in 4% of the study population. Mortality increased with increasing MEDS score and MEDS had the best prognostic test performance (AUC 0.85; CI 0.81–0.89), although the AUC overlapped with the other scores. Jones et al evaluated MEDS prediction of in-hospital mortality in a prospective cohort of patients enrolled in an early goal-directed therapy trial.[19] The cohort included 143 adult patients with suspected or confirmed infection and sepsis, severe sepsis, or septic shock. The average MEDS score was 10. In-hospital mortality occurred in 23% of patients. The MEDS score performed poorly (AUC 0.61; CI 0.50–0.72) and consistently underestimated patient mortality in the moderate-risk groups (MEDS score 5–15). Lee et al evaluated the MEDS score along with procalcitonin and C-reactive protein in ED patients with sepsis at an academic medical center in Taiwan.[20] They enrolled 525 consecutive adult ED patients with SIRS criteria with a presumed infectious cause, and excluded 66 patients due to age younger than 15 years, missing data or lost to follow-up, preexisting thyroid disease, or a noninfectious cause of SIRS. Outcomes included early (5-day) or late (30-day) mortality. The 30-day mortality rate was 10.5%. The MEDS score had superior prognostic accuracy for short- and long-term mortality over procalcitonin or C-reactive protein. Sankoff et al evaluated the MEDS score in 385 patients with SIRS at four academic EDs.[21] The primary outcome was 28-day mortality, which

Table 33.3 Mortality in Emergency Department Sepsis
(MEDS) score mortality estimate

Clinical category	MEDS score range	28-day mortality rate (%)
Very low risk	0–4	0.4–11
Low risk	5–7	3–5
Moderate risk	8–12	7–19
High risk	13–15	16–32
Very high risk	>15	39–40

Source: Data from [22].

occurred in 9%. The mortality rate increased correspondingly with the MEDS score and ranged from 0.6% to 40%. MEDS had better prognostic accuracy (AUC 0.88; CI 0.83–0.92) than lactate (0.78; CI 0.66–0.90). MEDS variables had excellent interrater reproducibility (kappa range 0.82–1.00), except terminal illness, which had moderate reliability (kappa = 0.64).

A detailed evidence-based review of the MEDS score was published by Carpenter et al in 2009.[22] They summarized the mortality rates associated with different MEDS scores, which are shown in Table 33.3. One study has been published subsequent to Carpenter's review. Nguyen et al compared the MEDS score to the Predisposition, Insult/Infection, Response, and Organ Dysfunction (PIRO) score and the APACHE II score.[23] They analyzed a prospectively maintained registry including adult patients with severe sepsis or septic shock meeting criteria for early goal-directed therapy over a 6-year period. Five hundred and forty-one patients were enrolled: 62% in septic shock, 47% with positive blood cultures, and 32% with in-hospital mortality. Median (25th and 75th percentile) MEDS scores were 12 (9 and 15), with predicted mortalities of 16% (9% and 39%). MEDS score was the least accurate (AUC 0.63, 0.60–0.70), although the AUCs of all three scores overlapped. The authors concluded that the PIRO may provide additional risk stratification in more severely ill patients.

Carpenter et al concluded that increasing MEDS scores are associated with increasing mortality, and that the score is accurate and reliable, except in patients with severe sepsis, where the scale may underestimate mortality. This is an example of spectrum bias (see Chapter 6), as the MEDS score performs better in populations of undifferentiated SIRS patients than in the sicker populations eligible for early goal-directed therapy. This is not surprising, as the MEDS score was derived in a cohort of ED patients getting blood cultures and admitted to the hospital, with an in-hospital mortality of approximately 5%.

Comment

Identifying patients at risk from sepsis and prognosticating short-term mortality are clinically important as they can help determine who should receive early aggressive therapies, disposition to ICUs, and guidance to family and other caregivers.

While many biomarkers and scoring systems have been evaluated to predict severity of sepsis, organ dysfunction, and mortality, few have been evaluated in the ED. Serum lactate either calculated in a central lab or using a point-of-care test is the most accurate single biomarker in predicting sepsis severity. Correspondingly, clearance of serum lactate in response to resuscitation appears to perform as well as $ScvO_2$. At this point, procalcitonin and other biomarkers do not have a clear additive benefit to serum lactate and we do not recommend their routine use in the emergent care of septic patients. We recommend use of the MEDS score to help identify which ED patients being admitted with infection are at risk of in-hospital mortality, as it is the only score that has been derived and multiply validated in ED populations. Clinicians should be aware that the MEDS may underestimate the likelihood of mortality in severely ill patients, such as those with severe sepsis or septic shock. In this group, use of aggressive interventions and ICU care is appropriate. In the future, new biomarkers and new prognostic tools are likely to emerge. Clinicians should be cautious before applying data from other settings, such as the ICU, to a general ED population.

References

1. Bone RC, Balk RA, Cerra FB *et al*. Definitions for sepsis and organ failure and guidelines for the use of innovative therapies in sepsis. The American College of Chest Physicians/Society of Critical Care Medicine (ACCP/SCCM) Consensus Conference Committee. Chest. 1992; 101(6): 1644–1655.
2. Dombrovskiy VY, Martin AA, Sunderram J *et al*. Rapid increase in hospitalization and mortality rates for severe sepsis in the United States: A trend analysis from 1993 to 2003. Critical Care Medicine. 2007; 35: 1244–50.
3. Wang HE, Shapiro NI, Angus DC *et al*. National estimates of severe sepsis in United States emergency departments. Critical Care Medicine. 2007; 35: 1928–36.
4. Winters BD, Eberlein M, Leung J *et al*. Long-term mortality and quality of life in sepsis: A systematic review. Critical Care Medicine. 2010; 38: 1276–83.
5. Rangel-Frausto MS, Pittet D, Costigan M *et al*. The natural history of the systemic inflammatory response syndrome (SIRS): A prospective study. Journal of the American Medical Association. 1995; 273: 117–23.
6. Rivers E, Nguyen B, Havstad S *et al*. Early goal-directed therapy in the treatment of severe sepsis and septic shock. New England Journal of Medicine. 2001; 345: 1368–77.

7. Jones AE, Heffner AC, Horton JM *et al.* Etiology of illness in patients with severe sepsis admitted to the hospital from the emergency department. Clinical Infectious Diseases. 2010; 50: 814–20.

8. Mikkelsen ME, Miltiades AN, Gaieski DF *et al.* Serum lactate is associated with mortality in severe sepsis independent of organ failure and shock. Critical Care Medicine. 2009; 37: 1670–7.

9. Shapiro NI, Fisher C, Donnino M *et al.* The feasibility and accuracy of point-of-care lactate measurement in emergency department patients with suspected infection. Journal of Emergency Medicine. 2010; 39: 89–94.

10. Jones AE, Shapiro NI, Trzeciak S *et al.* Lactate clearance vs. central venous oxygen saturation as goals of early sepsis therapy. Journal of the American Medical Association. 2010; 303: 739–46.

11. Tang BM, Eslick GD, Craig JC *et al.* Accuracy of procalcitonin for sepsis diagnosis in critically ill patients: Systematic review and meta-analysis. Lancet Infectious Diseases. 2007; 7: 210–17.

12. Jones AE, Fiechtl JF, Brown MD *et al.* Procalcitonin test in the diagnosis of bacteremia: A meta-analysis. Annals of Emergency Medicine. 2007; 50: 34–41.

13. Riedel S, Melendez JH, An AT *et al.* Procalcitonin as a marker for the detection of bacteremia and sepsis in the emergency department. American Journal of Clinical Pathology. 2011; 135: 182–9.

14. Lai CC, Tan CK, Chen SY *et al.* Diagnostic performance of procalcitonin for bacteremia in patients with bacterial infection at the emergency department. Journal of Infection. 2010; 61: 512–15.

15. Calle P, Cerro L, Valencia J *et al.* Usefulness of severity scores in patients with suspected infection in the emergency department: A systematic review. Journal of Emergency Medicine. 2011; 42(4): 374–91.

16. Shapiro NI, Wolfe RE, Moore RB *et al.* Mortality in Emergency Department Sepsis (MEDS) score: A prospectively derived and validated clinical prediction rule. Critical Care Medicine. 2003; 31: 670–5.

17. Chen CC, Chong CF, Liu YL *et al.* Risk stratification of severe sepsis patients in the emergency department. Emergency Medicine Journal. 2006; 23: 281–5.

18. Howell MD, Donnino MW, Talmor D *et al.* Performance of severity of illness scoring systems in emergency department patients with infection. Academic Emergency Medicine. 2007; 14: 709–14.

19. Jones AE, Saak K, Kline JA. Performance of the mortality in emergency department sepsis score for predicting hospital mortality among patients with severe sepsis and septic shock. American Journal of Emergency Medicine. 2008; 26: 689–92.

20. Lee CC, Chen SY, Tsai CL *et al.* Prognostic value of mortality in emergency department sepsis score, procalcitonin, and C-reactive protein in patients with sepsis at the emergency department. Shock. 2008; 29: 322–7.

21. Sankoff JD, Goyal M, Gaieski DF *et al.* Validation of the mortality in emergency department sepsis (MEDS) score in patients with systemic inflammatory response syndrome (SIRS). Critical Care Medicine. 2008; 36: 421–6.

22. Carpenter CR, Keim SM, Upadhye S *et al*. Risk stratification of the potentially septic patient in the emergency department: The mortality in the emergency department sepsis (MEDS) score. Journal of Emergency Medicine. 2009; 37: 319–27.

23. Nguyen HB, Van Ginkel C, Batech M *et al*. Comparison of predisposition, insult/infection, response, and organ dysfunction, acute physiology and chronic health evaluation II, and mortality in emergency department sepsis in patients meeting criteria for early goal-directed therapy and the severe sepsis resuscitation bundle. Journal of Critical Care. 2011 Oct 26; published online.

Chapter 34 **Septic Arthritis**

> **Highlights**
>
> - The prevalence of nongonococcal septic arthritis in adult ED patients with acute monoarticular arthritis is approximately 27%.
> - For the diagnosis of a septic joint in these patients, the most useful findings on history and physical exam are cellulitis overlying a prosthetic joint (LR+ 15) and recent (generally <3 months) joint surgery (LR+ 7).
> - Common laboratory tests such as peripheral WBC, ESR, and CRP do not accurately distinguish septic arthritis from other etiologies of monoarticular arthritis.
> - Synovial white blood cell counts >100,000 (LR+ 28) or >50,000 (LR+ 8) are the most useful tests to rule in the diagnosis of septic arthritis, while synovial lactate (LR− 0.14–0.16), LDH <250 U/L (LR− 0.09–0.11), and TNF_α < 36 pg/mL (LR− 0.07) may be useful to exclude the diagnosis.

Background

Acute monoarticular arthritis presenting to the emergency department (ED) can be due to a number of etiologies as summarized in Table 34.1.[1] Septic (bacterial) arthritis has an annual incidence of 10 per 100,000 individuals, but is more common among those with rheumatoid arthritis or a prosthetic joint (up to 70 cases per 100,000).[2,3] Septic arthritis most commonly affects the knees, which account for 50% of cases. In decreasing order of frequency, it also affects the hips, shoulders, and elbows, although virtually any articular surface can become infected.[4] Most cases result from hematogenous spread since bacterial organisms can easily enter the synovial fluid through synovial tissue, which lacks a basement membrane. Prompt diagnosis and appropriate antibiotic management of septic arthritis are essential since cartilage can be destroyed within days and the in-hospital mortality of treated infections can reach 15%.[5]

Evidence-Based Emergency Care: Diagnostic Testing and Clinical Decision Rules, Second Edition.
Jesse M. Pines, Christopher R. Carpenter, Ali S. Raja and Jeremiah D. Schuur.
© 2013 John Wiley & Sons, Ltd. Published 2013 by John Wiley & Sons, Ltd.

Table 34.1 Differential diagnosis of monoarticular arthritis

Infection (bacterial, fungal, mycobacterial, viral, and spirochete)
Rheumatoid arthritis
Gout/pseudogout
Lupus
Lyme disease
Sickle cell disease
Dialysis-related amyloidosis
Transient synovitis
Plant thorn synovitis
Metastatic carcinoma
Hemearthrosis
Pigmented villonodular synovitis
Neuropathic arthropathy
Intra-articular injury

Source: Data from [1].

Staphylococcal and streptococcal species produce 70% of nongonococcal septic arthritis cases. These Gram-positive species are isolated in both blood and synovial fluid in only 48% of cases.[4,6] Methicillin-resistant *Staphylococcus aureus* septic arthritis is being increasingly reported.[7] Patients with HIV are not at increased risk for septic arthritis.[8]

With an annual incidence of 3 per 100,000, gonococcal (GC) arthritis is another common cause of septic arthritis in the United States. Unlike nongonococcal septic arthritis, GC joint infections respond rapidly to appropriate antimicrobial management. Gonococcal septic arthritis is frequently accompanied by a tenosynovitis and, in the absence of pelvic symptoms, can be difficult to distinguish from non-GC septic arthritis. Gonococcal septic arthritis is more common in younger adults, with a 4:1 female-to-male predominance. Risk factors for GC arthritis are listed in Table 34.2. Gram

Table 34.2 Risk factors for gonococcal arthritis

Female
Pregnancy
Multiple sexual partners
Low socioeconomic status
Intravenous drug abuse
Mucosal infection (symptomatic or asymptomatic)
HIV
Lupus
Complement deficiencies
GC organism factors

Source: Data from [9].

stain (<50%), blood (<50%), and synovial cultures (~50%) are less often positive in GC septic arthritis, but genitourinary specimens will be positive in up about 90% of cases.[10]

Clinical question

What are the risk factors in the history and physical exam that are most associated with an increased probability of bacterial infection in monoarticular arthritis?

A recent meta-analysis summarized the accuracy of elements of the history, physical exam findings, and laboratory tests for ED patients with septic arthritis.[11] Only one study has prospectively assessed the prevalence of nongonococcal septic arthritis in ED patients with monoarticular arthritis, demonstrating an estimate of 27%.[12] The interval between joint surgery and septic arthritis exceeded 3 months in one-third of the cases. Table 34.3 summarizes septic arthritis risk factors from the past medical history, along with estimates of their diagnostic accuracy.[1,3,11] Notably, none of these findings, when absent, significantly reduced the probability of septic arthritis. No studies have evaluated physical exam findings for all patients with suspected septic arthritis, so likelihood ratios cannot be reported for the findings of joint pain, joint swelling, sweats, or rigors. However, fever has a LR+ 0.67 and LR− 1.7, making it unhelpful to rule in or rule out the diagnosis of septic arthritis.[13]

Table 34.3 Historical risk factors for non-gonococcal septic arthritis

Risk factor	Positive likelihood ratio	Negative likelihood ratio
Age >80 years	3.5 (1.7–6.4)	0.86 (0.70–0.96)
DM	2.7 (1.1–6.2)	0.93 (0.79–1.0)
Rheumatoid arthritis	2.5 (1.9–2.9)	0.45 (0.27–0.67)
Recent joint surgery	6.9 (3.7–11.6)	0.78 (0.63–0.90)
Hip or knee prosthesis	3.1 (1.9–4.5)	0.73 (0.55–0.88)
Skin infection	2.8 (1.7–4.2)	0.76 (0.58–0.91)
Prosthesis *and* skin infection	15.0 (8.0–26)	0.77 (0.62–0.88)
HIV infection	1.7 (0.76–1.5)	0.64 (0.23–1.37)

Reproduced from [11] with permission from John Wiley and Sons Ltd.

Clinical question

What are the diagnostic test characteristics of peripheral leukocytosis, sedimentation rate, C-reactive protein, and synovial cell counts or inflammatory markers for the diagnosis of septic arthritis?

Table 34.4 Serum inflammatory markers for non-gonococcal septic arthritis

Serum marker	Positive likelihood ratio	Negative likelihood ratio
WBC >10,000/mm^3	1.4 (1.1–1.8)	0.28 (0.07–1.10)
ESR >30 mm/hour	1.3 (1.1–1.8)	0.17 (0.20–1.3)
CRP >100 mg/L	1.6 (1.1–2.5)	0.44 (0.24–0.82)
Procalcitonin >0.3 ng/mL	11–13	0.3

Reproduced from [11] with permission from John Wiley and Sons Ltd.

Readily available serum inflammatory markers are not useful acutely (Table 34.4), although procalcitonin and inflammatory cytokines are promising in preliminary trials.[11] Since history and physical exam findings cannot significantly adjust the posttest probability of septic arthritis, synovial fluid analysis is essential for the diagnosis. Arthrocentesis can be safely performed in patients with therapeutic warfarin anticoagulation with a risk of clinically significant hemorrhage below 10%.[14] The American Rheumatologic Association suggests the following interpretation guidelines for synovial cell count interpretation: 200–2,000 WBC/mm^3 is non-inflammatory, 2,000–5,000 WBC/mm^3 is inflammatory, and >50,000 WBC/mm^3 is infectious. Four trials have prospectively assessed the diagnostic accuracy of synovial WBC, two trials have assessed low synovial glucose, and one trial each assessed LDH and tumor necrosis factor alpha (TNF$_\alpha$).[12,13,15–17] The range of LRs for each test is summarized in Table 34.5.

Table 34.5 Synovial Fluid Tests for Non-gonococcal Septic Arthritis

Test	Positive likelihood ratio	Negative likelihood ratio
sWBC >100,000 cell/mL	4.7–42.0	0.61–0.84
sWBC >50,000	2.2–19.0	0.33–0.57
sWBC >25,000	1.7–4.0	0.17–0.47
PMN >90%	1.8–4.2	0.10–0.63
Low glucose	2.5–4.2	0.43–0.74
Protein >3 g/dL	0.89–0.93	1.10
LDH >250 U/L	1.9	0.09–0.11
TNF$_\alpha$ > 36.2 pg/mL	3.3	0.07
Lactate		
>5.6 mmol/L	2.4	0.46
>12 mmol/L	19	0.14
>0.05 mmol/L	21	0.16

Reproduced from [11] with permission from John Wiley and Sons Ltd.

One recent diagnostic systematic review reported the summary LR+ of sWBC >100 and sWBC >50 of 28.0 and 7.7, respectively.[1] With the exception of LDH and TNF_α (which is generally not available in most EDs), none of these synovial tests is sufficient to exclude the diagnosis of septic arthritis. However, a sWBC > 100,000 is sufficient to rule in the diagnosis. Based upon these measures of sWBC diagnostic accuracy and evidence-based estimates of diagnostic test risk and treatment risk and benefit, the threshold below which emergency physicians should contemplate not performing an arthrocentesis is 5% and the threshold above which treatment should ensue without an arthrocentesis is 39% (see Chapter 1).[11,18]

Only one systematic review has reported the interval likelihood ratio (iLR) for sWBC: for the range of 0–25 cells/mL, the iLR is 0.33; for the range of 25–50 cells/mL, the iLR is 1.06; for the range of 50–100 cells/mL, the iLR is 3.59; and for the sWBC >100 cells/mL, the iLR is infinity.[11] Gram stain of synovial fluid is specific (approaching 100%) for nongonococcal septic arthritis, but its sensitivity is poor, with 40–55% false-negative rates.[19] Although synovial fluid should be evaluated for uric acid or calcium pyrophosphate crystals, telltale signs of crystalloid arthropathies, septic arthritis may still be present as it can coexist with gout or pseudogout in 1.5% of cases.[20]

Several retrospective series have explored the diagnostic accuracy of ESR and CRP in adults with monoarticular arthritis. Li et al assessed only cases of confirmed septic arthritis and demonstrated a sensitivity of 96% for ESR >30 mm/hour. Given the possibility of selection bias, this sensitivity may be falsely elevated.[21] In another retrospective review, Li et al demonstrated a ESR sensitivity of 75% and a specificity of 11% using the same definition of abnormal.[22] Hariharan only assessed confirmed septic arthritis cases and, using a threshold of ESR >10 mm/hour and CRP ≥ 20 mg/L, noted sensitivities of 98% and 92%, respectively.[23] Using ESR >15 mm/hour and CRP >0.8 mg/L, Ernst et al demonstrated sensitivities of 66% and 90%, respectively.[24] Söderquist et al demonstrated that both ESR (mean 81 mm/hour versus 54 mm/hour) and CRP (mean 182 mg/L versus 101 mg/L) were significantly higher on admission in patients with septic arthritis than in those with a crystalloid arthropathy.[17]

No clinical decision rules have been derived to assist with the diagnosis of adult septic arthritis. Single-center validation of a pediatric CDR identified four variables associated with increased risk of hip septic arthritis, with a receiver operating curve (ROC) area under the curve of 0.86: history of a fever, non-weight-bearing, ESR >40, and serum WBC >12.[25]

Comment

While a history of recent joint surgery (generally within 3 months) and the physical exam finding of cellulitis overlying a prosthetic knee or hip, other history, physical exam, and routine blood tests are not helpful in distinguishing septic arthritis from other forms of monoarticular arthritis. In other words, neither the presence nor the absence of any of these findings significantly changes the probability of septic arthritis. In contrast, the presence of a synovial WBC $>100,000$ will significantly increase the probability of septic arthritis from 27% to 91% based upon the dichotomous likelihood ratio. Future trials are needed to evaluate the value of inflammatory synovial markers such as lactate, LDH, TNF_α, IL-6, or IL-8, which may be useful to rule out septic arthritis. In addition, prospective trials enrolling consecutive patients with suspected septic arthritis are needed in adults and children to fully understand the sensitivity, specificity, and positive and negative likelihood ratios for elements of the history and physical exam. Diagnostic trials that only evaluate patients with disease will falsely increase the measured sensitivity.[26] Combinations of findings from the history and physical exam, serum, and synovial fluid labs may be more accurate than any single finding, so methodologically rigorous clinical decision rule derivation and validation trials are also needed. In the meantime, clinicians should be aware of the risk factors for gonococcal and nongonococcal septic arthritis and expeditiously select appropriate diagnostic and therapeutic options while consulting orthopedic surgery for early operative management in cases where the clinical evaluation remains less than definitive.

References

1. Margaretten M, Kohlwes J, Moore D, Bent S. Does this adult patient have septic arthritis? Journal of the American Medical Association. 2007; 297: 1478–788.
2. Goldenberg DL. Septic arthritis. Lancet 1998; 351: 197–202.
3. Kaandorp C, Van Schaardenburg D, Krijnen P, Habbema J, Van De Laar M. Risk factors for septic arthritis in patients with joint disease. Arthritis & Rheumatism. 1995; 38: 1819–25.
4. Kaandorp C, Dinant H, Van De Laar M, Moens H, Prins A, Dijkmans B. Incidence and sources of native and prosthetic joint infection: A community based prospective survey. Annals of the Rheumatic Diseases. 1997; 56: 470–5.
5. Gupta MN, Sturrock RD, Field M. A prospective 2-year study of 75 patients with adult-onset septic arthritis. Rheumatology. 2001; 40: 24–30.
6. Gupta MN, Sturrock RD, Field M. Prospective comparative study of patients with culture proven and high suspicion of adult onset septic arthritis. Annals of the Rheumatic Diseases. 2003; 62: 327–31.

7. Frazee BW, Fee C, Lambert L. How common is MRSA in adult septic arthritis? Annals of Emergency Medicine. 2009; 54: 695–700.

8. Saraux A, Taelman H, Blanche P et al. HIV infection as a risk factor for septic arthritis. British Journal of Rheumatology. 1997; 36: 333–7.

9. Bardin T; Gonococcal arthritis, Best Pract Research Clin Rheum 2003; 17: 201–208.

10. Angulo JM, Espinoza LR. Gonococcal arthritis. Comprehensive Therapy. 1999; 25: 155–62.

11. Carpenter CR, Schuur JD, Everett WW, Pines JM. Evidence-based diagnostics: Adult septic arthritis. Academic Emergency Medicine. 2011; 18: 781–96.

12. Jeng GW, Wang CR, Liu ST et al. Measurement of synovial tumor necrosis factor-alpha in diagnosing emergency patients with bacterial arthritis. American Journal of Emergency Medicine. 1997; 15: 626–9.

13. Kortekangas P, Aro H, Tuominen J, Toivanen A. Synovial fluid leukocytosis in bacterial arthritis vs. reactive arthritis and rheumatoid arthritis in the adult knee. Scandanavian Journal of Rheumatology. 1992; 21: 283–8.

14. Thumboo J, O'Duffy JD. A prospective study of the safety of joint and soft tissue aspirations and injections in patients taking warfarin sodium. Arthritis & Rheumatism. 1998; 41: 736–9.

15. Krey PR, Bailen DA. Synovial fluid leukocytosis: A study of extremes. American Journal of Medicine 1979; 67: 436–42.

16. Shmerling R, Delbanco T, Tosteson A, Trentham D. Synovial fluid tests: What should be ordered? Journal of the American Medical Association. 1990; 264: 1009–14.

17. Söderquist B, Jones I, Fredlund H, Vikerfors T. Bacterial or crystal-associated arthritis? Discriminating ability of serum inflammatory markers. Scandanavian Journal of Infectious Disease. 1998; 30: 591–6.

18. Pauker SG, Kassirer JP. The threshold approach to clinical decision making. New England Journal of Medicine. 1980; 302: 1109–17.

19. Faraj A, Omonbude O, Godwin P. Gram staining in the diagnosis of acute septic arthritis. Acta Orthopaedica Belgica. 2002; 68: 388–91.

20. Shah K, Spear J, Nathanson LA, Mccauley J, Edlow JA. Does the presence of crystal arthritis rule out septic arthritis? Journal of Emergency Medicine. 2007; 32: 23–6.

21. Li SF, Henderson J, Dickman E, Darzynkiewicz R. Laboratory tests in adults with monoarticular arthritis: Can they rule out a septic joint? Academic Emergency Medicine. 2004; 11: 276–80.

22. Li SF, Cassidy C, Chang C, Gharib S, Torres J. Diagnostic utility of laboratory tests in septic arthritis. Emergency Medicine Journal. 2007; 24: 75–7.

23. Hariharan P, Kabrhel C. Sensitivity of erythrocyte sedimentation rate and c-reactive protein for the exclusion of septic arthritis in emergency department patients. Journal of Emergency Medicine. 2011; 40: 428–31.

24. Ernst AA, Weiss SJ, Tracy LA, Weiss NR. Usefulness of CRP and ESR in predicting septic joints. Southern Medical Journal. 2010; 103: 522–6.

25. Kocher MS, Mandiga R, Zurakowski D, Barnewolt C, Kasser JR. Validation of a clinical prediction rule for the differentiation between septic arthritis and transient synovitis of the hip in children. Journal of Bone and Joint Surgery, American Volume. 2004; 86–A: 1629–35.

26. Newman TB, Kohn MA. Evidence-based diagnosis (practical guide to biostatistics and epidemiology). Cambridge: Cambridge University Press; 2009.

Chapter 35 **Osteomyelitis**

Highlights

- Very little research has been conducted on the diagnosis of nondiabetic foot osteomyelitis.
- Ulcer size >2 cm, a positive probe-to-bone test, or ESR >70 mm/hour each independently increases the likelihood of the diagnosis of diabetic osteomyelitis.
- Only a negative MRI significantly decreases the likelihood of diabetic foot osteomyelitis.
- Other history, physical exam, laboratory results, and imaging tests do not significantly reduce the posttest probability for diabetic foot osteomyelitis.

Background

Osteomyelitis is an infectious, inflammatory process that results in bony destruction. The infection can be isolated to the cortex or involve the periosteum and surrounding soft tissues (Figure 35.1).[1] The symptoms of acute osteomyelitis are typically noted over weeks, while chronic osteomyelitis can evolve over months or years. Gram-positive organisms, *Staphylococcus aureus* in particular, are the most common organisms involved, but the specific infective agent depends upon the site of infection and whether the joint is prosthetic or native (Figure 35.2). Since the inflammatory process destroys vascular channels, systemic antibiotics do not penetrate infections and are rarely effective alone. Surgical debridement with antibiotics has become the standard of care.[2]

Osteomyelitis affects all age groups. Although instrumentation-related (prosthetic joint) osteomyelitis is most common, hematogenous infections can occur in both the pediatric and geriatric populations.[3] Osteomyelitis can also result from direct inoculation or contiguous spread from an adjacent area

Evidence-Based Emergency Care: Diagnostic Testing and Clinical Decision Rules, Second Edition.
Jesse M. Pines, Christopher R. Carpenter, Ali S. Raja and Jeremiah D. Schuur.
© 2013 John Wiley & Sons, Ltd. Published 2013 by John Wiley & Sons, Ltd.

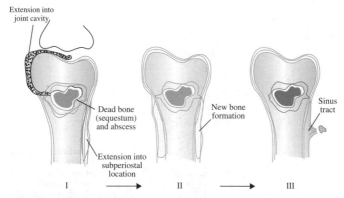

Figure 35.1 The progression of chronic osteomyelitis. Phase I: An area of devascularized dead bone is sequestered into an abscess cavity. Note that extension of intramedullary infection into an intracapsular location can result in septic arthritis, while progression into a periosteal location may produce periosteal elevation. Phase II: New bone formation results from periosteal elevation. Phase III: Extension of the abscess and necrotic material through cortical bone creates a fistula. (Reproduced from Jauregui LE et al. Diagnosis and management of bone infections (1995) with permission from Informa Healthcare).

of soft tissue infection. Risk factors for osteomyelitis include intravascular catheters, intravenous drug abuse, and nonbone foci of infections such as cellulitis, cutaneous abscesses, and urinary tract infections.[4] A history of sickle cell anemia can predispose children to osteomyelitis. Direct inoculation mechanisms include penetrating injuries such as open fractures or the internal fixation of long bone fractures.[4]

Foot ulcers can be venous, arterial, or diabetic, and the distinction can be challenging.[5] Generally, venous ulcers are proximal to the malleoli with irregular borders, whereas arterial ulcers involve the toes or shins with a pale and punched-out appearance. By comparison, diabetic ulcers typically occur in areas of increased pressure, such as the soles. Approximately 2.5% of diabetic patients also have Charcot neuropathy involving the tarsal or tarsometatarsal joints.[6] Charcot neuropathy can mimic diabetic osteomyelitis with a very similar clinical presentation, but the management for the two conditions is vastly different; the standard care for Charcot neuropathy is a cast and non-weight-bearing status rather than antibiotics and debridement. Distinguishing Charcot neuropathy from diabetic osteomyelitis is important for emergency physicians since catastrophic bony collapse in the ankle joint can occur in a short timeframe in Charcot neuropathy.[7]

Despite the fact that osteomyelitis of the foot or ankle is the primary or secondary reason for 75,000 hospitalizations in the United States each year,

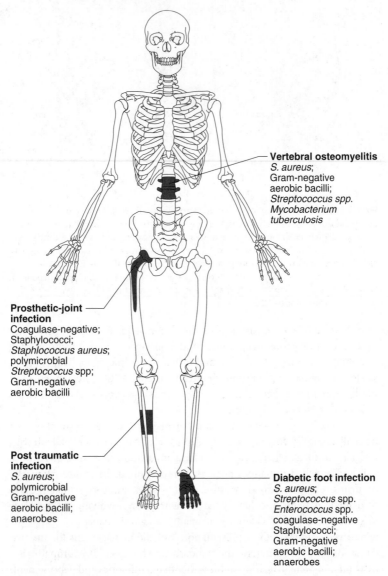

Vertebral osteomyelitis
S. aureus;
Gram-negative
aerobic bacilli;
Streptococcus spp.
Mycobacterium
tuberculosis

**Prosthetic-joint
infection**
Coagulase-negative;
Staphylococci;
Staphlococcus aureus;
polymicrobial
Streptococcus spp;
Gram-negative
aerobic bacilli

**Post traumatic
infection**
S. aureus;
polymicrobial
Gram-negative
aerobic bacilli;
anaerobes

Diabetic foot infection
S. aureus;
Streptococcus spp.
Enterococcus spp.
coagulase-negative
Staphylococci;
Gram-negative
aerobic bacilli;
anaerobes

Figure 35.2 The microbiology of osteomyelitis. The microorganisms of osteomyelitis in order of prevalence from high to low by site of infection. (Reprinted from [1] Lew DP, Waldvogel FA. Osteomyelitis. Lancet. 2004; 364(9431): 369–79. Copyright (2004), with permission from Elsevier).

clinicians often underestimate the likelihood of diabetic foot osteomyelitis.[8] Foot-related complications account for 20% of diabetes-related admissions in North America[9] and as many as 15% of patients with diabetic foot ulcers ultimately require amputations. One study found that, over a 3-year period, 61% of diabetic foot ulcers are likely to recur, 10% of ulcers will lead to amputation, and the overall survival rate for diabetic patients with foot ulcers was only 72% (compared to 87% for age- and gender-matched diabetic control patients).[10] The presence of diabetic foot osteomyelitis increases the risk of amputation with a 30-day postamputation perioperative mortality rate of 7–15%.[11–13]

A review of 2007 data from the Centers for Disease Control and the American Diabetic Association found that up to $38 billion was spent on diabetic foot ulcer-related problems in the United States that year. However, despite the expenses associated with diabetic foot ulcers, diagnostic cost-effectiveness models of osteomyelitis in these patients have yielded diverging recommendations. Eckman et al suggested that

> *noninvasive testing adds significant expense to the treatment of patients with non-insulin-dependent diabetes in whom pedal osteomyelitis is suspected and such testing may result in little improvement in health outcomes. In patients without systemic toxicity, a 10-week course of culture-guided oral antibiotic therapy following surgical debridement may be as effective as and less costly than other approaches.*[14]

On the other hand, Mushlin et al suggested that "when the likelihood of osteomyelitis is higher (10–20%), scanning results in outcomes and cost-effectiveness ratios comparable to those of immediate biopsy and is less invasive. When the probability of osteomyelitis is 50%, biopsy is quite cost-effective compared with all the other strategies ... and is preferred to the scan strategy."[15]

Clinical question

What is the diagnostic accuracy of X-ray, nuclear imaging, or magnetic resonance imaging (MRI) for the diagnosis of nondiabetic osteomyelitis?
Plain films can demonstrate joint space widening or narrowing, periosteal reaction, and bone destruction, although the latter is not apparent for up to 21 days after the onset of infection.[16] When metal is in close proximity to an area of osteomyelitis, image resolution is suboptimal due to beam-hardening artifact.[17] No studies have evaluated the diagnostic accuracy of plain films, nuclear imaging, or MRI for acute osteomyelitis. Narrative reviews have

reported unreferenced sensitivities for conventional X-ray of 43–75% and specificities of 75–83% for *acute* osteomyelitis.[17] Two studies totaling 33 patients summarized in one meta-analysis evaluated plain radiography for *chronic* osteomyelitis and found that sensitivity ranged from 60% to 78% and specificity from 67% to 100%.[18–20] Whalen et al assessed radiography for vertebral osteomyelitis only.[19] A systematic review has summarized only one study that assessed computed tomography to diagnosis chronic osteomyelitis. demonstrating a sensitivity of 67% and a specificity of 50%.[19,20]

Clinical question

What is the diagnostic accuracy of history, physical exam, or readily available labs for the diagnosis of diabetic foot osteomyelitis?

The best-estimate pretest probability for diabetic osteomyelitis in a patient with a clinically suspicious lesion is 15%.[21] Unfortunately, no findings on history or physical exam significantly *decrease* the probability of diabetic osteomyelitis (Table 35.1). Ulcer size >2 cm, bone exposure, a positive probe-to-bone test, a Wagner grade >2 (Table 35.1), or ESR >70 mm/h each significantly *increases* the likelihood of diabetic osteomyelitis.[22–26] A positive probe test is defined as when "on gentle probing, the evaluator detected a rock-hard, often gritty structure at the ulcer base without the apparent presence of any intervening soft tissue."[22] No studies have evaluated the role of serial white blood cell (WBC) counts, erythrocyte sedimentation rates (ESRs), or X-rays.

Clinical question

What is the diagnostic accuracy of X-ray, nuclear imaging, or MRI for the diagnosis of diabetic osteomyelitis?

X-ray criteria for osteomyelitis include focal loss of trabecular bone, periosteal reaction, and frank bone destruction. Plain film X-rays have been evaluated in 16 studies (six prospective) totaling 567 diabetic patients.[21] While positive x-ray findings can increase the probability of diabetic osteomyelitis, only a negative MRI can substantially reduce the likelihood of foot osteomyelitis in diabetic patients.[26] MRI criteria for osteomyelitis are generally defined as focally decreased marrow signal intensity in T1-weighted images and a focally increased signal intensity in fat-suppressed T2-weighted or short tau inversion recovery images (Figure 35.3a and b). One meta-analysis of 16 MRI studies reported a summary positive likelihood ratio of 3.8 (CI 2.5–5.8) and a negative likelihood ratio of 0.14 (CI 0.08–0.26), which was superior to the diagnostic accuracy of technetium-99m bone scanning using bone biopsy histology as the criterion standard.[26]

Table 35.1 Diagnostic test characteristics for diabetic osteomyelitis

Diagnostic test	Positive likelihood ratio	Negative likelihood ratio
Bone exposure	9.2	0.70
Probe to bone test	6.4	0.39
Ulcer area >2 cm^2	7.2	0.48
Ulcer inflammation	1.5	0.84
Clinical judgment (Wagner >2)	5.5	0.54
ESR >70 mm/h	11.0	0.34
Swab culture	1.0	1.0
X-ray	2.3	0.63
MRI	3.8	0.14

Note: Wagner Grading Scale:
- Grade 0 = No open lesions; may have evidence of healed lesions or deformities
- Grade 1 = Superficial ulcer
- Grade 2 = Deeper ulcer to tendon, bone, or joint capsule
- Grade 3 = Deeper tissues involved, with abscess, osteomyelitis, or tendonitis
- Grade 4 = Localized gangrene of toe or forefoot
- Grade 5 = Gangrene of foot.

Source: Data from [21].

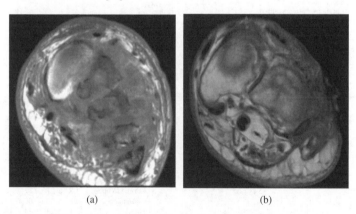

(a)   (b)

Figure 35.3 MRI appearance of (a) Charcot neuropathy compared with (b) osteomyelitis. (a) Neuropathic arthropathy. MRI demonstrating diffuse soft tissue swelling without an ulcer. Constellation of findings (soft tissue swelling, no ulcer, joint disorganization and bone fragmentation) characteristic of neuropathic arthropathy. (b) Osteomyelitis: MRI demonstrating large soft tissue ulcer in continuity with cuboid bone marrow edema and destruction, diagnostic of osteomyelitis on MRI. In the radiology of diabetic feet, no ulcer = no osteomyelitis. (Images courtesy of Dr. Jennifer Demertzis, Assistant Professor, Department of Radiology, Washington University in St. Louis).

Another meta-analysis evaluated the diagnostic accuracy of various nuclear imaging studies for diabetic foot infections, including technetium and tagged WBC scans.[27] Sensitivities range from 80.7% to 96.8%, but specificities were lower (46.4–88.5%). The optimal nuclear imaging test appeared to be the ^{99m}Tc/^{111} In-WBC scan with a positive likelihood ratio of 7.0 and a negative likelihood ratio of 0.22, but the human immunoglobulin study had a negative likelihood ratio of 0.05.[27] Bone scintigraphy can yield false-positive results with Charcot arthropathy, gout, trauma, or surgery.[1]

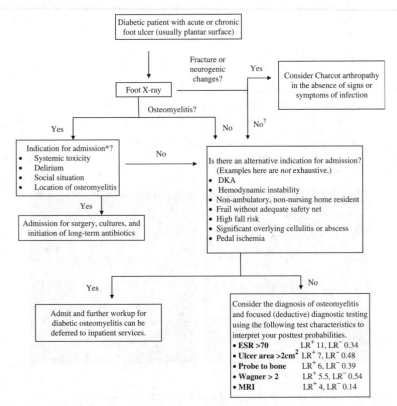

*Osteomyelitis diagnosis by itself may not automatically require admission. For example, chronic osteomyelitis or isolated toe osteomyelitis can be managed as an outpatient. In general, the more proximal the osteomyelitis is (i.e., forefoot < midfoot or rear-foot < ankle), the higher the risk of limb loss and progression.
†Charcot osteoarthropathy can exist without apparent fracture on X-ray. Therefore, if the patient has a warm, swollen foot with or without pain and without other evidence of infection, Charcot should still be considered even if X-rays are nondiagnostic.

Figure 35.4 Diagnostic algorithm for diabetic foot osteomyelitis in the emergency department.

Comment

No research describing the diagnostic accuracy for history, physical exam, or laboratory evaluation for adult osteomyelitis in nondiabetic patients was identified. Similarly, very little diagnostic imaging accuracy research has been identified in systematic reviews of nondiabetic osteomyelitis.

Although the probe-to-bone test offers one potential, biologically plausible, and low-cost option to quickly diagnose probable osteomyelitis of diabetic foot ulcers, further research is needed to verify the reliability and diagnostic accuracy of this test in the hands of emergency providers. In addition, the willingness of emergency physicians and specialists to incorporate the results of probe testing into diagnostic and therapeutic algorithms to obviate the need for expensive and time-consuming imaging modalities such as bone scan and MRI would be determined only by a randomized controlled trial.[28] If consultants require an MRI regardless of the results of the probe-to-bone test, then there would be minimal value to performing the probe test. Figure 35.4 provides an algorithm based upon the best available evidence to guide the diagnostic evaluation of diabetic foot ulcers with suspected osteomyelitis in the emergency department.

Future research is needed to understand the usefulness and reliability of combinations of history, physical exam, labs, and imaging tests for the risk stratification of osteomyelitis in ED patients with diabetic foot lesions. Ultimately, a clinical decision rule may help to efficiently and reliably risk-stratify diabetic foot lesions for osteomyelitis in the ED.

References

1. Lew DP, Waldvogel FA. Osteomyelitis. Lancet. 2004; 364(9431): 369–79.
2. Conterno LO, da Silva Filho CR. Antibiotics for treating chronic osteomyelitis in adults. Cochrane Database Systematic Reviews. 2009(3): CD004439.
3. Haas DW, McAndrew MP. Bacterial osteomyelitis in adults: Evolving considerations in diagnosis and treatment. American Journal of Medicine. 1996; 101(5): 550–61.
4. Wald ER. Risk factors for osteomyelitis. American Journal of Medicine. 1985; 78(6B): 206–12.
5. London NG, Donnelly R. ABC of arterial and venous disease: Ulcerated lower limb. British Medical Journal. 2000; 320(7249): 1589–91.
6. Gierbolini R. Charcot's foot: Often overlooked complication of diabetes. Journal of the American Academy of Physician Assistants. 1999; 12(6): 62–8.
7. van der Ven A, Chapman CB, Bowker JH. Charcot neuroarthropathy of the foot and ankle. Journal of the American Academy of Orthopaedic Surgeons. 2009; 17(9): 562–71.

8. Newman LG, Waller J, Palestro CJ, Schwartz M, Klein MJ, Hermann G *et al.* Unsuspected osteomyelitis in diabetic foot ulcers: Diagnosis and monitoring by leukocyte scanning with indium in 111 oxyquinoline. Journal of the American Medical Association. 1991; 266(9): 1246–51.

9. Berard LD, Booth G, Capes S, Quinn K, Woo V. Canadian Diabetes Association 2008 Clinical Practice Guidelines for the prevention and management of diabetes in Canada. Canadian Journal of Diabetes. 2008; 32(Suppl 1): 1–215.

10. Apelqvist J, Larsson J, Agardh CD. Long-term prognosis for diabetic patients with foot ulcers. Journal of Internal Medicine. 1993; 233(6): 485–91.

11. Bamberger DM, Daus GP, Gerding DN. Osteomyelitis in the feet of diabetic patients: Long-term results, prognostic factors, and the role of antimicrobial and surgical therapy. American Journal of Medicine. 1987; 83(4): 653–60.

12. Subramaniam B, Pomposelli F, Talmor D, Park KW. Perioperative and long-term morbidity and mortality after above-knee and below-knee amputations in diabetics and nondiabetics. Anesthesia & Analgesia. 2005; 100(5): 1241–7.

13. Stone PA, Flaherty SK, Aburahma AF, Hass SM, Jackson JM, Hayes JD *et al.* Factors affecting perioperative mortality and wound-related complications following major lower extremity amputations. Annals of Vascular Surgery. 2006; 20(2): 209–16.

14. Eckman MH, Greenfield S, Mackey WC, Wong JB, Kaplan S, Sullivan L *et al.* Foot infections in diabetic patients: Decision and cost-effectiveness analyses. Journal of the American Medical Association. 1995; 273(9): 712–20.

15. Mushlin AI, Littenberg B. Diagnosing pedal osteomyelitis: Testing choices and their consequences. Journal of General Internal Medicine. 1994; 9(1): 1–7.

16. Gold RH, Hawkins RA, Katz RD. Bacterial osteomyelitis: Findings on plain radiography, CT, MR, and scintigraphy. American Journal of Roentgenology. 1991; 157(2): 365–70.

17. Pineda C, Espinosa R, Pena A. Radiographic imaging in osteomyelitis: The role of plain radiography, computed tomography, ultrasonography, magnetic resonance imaging, and scintigraphy. Seminars in Plastic Surgery. 2009; 23(2): 80–9.

18. Al-Sheikh W, Sfakianakis GN, Mnaymneh W, Hourani M, Heal A, Duncan RC *et al.* Subacute and chronic bone infections: Diagnosis using In-111, Ga-67 and Tc-99m MDP bone scintigraphy, and radiography. Radiology. 1985; 155(2): 501–6.

19. Whalen JL, Brown ML, McLeod R, Fitzgerald RH. Limitations of indium leukocyte imaging for the diagnosis of spine infections. Spine. 1991; 16(2): 193–7.

20. Termaat MF, Raijmakers PG, Scholten HJ, Bakker FC, Patka P, Haarman HJ. The accuracy of diagnostic imaging for the assessment of chronic osteomyelitis: A systematic review and meta-analysis. Journal of Bone and Joint Surgery, American Volume. 2005; 87(11): 2464–71.

21. Butalia S, Palda VA, Sargeant RJ, Detsky AS, Mourad O. Does this patient with diabetes have osteomyelitis of the lower extremity? Journal of the American Medical Association. 2008; 299(7): 806–13.

22. Grayson ML, Gibbons GW, Balogh K, Levin E, Karchmer AW. Probing to bone in infected pedal ulcers: A clinical sign of underlying osteomyelitis in diabetic patients. Journal of the American Medical Association. 1995; 273(9): 721–3.

23. Wagner FW. The dysvascular foot: A system for diagnosis and treatment. Foot Ankle. 1981; 2(2): 64–122.

24. Enderle MD, Coerper S, Schweizer HP, Kopp AE, Thelen MH, Meisner C *et al*. Correlation of imaging techniques to histopathology in patients with diabetic foot syndrome and clinical suspicion of chronic osteomyelitis: The role of high-resolution ultrasound. Diabetes Care. 1999; 22(2): 294–9.

25. Vesco L, Boulahdour H, Hamissa S, Kretz S, Montazel JL, Perlemuter L *et al*. The value of combined radionuclide and magnetic resonance imaging in the diagnosis and conservative management of minimal or localized osteomyelitis of the foot in diabetic patients. Metabolism. 1999; 48(7): 922–7.

26. Kapoor A, Page S, Lavalley M, Gale DR, Felson DT. Magnetic resonance imaging for diagnosing foot osteomyelitis: A meta-analysis. Archives of Internal Medicine. 2007; 167(2): 125–32.

27. Capriotti G, Chianelli M, Signore A. Nuclear medicine imaging of diabetic foot infection: Results of meta-analysis. Nuclear Medicine Communications. 2006; 27(10): 757–64.

28. Lord SJ, Irwig L, Simes RJ. When is measuring sensitivity and specificity sufficient to evaluate a diagnostic test, and when do we need randomized trials? Annals of Internal Medicine. 2006; 144(11): 850–5.

Chapter 36 **Sexually Transmitted Diseases (STDs)**

Highlights

- Sexually transmitted diseases (STDs) are frequent causes of ED visits, either for genitourinary symptoms, such as dysuria or discharge, or for nonspecific symptoms, such as abdominal pain.
- There is not a validated clinical decision rule to reliably distinguish a urinary tract infection from an STD in women with dysuria, so clinicians should have a low threshold for testing and treating for STDs.
- Nucleic acid amplification–based tests for chlamydia and gonorrhea perform as well on first-catch urine samples as on endocervical or urethral swabs, allowing patients to avoid these more painful collection procedures.

Background

Sexually transmitted diseases (STDs) cause a significant number of emergency department (ED) visits and are prevalent in the population visiting the ED. The most common presenting complaints associated with STDs are urethritis or cervicitis, but patients with STDs can present with complaints due to sequellae of STDs such as pelvic inflammatory disease (PID), tubo-ovarian abscesses, orchitis, or nonspecific complaints such as abdominal pain. Pelvic inflammatory disease (PID) is the most frequent gynecologic cause of ED visits, with approximately 250,000 ED visits per year.[1] Additionally, a small but significant proportion of ED patients (5% – 10%) have been found to have asymptomatic STDs during routine screening programs.[2,3]

In the ED, diagnosis and treatment of STDs are particularly important, as many ED patients are at risk, do not have regular access to healthcare, and may not follow up with primary care providers. If the diagnosis and appropriate treatment are not made during or directly out of the ED visit, an STD may smolder, leaving the patient at risk of the sequelae of an untreated STD,

Evidence-Based Emergency Care: Diagnostic Testing and Clinical Decision Rules, Second Edition. Jesse M. Pines, Christopher R. Carpenter, Ali S. Raja and Jeremiah D. Schuur.
© 2013 John Wiley & Sons, Ltd. Published 2013 by John Wiley & Sons, Ltd.

including PID, infertility, ectopic pregnancy, and transmission to others. Studies have found that emergency providers do not accurately diagnose STDs. A study by Yealy et al found that among 148 female ED patients with culture-proven gonorrhea or chlamydia, 53% were treated with a regimen suggested by the CDC prior to ED release.[4] Of those not treated, one-quarter were lost to follow-up and 20% had delays to treatment of 14–60 days. On the other hand, studies have shown that only 10–20% of patients diagnosed with cervictis or PID in the ED ultimately have positive diagnostic tests for STDs.[5,6] Due to a lack of definitive diagnostic test results in the ED and lack of continuity of care, having a low threshold to treat is more reasonable. In this chapter, we address the clinical presentation of urethritis, and laboratory diagnostic tests for *Chlamydia trachomatis* and *N. gonorrhea*. We do not address other STDs including HIV, herpes, and syphilis. We do not address the diagnosis of PID, as this is a clinical diagnosis, and clinical studies have not consistently shown a preferred diagnostic algorithm.[7] For additional information, readers can review the Centers for Disease Control and Prevention (CDC), "Sexually Transmitted Diseases Treatment Guidelines, 2010."[8]

Clinical question

Can the history, physical exam, and urinalysis reliably differentiate a urinary tract infection (UTI) from a STD?

Urinary symptoms such as dyusuria, frequency, and discharge are common chief complaints in the ED and can represent a simple UTI or an STD, such as gonorrhea or chlamydia (see Chapter 32). Clinicians typically take a history and a physical and obtain urinalysis including urine dipstick and microscopy when evaluating such patients. Historically, emergency providers would use microscopy and Gram stain of urethral discharge or swab material to identify the presence of *N. gonorrhea*, but the Gram stain in isolation lacks sufficient diagnostic ability to detect either *C. trachomatis* or *N. gonorrhea* infection in the ED.[9] Differentiating between a UTI and urethritis or cervicitis from an STD is an important clinical question. As the definitive diagnostic tests for STDs do not generally come back during the course of an ED visit, clinicians must decide which patients to treat for STDs. A number of studies have examined the prevalence of UTIs and STDs in ED patients with symptoms of a UTI. These studies have focused on women, and most have focused on adolescent women in inner-city EDs; they have found that among patients with symptoms of a UTI, the prevalence of an STD ranges from 17% to 33%.

Shapiro et al analyzed a prospective cohort of 92 adult female ED patients with urinary frequency, urgency, dysuria, and no new vaginal discharge or change in discharge. They found that using the history, examination, and urine dip results, clinicians were 50% sensitive (CI 23–77%) and 86% specific (CI 76–93%) for an STD.[10] They also found that the only independent predictor of an STD was a history of having more than one sex partner during the preceding year. Huppert et al analyzed a cross-sectional sample of 296 sexually active females aged 14–22 years in a hospital-based teen health center or ED, including 154 with urinary symptoms. They found that the presence or absence of a UTI was not predictive of an STD and that likelihood of an STD was increased in subjects reporting more than one sexual partner within the past 3 months (OR 4.5) and in those reporting a prior history of STD (OR 3.0).[11] Berg et al reviewed the charts of 94 female ED patients who had pelvic examinations and were released from the ED with a sole diagnosis of UTI.[12] They found that 53% had proven STDs (19% gonorrhea, 22% chlamydia, and 33% trichomonas) and that complaints, physical findings, and laboratory results did not predict which patients did or did not have STDs.

Reed et al analyzed a cross-sectional sample of 250 adolescent females with symptoms leading the clinician to perform STD testing, in order to develop a decision rule to identify adolescent females with cervical infections.[13] Predictors of an STD were African American race (OR = 3.2), new partner within 3 months (OR = 1.9), cervical discharge (OR = 2.0), absence of yeast forms (OR = 3.3), and >10 white blood cells (OR = 2.5) on vaginal Gram stain. Yet, an algorithm using these variables was only 75% sensitive and 71% specific, with a negative predictive value of 85%. Prentiss et al performed a prospective cross-sectional study of 233 females aged 13 to 21 years who presented to an urban pediatric ED with urinary symptoms.[14] Pediatric emergency physicians' diagnoses of STD or UTI were compared with the criterion standard diagnosis. Of the 211 patients with complete data, 120 (57%) patients had UTIs and 19 patients (9%) had STDs. Physicians predicted STDs in 35 patients (17%), of which 9 (25%) had laboratory-proven infections. STDs in 10 patients (53%) were undiagnosed, in 26 patients (74%) were misdiagnosed, and in 9 patients (26%) were correctly diagnosed. Thirteen patients (6%) had co-infection with both an STD and a UTI. The authors of these studies concluded that all adolescent patients presenting with urinary symptoms and STD risk factors should be tested for STDs and UTIs and either have adequate follow-up established to ensure timely treatment or should be treated from the ED.

Clinical question

Can urine tests reliably diagnose gonorrhea and chlamydia?

Multiple tests are available to diagnose gonorrhea and chlamydia. Diagnostic tests available for chlamydia include culture, direct immunofluorescence, enzyme-linked immunosorbent assay (ELISA), and nucleic acid amplification techniques (NAATs). Until the development of nucleic acid–based diagnostic tests, the criterion standard for diagnosing chlamydia was tissue culture of urethral or cervical swab specimens, a timely and expensive test, with sensitivity of only 50–85%.[15] Nucleic acid–based diagnostic tests can be performed on an endocervical sample (obtained by rotating a swab within the endocervical canal during a speculum exam), on a vaginal swab specimen, or on urine. The latter two can be collected without performing a pelvic exam. Using the "first-void urine" specimen, the initial urine sample voided after awakening, increases sensitivity. In the ED, this should be the first catch of the first urine sample produced.

Cook et al performed a systematic review of studies that assessed the sensitivity and specificity of three commercially available nucleic acid amplification tests (polymerase chain reaction, transcription-mediated amplification, and strand displacement amplification assays) for *C. trachomatis* and *N. gonorrhea* in urine specimens.[15] They identified 29 eligible studies and calculated separate summary estimates for men and women and for chlamydial and gonococcal infections for each assay. The test characteristics are summarized in Table 36.1.

The pooled specificities of each of the three assays on urine samples were higher than 97% for both chlamydial infection and gonorrhea. The sensitivities did not vary according to the prevalence of infection or the presence of symptoms. The authors concluded that the results of nucleic acid amplification tests on urine samples for chlamydia are comparable to those obtained on samples collected directly from the cervix or urethra, but that the sensitivity of the polymerase chain reaction assay for gonorrhea in women's urine is much lower than in urethral swabs and should not be used.

While nucleic acid amplification techniques generally are not available during the course of an ED visit, several point-of-care (POC) tests exist for chlamydia. Hislop et al conducted a systematic review of the clinical effectiveness of rapid POC tests for the diagnosis of genital chlamydia infection.[16] They included 13 studies enrolling 8,817 participants and calculated summary test characteristics. The pooled estimates for the chlamydia rapid test (CRT) on vaginal swab specimens were a sensitivity of 80% (CI 73–85%) and specificity of 99% (CI 99–100%); for first void urine (FVU), specimen's sensitivity was 77% (CI 59–89%) and specificity was 99% (CI 98–99%). The pooled

Table 36.1 Diagnostic characteristics of nucleic acid amplification tests for STDs

| | *Chlamydia trachomatis* | | | |
| | Urine samples | | Urethral samples | |
Test	Sensitivity (%)	Specificity (%)	Sensitivity (%)	Specificity (%)
Polymerase chain	M: 84%	M: 99%	M: 88%	M: 99%
reaction (PCR)	F: 83%	F: 99%	F: 86%	F: 99%
Transcription-mediated	M: 88%	M: 99%	M: 96%	M: 99%
amplification (TMA)	F: 93%	F: 99%	F: 97%	F: 99%
Strand displacement	M: 93%	M: 94%	M: 92%	M: 96%
amplification (SDA)	F: 80%	F: 99%	F: 94%	F: 98%
	Neisseria gonorrhea			
	Urine samples		Urethral samples	
Test	Sensitivity (%)	Specificity (%)	Sensitivity (%)	Specificity (%)
PCR	M: 90%	M: 99%	M: 96%	M: 99%
	F: 56%	F: 99%	F: 94%	F: 99%
TMA	M: n/a	M: n/a	M: n/a	M: n/a
	F: 91%	F: 99%	F: 99%	F: 99%
SDA	M: n/a	M: n/a	M: n/a	M: n/a
	F: 85%	F: 99%	F: 97%	F: 99%

Note: n/a = no studies met inclusion criteria; M = males; and F = females.
Source: Data from [15].

estimates of a second test, Clearview Chlamydia, on vaginal, cervical, and urethral swab specimens combined, were a sensitivity of 52% (CI 39–65%) and specificity of 97% (CI 94–100%). The authors concluded that as both POC tests were more costly and less effective than nucleic acid amplification techniques, nucleic acid tests should still be the diagnostic test of choice.

Comment

In patients with genitourinary symptoms suggestive of UTI or PID, testing and treatment should be based upon the clinical probability of the patient having an STD and their likelihood of following up for outpatient care. There is not yet a reliable clinical decision rule using history, physical, and urinalysis results that can differentiate between UTI and STD among patients with dysuria. One clinical decision rule has been derived for adolescent women, but it has low sensitivity and specificity.[13] Individuals with the possibility of an STD should undergo testing with a nucleic acid amplification testing for gonorrhea and chlamydia. Clinicians should identify which test their local lab uses, as it affects diagnostic test performance. All nucleic acid tests are comparable for testing for chlamydia in urine samples or urethral swabs.

The sensitivity of the polymerase chain reaction assay for gonorrhea in women's urine is much lower than in cervical swabs and should not be used. Antibiotic treatment should be given in the ED to patients with moderate to high risk of an STD, and to patients in whom the clinician has any suspicion, if follow-up cannot be reliably arranged. All patients at risk for an STD should be referred for outpatient HIV testing.

References

1. Sutton MY, Sternberg M, Zaidi A *et al.* Trends in pelvic inflammatory disease hospital discharges and ambulatory visits, United States, 1985–2001. Sexually Transmitted Diseases. 2005; 32: 778–84.

2. Todd CS, Haase C, Stoner BP. Emergency department screening for asymptomatic sexually transmitted infections. American Journal of Public Health. 2001 Mar; 91(3): 461–4.

3. Mehta SD, Hall J, Lyss SB *et al.* Adult and pediatric emergency department sexually transmitted disease and HIV screening: Programmatic overview and outcomes. Academic Emergency Medicine. 2007; 14: 250–8.

4. Yealy DM, Greene TJ, Hobbs GD. Underrecognition of cervical *Neisseria gonorrhoeae* and *Chlamydia trachomatis* infections in the emergency department. Academic Emergency Medicine. 1997; 4: 962–7.

5. Burnett AM, Anderson CP, Zwank MD. Laboratory-Confirmed Gonorrhea and/or Chlamydia Rates in Clinically Diagnosed Pelvic Inflammatory Disease and cervicitis. *American Journal of Emergency Medicine.* 2012 Sep; 30(7): 1114–7.

6. Parker CA, Topinka MA. The incidence of positive cultures in women suspected of having PID/salpingitis. Academic Emergency Medicine. 2000; 7: 1170.

7. Blenning CE, Muench J, Judkins DZ *et al.* Clinical inquiries: Which tests are most useful for diagnosing PID? Journal of Family Practice. 2007; 56: 216–20.

8. Workowski KA, Berman S, Centers for Disease Control and Prevention (CDC). Sexually transmitted diseases treatment guidelines, 2010. MMWR Recommendations and Reports. 2010; 59: 1–110.

9. Stefanski P, Hafner JW, Riley SL *et al.* Diagnostic utility of the genital Gram stain in ED patients. American Journal of Emergency Medicine. 2010; 28: 13–18.

10. Shapiro T, Dalton M, Hammock J *et al.* The prevalence of urinary tract infections and sexually transmitted disease in women with symptoms of a simple urinary tract infection stratified by low colony count criteria. Academic Emergency Medicine. 2005; 12: 38–44.

11. Huppert JS, Biro F, Lan D *et al.* Urinary symptoms in adolescent females: STI or UTI? Journal of Adolescence Health. 2007; 40: 418–24.

12. Berg E, Benson DM, Haraszkiewicz P *et al.* High prevalence of sexually transmitted diseases in women with urinary infections. Academic Emergency Medicine. 1996; 3: 1030–4.

13. Reed JL, Mahabee-Gittens EM, Huppert JS. A decision rule to identify adolescent females with cervical infections. Journal of Women's Health (Larchmont). 2007; 16: 272–80.

14. Prentiss KA, Newby PK, Vinci RJ. Adolescent female with urinary symptoms: A diagnostic challenge for the pediatrician. Pediatric Emergency Care. 2011; 27: 789–94.

15. Cook RL, Hutchison SL, Ostergaard L *et al.* Systematic review: Noninvasive testing for *Chlamydia trachomatis* and *Neisseria gonorrhoeae*. Annals of Internal Medicine. 2005; 142: 914–25.

16. Hislop J, Quayyum Z, Flett G *et al.* Systematic review of the clinical effectiveness and cost-effectiveness of rapid point-of-care tests for the detection of genital chlamydia infection in women and men. Health Technology Assessment. 2010; 14: 1–97, iii–iv.

Chapter 37 **Influenza**

Highlights

- Assessing the current regional pretest probability of influenza is essential to distinguishing influenza from influenza-like illness mimics.
- Taken alone, no signs or symptoms accurately rule in or rule out the diagnosis of influenza.
- Rapid influenza tests can effectively rule in, but not rule out, the diagnosis of influenza and are superior to clinical gestalt. However, they are cost-effective only within a narrow range of disease prevalence.

Background

Each year, up to 20% of residents in the United States and United Kingdom develop influenza, resulting in over 134,000 hospitalizations.[1] Influenza increases morbidity and mortality for a number of specific patient populations, including the very young, the elderly, and those with chronic lung disease.[2–5] Geriatric patients (>65 years) account for 90% of the 3,000–48,000 annual influenza deaths in the United States.[6] In general, healthy children and young adults do not experience life-threatening complications from influenza, but antigenic shifts in 1918, 1957, and 1968 were associated with viral pneumonia, acute respiratory distress syndrome, and multiorgan failure in these populations. Interpandemic influenza is an extremely unpleasant experience even for healthy individuals, with significant costs accrued due to diminished productivity, absenteeism, and related healthcare expenditures. In the United States, influenza results in $10.4 billion (2003 US$) in direct healthcare costs and $16.3 billion in lost earnings each year.[1,7]

Emergency department (ED) resources are occasionally strained by influenza-like illness (ILI) pandemics such as severe acute respiratory syndrome (SARS) in 2003 and H1N1 swine flu in 2009. Since infectious patients

---

Evidence-Based Emergency Care: Diagnostic Testing and Clinical Decision Rules, Second Edition. Jesse M. Pines, Christopher R. Carpenter, Ali S. Raja and Jeremiah D. Schuur.
© 2013 John Wiley & Sons, Ltd. Published 2013 by John Wiley & Sons, Ltd.

need to be sequestered during such pandemics in order to limit the exposure of the general population, diagnostic testing may be unavailable, emphasizing the importance of emergency clinicians' understanding of the diagnostic accuracy of bedside testing to distinguish influenza from ILI.[8] ILI is defined by the Centers for Disease Control (CDC) as a temperature higher than 37.8°C with a cough or sore throat, but patients with influenza may present to the ED with a variety of atypical manifestations including delirium, falls, vomiting, incontinence, or diarrhea. Clinicians must integrate the chief complaint with a thorough review of systems within the context of their own regional influenza prevalence.[9]

Two strains of influenza exist (Type A and Type B) and are clinically indistinguishable. However, the distinction remains relevant because older antiviral agents (amantadine and rimantadine) are effective for Type A only. Newer antiviral medications like oseltamivir are effective against both types, but only if used within 48 hours of symptom onset, emphasizing the importance of early diagnosis.[10] Unfortunately, the "viral syndrome" is not unique to influenza and may be the presentation for a variety of viral (rhinovirus, adenovirus, and parainfluenza) and bacterial (Legionella, Mycoplasma, and Streptococccal) respiratory infections that do not respond to anti-influenza therapy.

The prevalence of influenza is in a constant state of flux, influenced by the geographical region, time of year, and patient population. In the United States, the CDC maintains a weekly report of influenza activity stratified by region and influenza subtype (http://www.cdc.gov/flu/weekly/). Although these estimates are derived from office-based practices rather than the ED, they can be used to estimate regional influenza pretest probabilities while interpreting physical exam findings and contemplating viral testing and therapy. For example, in the week of 14 November 2011, the proportion of tested specimens that demonstrated influenza was 0.6% and ILI represented 1.3% of office visits. Therefore, the prevalence of influenza was $0.6\% \times 1.3\% = 0.0078\%$ (the pretest probability). Similar influenza epidemiological data outside the United States are also available at http://www.cdc.gov/flu/weekly/intsurv.htm.

Clinical question

What is the diagnostic accuracy of the history and physical exam for influenza?
One diagnostic meta-analysis intentionally neglected manuscripts in the immediate post-SARS period, focusing instead on influenza. Based upon six studies of 7,105 patients (five prospective, none ED based),[11–16] they reported the summary estimates as shown in Table 37.1.[17] Another systematic review

Table 37.1 Diagnostic accuracy of signs or symptoms for influenza

Sign or symptom	Positive likelihood ratio	Negative likelihood ratio
Chills		
All ages	1.1	0.68
Only ≥60 years	2.6	0.66
Cough		
All ages	1.1	0.42
Only ≥60 years	2.0	0.57
Fever		
All ages	1.8	0.40
Only ≥60 years	3.8	0.72
Fever and cough		
All ages	1.9	0.54
Only ≥60 years	5.0	0.75
Fever, cough, and acute onset		
All ages	2.0	0.54
Only ≥60 years	5.4	0.77
Headache		
All ages	1.0	0.75
Only ≥60 years	1.9	0.70
Malaise		
All ages	0.98	1.1
Only ≥60 years	2.6	0.55
Myalgia		
All ages	0.93	1.2
Only ≥60 years	2.4	0.68
Sneezing		
All ages	1.2	0.87
Only ≥60 years	0.47	2.1
Sore throat		
All ages	1.0	0.96
Only ≥60 years	1.4	0.77
Vaccine history		
All ages	0.63	1.1

Source: Data from [17].

that included two additional studies[18,19] reported several more elements of the history that may be useful to rule in (rigors LR+ 7.2, fever and presenting within 3 days LR+ 4.0, and sweating LR+ 3.0) or rule out (any systemic symptoms LR− 0.36, coughing LR− 0.38, and inability to cope with daily activities LR− 0.39) influenza.[20]

Another systematic review evaluated the accuracy of clinical decision rules or combinations of signs and symptoms known as *heuristics*.[21] Based upon 12

Table 37.2 Diagnostic accuracy for combinations of signs or symptoms for influenza

Sign or symptom	Number of studies	Positive likelihood ratio (range)	Negative likelihood ratio (range)
Fever and cough	5	1.7–5.1	0.4–0.7
Fever, cough, and acute onset	4	2.0–6.5	0.3–0.8
Cough, headache, and pharyngitis	1	3.7	0.26

Source: Data from [21].

heterogeneous studies, none of which assessed the internal or external validity of their models, the authors reported no clinical decision rules. Three simple heuristics for influenza diagnosis that have been evaluated in seven studies were identified (Table 37.2).[12,14,22–25] Two of these studies were ED-based.

Stein et al evaluated 258 consecutive adult ED or urgent care patients with respiratory tract infections during the 2002 flu season, testing clinician gestalt against the "cough and fever" heuristic and using polymerase chain reaction (PRC) as the criterion standard. The prevalence of influenza was 21%. The heuristic had LR+ 5.1 and LR− 0.7 versus gestalt LR+ 3.6 and LR− 0.77. However, when stratified by how soon patients presented after symptom onset, clinical gestalt had LR+ 17.3 and LR− 0.4 if symptom onset was less than 48 hours prior to evaluation.[24] Friedman and Attia evaluated 128 children (ages 0–17 years) with ILI, defined as a temperature >38°C in the ED and at least one additional symptom (coryza, cough, headache, sore throat, or muscle aches), during the 2002 influenza season. The prevalence of influenza in their population was 35%, and the heuristic of cough–headache–pharyngitis was evaluated using viral cultures as the criterion standard, yielding LR+ 3.7 (CI 2.3–6.3) and LR− 0.26 (CI 0.14–0.44).[23] Another prediction rule has been derived to estimate the probability of hospitalization or all-cause mortality with the diagnosis of influenza. This score-based rule assesses age, gender, pre-illness outpatient visit rate, comorbidities, and prior pneumonia or influenza hospitalizations, yielding LR+ 8.1 (CI 5.0–13.3) and LR− 0.12 (CI 0.08–0.2) with a cutoff score of 50.[26]

Clinical question

What is the diagnostic accuracy of rapid influenza test kits?
The CDC maintains a summary of diagnostic accuracy information on rapid influenza tests for lab directors and clinicians (http://www.cdc.gov/flu/professionals/diagnosis/rapidlab.htm). One industry-sponsored meta-analysis of QuickVue® influenza tests summarized the diagnostic accuracy

Table 37.3 Diagnostic accuracy of rapid influenza tests and clinical gestalt

Patient population	Diagnostic test	Number of studies	Positive likelihood ratio	Negative likelihood ratio
Age 15 years	QuickVue®	14	10.5	0.39
	Gestalt	5	1.8	0.49
Age ≥15 years	QuickVue®	5	15.3*	0.41
	Gestalt	11	1.7	0.62

*Significant statistical heterogeneity, so random effects model used.
Source: Data from [27].

of the rapid test and compared it with clinical gestalt from six studies for two age groups (<15 years old and ≥15 years old), yielding the likelihood ratios in Table 37.3. In general, a negative result does not exclude the diagnosis, but a positive result does rule it in for all age groups. Compared with the QuickVue® test, clinical gestalt is not useful to rule in or rule out the diagnosis in either age group. These authors also evaluated 10 studies in which rapid influenza testing reduced overall diagnostic testing, antibiotic use, ED length of stay, and increased antiviral prescribing.[27]

Another diagnostic meta-analysis in 2005 identified five studies that compared one rapid test against a viral culture.[17] Only one trial evaluated multiple rapid influenza tests head to head. These investigators evaluated the Directigen Flu A, FLU OIA, Zstat Flu A/B, and QuickVue® influenza tests in children during the 1999 epidemic (49% prevalence). Each test had statistically equivalent LR+ (summary LR+ 4.7, CI 3.6–6.2). The Zstat Flu A/B did not rule out influenza as accurately as the other three tests. The summary LR− for the Directigen Flu A, FLU OIA, and QuickVue® was 0.06 (CI 0.03–0.12).[28]

Comment

History and physical exam are insufficient to rule in or rule out the diagnosis of influenza. Rapid tests are now available, but they cannot be used to rule out the diagnosis. If rapid test sensitivities range from 59% to 81% and specificities range from 70% to 99%, then rapid testing is less cost-effective in unvaccinated patients than empirical antiviral therapy unless the pretest probability of influenza is approximately 5–14%.[29,30] This diagnostic challenge highlights the importance of emergency care providers understanding their regional influenza prevalence while deciding upon ancillary influenza testing, antiviral therapy, or symptom management. Various patient-specific factors should influence antiviral treatment thresholds including symptom duration, vaccination status and anticipated vaccine efficacy, comorbid illness burden, and age-related susceptibility to suboptimal outcomes.

References

1. Thompson WW, Shay DK, Weintraub E, Brammer L, Bridges CC, Cox NJ *et al.* Influenza-associated hospitalizations in the United States. Journal of the American Medical Association. 2004; 292(11): 1333–40.

2. Neuzil KM, Reed GW, Mitchel EF, Griffin MR. Influenza-associated morbidity and mortality in young and middle-aged women. Journal of the American Medical Association. 1999; 281(10): 901–7.

3. Neuzil KM, Wright PF, Mitchel EF, Griffin MR. The burden of influenza illness in children with asthma and other chronic medical conditions. Journal of Pediatrics. 2000; 137(6): 856–64.

4. Griffin MR, Coffey CS, Neuzil KM, Mitchel EF, Wright PF, Edwards KM. Winter viruses: Influenza- and respiratory syncytial virus-related morbidity in chronic lung disease. Archives of Internal Medicine. 2002; 162(11): 1229–36.

5. Ellis SE, Coffey CS, Mitchel EF, Dittus DS, Griffin MR. Influenza- and respiratory syncytial virus-associated morbidity and mortality in the nursing home population. Journal of the the American Geriatric Society. 2003; 51(6): 761–7.

6. Estimates of deaths associated with seasonal influenza: United States, 1976–2007. Morbidity and Mortality Weekly Report. 2010; 59(33): 1057–60.

7. Molinari NA, Ortega-Sanchez IR, Messonnier ML, Thompson WW, Wortley PM, Weintraub E *et al.* The annual impact of seasonal influenza in the US: Measuring disease burden and costs. Vaccine. 2007; 25(27): 5086–96.

8. Lee TT, Taggart LR, Mater B, Katz K, Mcgeer A. Predictors of pandemic influenza infection in adults presenting to two urban emergency departments, Toronto, 2009. Canadian Journal of Emergency Medicine. 2011; 13(1): 7–12.

9. Monmany J, Rabella N, Margall N, Domingo P, Gich I, Vazquez G. Unmasking influenza virus infection in patients attended to in the emergency department. Infection. 2004; 32(2): 89–97.

10. Jefferson T, Jones M, Doshi P, Del Mar C, Dooley L, Foxlee R. Neuraminidase inhibitors for preventing and treating influenza in healthy adults. Cochrane Database Systematic Reviews. 2010; 17(2): Cd001265.

11. Nicholson KG, Kent J, Hammersley V, Cancio E. Acute viral infections of upper respiratory tract in elderly people living in the community: Comparative, prospective, population based study of disease burden. British Medical Journal. 1997; 315(7115): 1060–4.

12. Govaert TM, Dinant GJ, Aretz K, Knottnerus JA. The predictive value of influenza symptomatology in elderly people. Family Practice. 1998; 15(1): 16–22.

13. Carrat F, Tachet A, Rouzioux C, Housset B, Valleron AJ. Evaluation of clinical case definitions of influenza: Detailed investigation of patients during the 1995–1996 epidemic in France. Clinical Infectious Disease. 1999; 28(2): 283–90.

14. Monto AS, Gravenstein S, Elliott M, Colopy M, Schweinle J. Clinical signs and symptoms predicting influenza infection. Archives of Internal Medicine. 2000; 160(21): 3243–7.

15. Hulson TD, Mold JW, Scheid D, Aaron M, Aspy CB, Ballard NL *et al.* Diagnosing influenza: The value of clinical clues and laboratory tests. Journal of Family Practice. 2001; 50(12): 1051–6.

16. Van Elden LJR, Van Essen GA, Boucher CAB, Van Loon AM, Nijhuis M, Schipper P *et al.* Clinical diagnosis of influenza virus infection: Evaluation of diagnostic tools in general practice. British Journal of General Practice. 2001; 51(469): 630–4.

17. Call SA, Vollenweider MA, Hornung CA, Simel DL, Mckinney WP. Does this patient have influenza? Journal of the American Medical Association. 2005; 293(8): 987–97.

18. Lina B, Valette M, Foray S, Luciani J, Stagnara J, Lee DM *et al.* Surveillance of community-acquired viral infections due to respiratory viruses in Rhone-Alpes (France) during winter 1994 to 1995. Journal of Clinical Microbiology. 1996; 34(12): 3007–11.

19. Long CE, Hall CB, Cunningham CK, Weiner LB, Alger KP, Gouveia M *et al.* Influenza surveillance in community-dwelling elderly compared with children. Archives of Family Medicine. 1997; 6(5): 459–65.

20. Ebell MH, White LL, Casault T. A systematic review of the history and physical examination to diagnose influenza. Journal of the American Board of Family Practice. 2004; 17(1): 1–5.

21. Ebell MH, Afonso A. A systematic review of clinical decision rules for the diagnosis of influenza. Annals of Family Medicine. 2011; 9(1): 69–77.

22. Boivin G, Hardy I, Teller G, Maziade J. Predicting influenza infections during epidemics with use of a clinical case definition. Clinical Infectious Disease. 2000; 31(5): 1166–9.

23. Friedman MJ, Attia MW. Clinical predictors of influenza in children. Archives of Pediatrics and Adolescent Medicine. 2004; 158(4): 391–4.

24. Stein J, Louie J, Flanders S, Maselli J, Hacker JK, Drew WL *et al.* Performance characteristics of clinical diagnosis, a clinical decision rule, and a rapid influenza test in the detection of influenza infection in a community sample of adults. Annals of Emergency Medicine. 2005; 46(5): 412–9.

25. Van Den Dool C, Hak E, Wallinga J, Van Loon AM, Lammers JWJ, Bonten MJM. Symptoms of influenza virus infection in hospitalized patients. Infectious Control and Hospital Epidemiology. 2008; 29(4): 314–9.

26. Hak E, Wei F, Nordin J, Mullooly J, Poblete S, Nichol KL. Development and validation of a clinical prediction rule for hospitalization due to pneumonia or influenza or death during influenza epidemics among community-dwelling elderly persons. Journal of Infectious Disease. 2004; 189(3): 450–8.

27. Petrozzino JJ, Smith C, Atkinson MJ. Rapid diagnostic testing for seasonal influenza: An evidence-based review and comparison with unaided clinical diagnosis. Journal of Emerg Medicine. 2010; 39(4): 476–90.

28. Rodriguez WJ, Schwartz RH, Thorne MM. Evaluation of diagnostic tests for influenza in a pediatric practice. Pediatric Infectious Disease Journal. 2002; 21(3): 193–6.

29. Smith KJ, Roberts MS. Cost-effectiveness of newer treatment strategies for influenza. American Journal of Medicine. 2002; 113(4): 300–7.

30. Rothberg MB, Bellantonio S, Rosee DN. Management of influenza in adults older than 65 years of age: Cost-effectiveness of rapid testing and antiviral therapy. Annals of Internal Medicine. 2003; 139(5Pt 1): 321–9.

Chapter 38 **Pediatric Fever in Children Aged 3–36 Months**

Highlights

- Ill-appearing or hemodynamically unstable children with fevers should be fully evaluated for serious bacterial infection with laboratory tests; chest X-ray; cultures of the blood, urine, and CSF (if indicated); and empiric antibiotic therapy.
- Well-appearing children with a fever without a source (FWS) between 3 and 36 months of age should be stratified by whether or not they have been fully immunized for *Haemophilus influezae* type b and pneumococcal disease.
- Incompletely immunized children with FWS should have a urinalysis and culture sent, a CBC drawn and blood cultures obtained if the WBC is $\geq 15,000/microL$, and a chest X-ray obtained if the WBC is $\geq 20,000/microL$. Any positive findings or a WBC $\geq 15,000/microL$ should prompt treatment with empiric antibiotics.
- Immunized children with FWS should have a urinalysis and urine culture for girls younger than 24 months, uncircumcised boys younger than 12 months, or circumcised boys younger than 6 months old. Any positive findings should prompt treatment for a UTI.

Background

Fever is one of the most common reasons for children to present to the emergency department (ED). While the evaluation for neonates and young infants is outlined in Chapter 26, the evaluation of older children between the ages of 3 and 36 months is more complex and depends on their general appearance as well as whether they have completed a full series of vaccinations for *Haemophilus influenzae* type b and pneumococcal disease. Since the primary booster series is not complete until 6 months of age, all children younger than 6 months are also considered incompletely immunized.

Evidence-Based Emergency Care: Diagnostic Testing and Clinical Decision Rules, Second Edition. Jesse M. Pines, Christopher R. Carpenter, Ali S. Raja and Jeremiah D. Schuur. © 2013 John Wiley & Sons, Ltd. Published 2013 by John Wiley & Sons, Ltd.

The initial decision when presented with a febrile child is the determination of whether or not the child is ill appearing or hemodynamically unstable. If there is either an ill-appearing child or hemodynamic instability, the child should be fully evaluated with laboratory tests (including a complete blood count (CBC) and blood cultures, a urinalysis and culture, a chest X-ray, and possibly a lumbar puncture if meningitis is under consideration), resuscitated with intravenous fluids, and treated with prompt antibiotics (see Chapter 26). Antibiotic coverage should be directed towards any obvious source of infection (e.g., pneumonia). However, some children who are not ill appearing or clinically unstable will nevertheless still have serious occult infections that require antibiotic treatment and possible hospitalization. The emergency physician's role is to identify those children through clinical judgment and diagnostic testing.

Clinical question

Which laboratory tests should be performed on the well-appearing but incompletely immunized child between 3 and 36 months of age?

Unimmunized (or incompletely immunized) children are at higher risk of bacterial infection than their immunized counterparts. Lee et al evaluated 11,911 pediatric ED patients considered to be at risk for bacteremia.[1] Of these, blood cultures were positive in 149 (1.6%). In univariate analysis, temperature, absolute neutrophil count, and absolute band count were not found to be associated with occult bacteremia while white blood cell (WBC) count $\geq 15,000$/microL did show an association, with a sensitivity of 86%, a specificity of 77%, and a positive predictive value of 5.1%. Similarly, Kuppermann et al found that a WBC $\geq 15,000$/microL had a sensitivity of 80% and a specificity of 69% for occult bacteremia in an observational study of 6,579 children between 3 and 36 months of age.[2] This association of leukocytosis with occult bacteremia, while imperfect, serves as the basis for the current recommendation for empiric treatment in unimmunized children with WBC counts $\geq 15,000$/microL.

Pneumonia can be apparent in the tachypneic, hypoxemic, or dyspneic child; however, it can be present even in well-appearing children. In a study that included 225 patients who underwent chest X-ray (79 because of respiratory symptoms and 146 because of leukocytosis with no identifiable source), Bachur et al found that while 40% (CI 20–52%) of the children with respiratory symptomatology had pneumonias, 26% (CI 19–34%) of the children with isolated leukocytosis did as well.[3] This finding was confirmed by Brauner et al in 2010 when they studied 146 patients with "extreme leukocytosis" (WBC $\geq 25,000$/microL) and found that 28% of them had segmental or lobar pneumonia, even in the post–conjugate pneumococcal vaccine era.[4]

Unimmunized children with fever without source (FWS) and WBC $\geq 15,000/\text{microL}$, a positive urinalysis (discussed in this chapter), or a finding on chest X-ray should be treated with emperic antibiotics (typically ceftriaxone 50 mg/kg intramuscularly) pending the results of blood and urine cultures. The primary source of evidence for this strategy is a meta-analysis involving four trials, which included 7,899 children, all of whom had FWS and were between 3 and 36 months of age.[5] Treatment with intramuscular ceftriaxone reduced the incidence of serious bacterial infection by approximately 75%.

Clinical question

Which laboratory tests should be performed on the well-appearing immunized child between 3 and 36 months of age with a fever without a source?

Since the implementation of routine immunization in infants, the incidence of occult bacteremia has decreased from 5% to less than 1%, and a decision analytic model by Lee et al suggests that, at this low incidence of bacteremia, routine laboratory evaluation and empirical antibiotic therapy for FWS are not cost-effective.[6]

Nevertheless, urinary tract infections (UTIs) are still common in children between the ages of 3 and 36 months, especially girls younger than 24 months. Additionally, in male patients, a meta-analysis by Shaikh et al found that lack of circumcision increased the likelihood of a UTI (LR+ 2.8, CI 1.9–4.3).[7] For this reason, immunized girls younger than 24 months, immunized uncircumcised boys younger than 12 months, and circumcised boys younger than 6 months should have urinalyses and urine cultures obtained.

Comment

While no clinical decision rules exist to help guide the evaluation of well-appearing patients with FWS between the ages of 3 and 36 months, there are a number of guidelines based on relatively good evidence that can guide management. In immunized children, most testing can be avoided as no tests or empirical antibiotics have been shown to improve outcomes except urinalyses and cultures in the populations outlined in this chapter. Incompletely immunized children require a urinalysis and culture as well as a screening CBC and, if appropriate, blood cultures (if their WBC $\geq 15,000/\text{microL}$), a chest X-ray (if their WBC $\geq 20,000/\text{microL}$), and empirical ceftriaxone if blood cultures are sent.

Nevertheless, despite these recommendations being promulgated nationwide, a recent analysis by Simon et al found that they were poorly followed; no testing at all was performed in 59% of immunized febrile children in the United States between 6 and 36 months of age (which included not obtaining urinalyses in 60% of girls with fevers ≥39°C); CBCs were obtained in 21%; and antibiotics were prescribed in approximately 20% of the patients in whom no testing was obtained, underscoring the need for appropriate education measures as adjuncts to guideline development.[8]

References

1. Lee GM, Harper MB. Risk of bacteremia for febrile young children in the post-*Haemophilus influenzae* type b era. Archives of Pediatrics and Adolescent Medicine. 1998 Jul; 152(7): 624–8.

2. Kuppermann N, Fleisher GR, Jaffe DM. Predictors of occult pneumococcal bacteremia in young febrile children. Annals of Emergency Medicine. 1998 Jun; 31(6): 679–87.

3. Bachur R, Perry H, Harper MB. Occult pneumonias: Empiric chest radiographs in febrile children with leukocytosis. Annals of Emergency Medicine. 1999 Feb; 33(2): 166–73.

4. Brauner M, Goldman M, Kozer E. Extreme leucocytosis and the risk of serious bacterial infections in febrile children. Archives of Diseases in Childhood. 2010 Mar; 95(3): 209–12.

5. Bulloch B, Craig WR, Klassen TP. The use of antibiotics to prevent serious sequelae in children at risk for occult bacteremia: A meta-analysis. Academic Emergency Medicine. 1997 Jul; 4(7): 679–83.

6. Lee GM, Fleisher GR, Harper MB. Management of febrile children in the age of the conjugate pneumococcal vaccine: A cost-effectiveness analysis. Pediatrics. 2001 Oct; 108(4): 835–44.

7. Shaikh N, Morone NE, Lopez J, Chianese J, Sangvai S, D'Amico F *et al*. Does this child have a urinary tract infection? Journal of the American Medical Association. 2007 Dec 26; 298(24): 2895–904.

8. Simon AE, Lukacs SL, Mendola P. Emergency department laboratory evaluations of fever without source in children aged 3 to 36 months. Pediatrics. 2011 Dec; 128(6): e1368–75.

SECTION 5
Surgical and Abdominal Complaints

Chapter 39 **Acute, Nonspecific, Nontraumatic Abdominal Pain**

Highlights

- Plain abdominal X-rays are not helpful in ruling out serious abdominal diagnoses in patients with abdominal pain.
- Compared to plain abdominal X-rays, noncontrast abdominal CT identifies intra-abdominal pathologies with higher sensitivity and specificity.

Background

Acute abdominal pain is one of the most common presenting complaints to the emergency department (ED), accounting for about 5% of all ED visits. Developments in imaging techniques have dramatically changed the ED evaluation of abdominal pain. Twenty years ago, ED patients with abdominal pain were routinely evaluated by surgical consultants who decided whether to take the patient to the operating room (OR), admit and observe, or discharge the patient from the ED. Now, because of improvements in laboratory tests and imaging technology in the ED, the majority of abdominal pain evaluations in the ED are completed without surgical consultation and about 80% result in discharge home.[1] Surgeons are generally involved only if the patient is unstable, has had a recent operation, or has a clear indication for an operation (e.g., peritonitis or CT-confirmed diagnosis of appendicitis) after the results of laboratory tests and diagnostic studies are available. Nearly 90% of most presentations of acute abdominal pain fall into one of eight diagnoses: appendicitis, bowel obstruction, cholecystitis, renal colic, peptic ulcer disease, pancreatitis, diverticular disease, and nonspecific abdominal pain. With such a wide array of potential etiologies for abdominal pain, the clinician must decide how to rationally use diagnostic tests and balance the

Evidence-Based Emergency Care: Diagnostic Testing and Clinical Decision Rules, Second Edition. Jesse M. Pines, Christopher R. Carpenter, Ali S. Raja and Jeremiah D. Schuur. © 2013 John Wiley & Sons, Ltd. Published 2013 by John Wiley & Sons, Ltd.

pressure not to miss any serious diagnoses against concerns about costs of testing and adverse effects of imaging.

Laboratory tests, such as complete blood count, urinalysis, liver function tests and tests for pancreatic enzymes are frequently ordered on ED patients with acute nontraumatic abdominal pain.[2] While many studies have evaluated the usefulness of lab tests in the diagnosis of specific conditions (e.g., appendicitis), we found few studies that evaluated laboratory tests among all acute undifferentiated abdominal pain. As none of these studies reliably determined whether a lab test changed the diagnosis or if other factors such as imaging or prolonged observation did, we do not discuss lab testing for undifferentiated abdominal pain patients, rather discussing it for specific conditions in subsequent chapters.

Radiographic imaging modalities available in many EDs include plain abdominal radiography, CT (with or without intravenous and oral contrast), and ultrasound, leaving clinicians with a choice of which tests to order and in what sequence. While it seems that a clinical decision rule could be helpful with this decision, nontraumatic abdominal pain is an extremely heterogeneous presenting complaint, and to date no rule has been validated. In this section the discussion will focus on eight of the common and serious clinical entities presenting as acute abdominal pain: bowel obstruction, acute pancreatitis, acute appendicitis, acute cholecystitis, aortic emergencies, ovarian torsion, kidney stones, and testicular torsion. To begin, we address the role of imaging in undifferentiated acute abdominal pain. In subsequent chapters, we address tests for the most common causes of acute nontraumatic abdominal pain.

Clinical question

Which diagnostic imaging modality is most sensitive in diagnosing patients with undifferentiated acute abdominal pain?

A British study from 2002 randomized 118 patients to either those with acute abdominal pain not requiring immediate surgery or those requiring immediate CT scanning to undergo early (within the first 24 hours) abdominal CT with contrast (oral, IV and rectal) or standard care, which in Britain was plain X-rays followed when necessary by ultrasound, CT and/or fluoroscopy.[3] Routine CT reduced initially missed "serious" diagnoses by 17% compared to the standard management pathway (4% vs. 21%). Average hospital length of stay was 1.1 days shorter in the early CT group, but was not statistically significant. All seven deaths in the series occurred in patients in the standard care group (three were diagnosed with bowel perforation and one with a ruptured abdominal aortic aneurysm). The authors conclude that early CT scanning in patients with acute abdominal pain improves diagnostic accuracy, and might reduce the duration of hospitalization and mortality.

Several studies have evaluated how abdominal CT changes diagnoses, admission decision and the need for surgery in ED patients. Rosen et al prospectively evaluated the added value of CT in 536 consecutive patients presenting with nontraumatic acute abdominal pain.[4] Physicians responded to five questions prior to ordering the CT scan, including their pretest diagnostic impression and level of certainty about intended management before CT results were available. Results were compared to the post-CT diagnosis and management. The majority of CT scans were ordered by interns and residents (87%) and the remainder by attending physicians. Pre- and posttest diagnoses were concordant for only 37% of the patients. CT scanning was associated with a reduction in rates of planned immediate surgical intervention from 13% to 5% and reduced the perceived need for admission by 17%. The authors concluded that ED use of CT was associated with increased diagnostic certainty, reduced unnecessary surgery and hospital admissions, and that the value of CT is greater than its direct costs.

Older adults with abdominal pain are at higher risk for adverse events as they are more likely to have life-threatening etiologies, confounding overlying comorbidities, and often present later in the course of disease with nonspecific symptoms. Esses et al prospectively studied the value of CT in 104 stable older adults with abdominal pain in the ED.[5] They asked ordering clinicians questions about the need for admission, surgery and antibiotics and compared the answers to the post CT management. They found that the post-CT decisions around admission were changed for 26% of the patients, decisions about a need for surgery were changed for 12%, and decisions about antibiotic therapy were changed for 21% of the patients. Hustey et al[6] prospectively evaluated an observational cohort of 337 patients aged 60 years and older. History was obtained prospectively, charts were reviewed retrospectively for radiographic findings clinical course, and disposition, and patients were contacted at 2 weeks for additional outcomes. Among older adults with acute nontraumatic abdominal pain, 37% had abdominal CT. The leading diagnoses were diverticulitis (18%), bowel obstruction (18%), nephrolithiasis (10%), and gallbladder disease (10%). CT was diagnostic in 57% of patients overall, in 75% of patients requiring acute intervention, and 85% of patients requiring acute surgical intervention. The authors of both studies concluded that the increase in diagnostic certainty and improved management both support the early use of CT in the ED for older adults with abdominal pain.

MacKersie et al performed a prospective study of ED patients presenting with acute abdominal pain in which they compared *noncontrast* abdominal CT with three-view plain abdominal radiography. They examined the test characteristics and diagnostic accuracy of the two imaging modalities compared to the final diagnosis made by surgical, pathological, and clinical follow-up at 6 months. Patients were enrolled if they had onset of acute abdominal pain within the previous 7 days. Patients were excluded if they were pregnant, were intoxicated, lacked the mental capacity for decision making, had vaginal bleeding, had penile discharge, had dysuria, or had hematuria without flank pain. Interpreting radiologists were blinded to the study and to the clinical history for each patient. Over a 7-month period, 103 patients were enrolled with 91 patients undergoing both studies. They found CT to have a sensitivity of 96% (CI 86–100%), specificity of 95% (CI 83–99%), and accuracy 96%. The acute abdominal series had a sensitivity of 30% (CI 18–45%), specificity of 88% (CI 74–96%), and accuracy of 56%. The final diagnoses included gastrointestinal diseases (n = 35) including acute appendicitis, acute cholecystitis, acute pancreatitis, diverticulitis, inflammatory bowel disease, hernias, and bowel obstructions, gynecological disease (n = 3), genitourinary disease (n = 8), metastatic disease (n = 4), and nonspecific abdominal pain (n = 41).

This study demonstrated that the *noncontrast* abdominal CT revealed the cause of acute abdominal pain, including many of the concerning surgical or medically emergent or urgent causes of acute abdominal pain, better than plain films. In many cases the CT led to the discovery of pathology that was not identified using plain radiography. This study also demonstrates that noncontrast CT has sufficiently high sensitivity, specificity, and accuracy to make it a clinically useful study, thus avoiding the risks of allergic reactions and contrast induced nephropathy.

A subset of patients from another study of undifferentiated acute abdominal pain patients presenting to an ED compared the diagnostic yields in patients undergoing both abdominal plain radiography and abdominal CT scanning.[7] Out of 1,000 patients, only 120 had both plain abdominal imaging and abdominal CTs performed. They compared imaging diagnoses to the final diagnosis, either at the time of ED discharge or hospital discharge, for the following six diagnoses: bowel obstruction, urolithiasis, appendicitis, pyelonephritis, pancreatitis, and diverticulitis. There were 25 cases of urolithiasis, nine cases of diverticulitis, two cases of pyelonephritis, and three cases each for bowel obstruction, appendicitis, and pancreatitis. Plain abdominal radiography had sensitivities of 0% (CI ranges 0–84%) for all but bowel obstruction (sensitivity 33%, CI 25–42%). The specificity for all of the diagnoses was 100% (CI range 96–100%). The diagnostic accuracy of abdominal radiography ranged from 80% to 98%. Abdominal CT had sensitivities across all of the diagnoses of 33–68% (CI 25–76%) with specificities ranging from 91% to 100% (CI 85–100%). The diagnostic accuracy of abdominal CT ranged from 86% to 98%. The authors of this small study concluded that plain abdominal radiography was insufficiently sensitive in the evaluation of acute nontraumatic abdominal pain.

Because of the difficulty of knowing exactly which lab tests, imaging studies, and history and physical exam findings are predictive of the need for acute medical or surgical interventions, defined as surgery or need for inpatient hospitalization, Gerhardt et al examined 165 patients undergoing acute abdominal imaging and non-contrast helical CT scanning of the abdomen with nontraumatic nonspecific abdominal pain.[8] Patients with abdominal pain for a week or less, nontraumatic in nature, and older than 18 years were included. The prevalence of urgent intervention within 24 hours of presentation was 13%, and an additional 34% underwent elective interventions that mitigated morbidity or mortality. They found that when all of the data was aggregated, including the acute abdominal series results, the noncontrast abdominal CT was the most accurate clinical variable for an acute medical or surgical intervention. In a classification and regression tree analysis, the combination of history, physical exam, acute abdominal series imaging, and noncontrast abdominal CT imaging yielded the best test characteristics to predict the need for medical or surgical intervention (sensitivity 92%, specificity 90%, a LR+ of 9.2, and a LR− of 0.09). Other models that did not include CT imaging had lower sensitivities and specificities and were felt to be clinically unacceptable. The authors of this derivation study concluded that the noncontrast abdominal CT was useful and the imaging study of choice when faced with nonspecific abdominal pain.

While diagnostic ultrasound has been studied for specific abdominal diagnoses (e.g., gallstones), its use in acute undifferentiated abdominal pain has only been studied recently, and has included ultrasound performed or interpreted by radiologists, not emergency physicians. A prospective study in the Netherlands evaluated eleven possible diagnostic strategies in 1,021 non-pregnant adults who presented to six EDs with acute abdominal pain whom a physician in the ED thought required some type of imaging.[9] The strategies included clinical evaluation alone or in combination with plain X-rays, ultrasound, and/or CT scanning. Physician reviewers later classified the patients as having had an urgent or a non-urgent condition (treatment within 24 hours not required) based on 6-month follow-up. The prevalence of urgent conditions was 65%. Clinical diagnosis alone was 88% sensitive and 41% specific for an "urgent" condition, while US in all patients would have been less sensitive (70%), but more specific (85%). Two strategies that involved doing ultrasound in all patients were the most sensitive: ultrasound followed by CT scanning if the ultrasound is negative or inconclusive (sensitivity 94%, specificity 68%), or CT only if the ultrasound is negative (sensitivity 85%, specificity 76%). These two strategies would result in the lowest use of CT (49% and 27% of patients, respectively). The authors concluded that in nonpregnant adults with acute abdominal pain, if a clinician thinks imaging is required, then ultrasound should be the initial modality, followed by CT, as ultrasound has high sensitivity and can reduce the use of CT by about half.

Comment

Acute abdominal pain is a common presenting complaint in the ED, frequently represents serious pathology and is difficult to diagnose clinically. A thorough history and physical exam are critical for clinicians to develop a differential diagnosis and corresponding pretest probabilities. While laboratory tests can be useful for the diagnosis of specific disorders, the routine

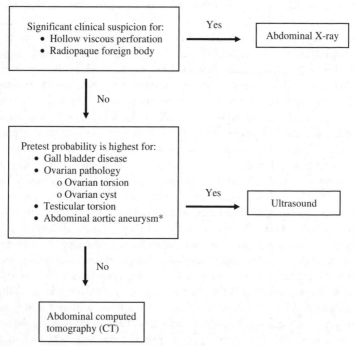

* The decision on which test to utilize first will depend on test availability. If it is possible to obtain ultrasound more rapidly than CT, for example emergency physician performed bedside ultrasound, or if CT requires a significant delay, then ultrasound should occur first.

Figure 39.1 Algorithm for diagnostic imaging in acute nontraumatic abdominal pain.

use of broad laboratory panels (e.g., "belly labs") for patients with nontraumatic abdominal pain is costly, has not been proven to increase diagnostic
accuracy, and is not recommended. Rather, clinicians should tailor their
laboratory ordering to specific diagnoses for which they have a moderate
to high pretest probability. Figure 39.1 presents an algorithm for selecting
the initial diagnostic imaging test in the patient with acute nontraumatic
abdominal pain. Of note, as multiple studies show that CT scanning is the
most sensitive and specific diagnostic imaging modality for acute abdominal
pain, it is likely to be the most useful initial test in patients in whom there
is not a clear leading diagnosis and in high-risk patient populations, such
as the elderly and immunosuppressed. Due to its diagnostic accuracy and
availability, CT use has increased exponentially in US EDs over the last 15
years, leading to concerns that it is used inappropriately in the ED. Further
research is needed to define a subset of abdominal pain patients that can safely
be evaluated without CT. Additionally, some centers may adopt protocols
using ultrasound as a first imaging modality of choice, followed by CT when
the ultrasound is equivocal or negative. While this will reduce the use of CT,
the vast majority of EDs do not have access to skilled ultrasonographers at
all times of day and night. For now, individual clinicians will continue to use
their judgment in ordering CT.

References

1. Bhuiya FA, Pitts SR, McCaig LF. Emergency department visits for chest pain and
   abdominal pain: United States, 1999–2008. NCHS Data Brief. 2010;(43): 1–8.
2. Nagurney JT, Brown DF, Chang Y et al. Use of diagnostic testing in the emergency
   department for patients presenting with non-traumatic abdominal pain. Journal
   of Emergency Medicine. 2003; 25: 363–71.
3. Ng CS, Watson CJ, Palmer CR et al. Evaluation of early abdominopelvic computed
   tomography in patients with acute abdominal pain of unknown cause: Prospective
   randomised study. British Medical Journal. 2002; 325: 1387.
4. Rosen MP, Siewert B, Sands DZ et al. Value of abdominal CT in the emergency
   department for patients with abdominal pain. European Radiology. 2003; 13:
   418–24.
5. Esses D, Birnbaum A, Bijur P et al. Ability of CT to alter decision making in elderly
   patients with acute abdominal pain. American Journal of Emergency Medicine.
   2004; 22: 270–2.
6. Hustey FM, Meldon SW, Banet GA et al. The use of abdominal computed
   tomography in older ED patients with acute abdominal pain. American Journal of
   Emergency Medicine. 2005; 23: 259–65.
7. Ahn SH, Mayo-Smith WW, Murphy BL et al. Acute nontraumatic abdominal
   pain in adult patients: Abdominal radiography compared with CT Evaluation1.
   Radiology. 2002; 225: 159–64.

8. Gerhardt RT, Nelson BK, Keenan S *et al*. Derivation of a clinical guideline for the assessment of nonspecific abdominal pain: The guideline for abdominal pain in the ED setting (GAPEDS) phase 1 study. American Journal of Emergency Medicine. 2005; 23: 709–77.
9. Lameris W, van Randen A, van Es HW *et al*. Imaging strategies for detection of urgent conditions in patients with acute abdominal pain: Diagnostic accuracy study. British Medical Journal. 2009; 338: b2431.

Chapter 40 **Small Bowel Obstruction**

Highlights

- Abdominal CT identifies small bowel obstructions with higher sensitivity, specificity, and accuracy than plain abdominal X-rays.
- Abdominal CT can typically identify the level and cause of the obstruction.
- Bedside abdominal ultrasound can be used as an initial screening tool by emergency physicians to rule in small bowel obstructions.

Background

Mechanical small bowel obstruction (SBO) is a surgical disorder of the small intestine, and is most commonly caused by intra-abdominal adhesions (75% of cases). Bowel strangulation, which occurs when bowel wall edema compromises perfusion to the intestine and necrosis ensues, is the most severe complication of SBO and is a surgical emergency. Left untreated, strangulated bowel will perforate, leading to peritonitis with a high rate of mortality. It is estimated that more than 300,000 patients undergo surgery every year in the United States for adhesion-induced SBO; however, SBOs can also occur for a number of other reasons including hernias, malignancies, volvulus, inflammatory conditions, foreign bodies, gallstones, pancreatitis, and intussusceptions. Their typical presentation is abdominal pain, distension, vomiting, and sometimes constipation. In the emergency department (ED), a frequently asked question is how to approach the diagnosis of SBO, particularly regarding the choice of the initial abdominal imaging study.

Clinical question

Which diagnostic imaging modality is most sensitive in diagnosing SBO?
SBOs can be categorized as either partial or complete obstructions, depending on whether any gas or liquid can pass through the point at which the small

Evidence-Based Emergency Care: Diagnostic Testing and Clinical Decision Rules, Second Edition.
Jesse M. Pines, Christopher R. Carpenter, Ali S. Raja and Jeremiah D. Schuur.
© 2013 John Wiley & Sons, Ltd. Published 2013 by John Wiley & Sons, Ltd.

bowel is narrowed. A small bowel follow-through series is typically used to differentiate between the two, but the 24-hour time course required to conduct this test makes it inappropriate for ED use.[1] This leaves other imaging modalities such as abdominal X-rays, computed tomography (CT), and ultrasound as the primary choices available to the emergency physician.

An early study by Frager et al was among the first to compare abdominal CT with abdominal X-rays for diagnosing SBO.[2] They studied 85 patients who obtained 90 acute abdominal X-ray series (supine and upright X-rays; Figures 40.1 and 40.2) as well as abdominal CTs with intravenous (IV) and oral contrast. The comparison criterion standard was surgical in 61 cases and clinical in 29 cases. In the cases with no obstruction (n = 24), X-ray was 88% specific (CI 66–100%), while CT was only 83% specific (CI 63–100%). However, for cases of partial and complete SBO (n = 20 and 46, respectively), CT had a sensitivity of 100% for both (CI 78–100% for partial SBO, and 92–100% for complete SBO), while X-ray had a sensitivity of 30% (CI 8–52%) for partial SBO and 46% (CI 32–60%) for complete SBO. The authors concluded that abdominal CT identified all partial and complete SBO better than plain abdominal films. CT also provided additional information regarding the degree and location of the obstruction that helped guide management in those cases requiring surgical intervention.

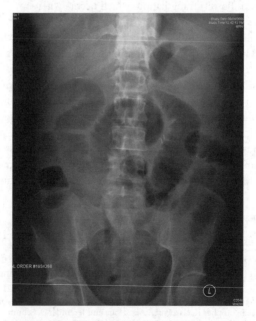

Figure 40.1 Supine abdominal X-ray with multiple dilated loops of bowel.

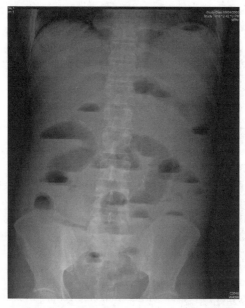

Figure 40.2 Upright abdominal X-ray with multiple air-fluid levels in dilated loops of bowel.

Additional studies retrospectively reviewed patients imaged with both abdominal x-rays and CTs. These studies found that a large proportion of patients with both normal and abnormal X-rays went on to obtain CTs[3,4] because x-rays were typically nonspecific and only 33% (CI 8–52%) sensitive for bowel obstruction.[5] Given this, CT has become the imaging modality of choice for patients with suspected bowel obstruction.[6]

The use of ultrasound imaging for evaluation of patients with suspected SBO was first described in a small study in 1999 in which 32 patients with acute abdominal pain received an abdominal X-ray series, CT with oral and IV contrast (+/− rectal contrast), and abdominal ultrasound.[7] The study sought to compare the sensitivities, specificities, and accuracies of each imaging modality compared with the outcomes at surgery (n = 25) and clinical follow-up (n = 7). The interpreting radiologists were blinded to the findings from the other imaging studies, and all imaging occurred within 6–36 hours after presentation. There were a total of 30 bowel obstructions, and the imaging results are shown in Table 40.1.

The authors concluded that CT yielded a significantly higher sensitivity with 100% specificity in diagnosing bowel obstruction, but that ultrasound

Table 40.1 Test characteristics for bowel obstruction evaluation using X-ray, computed tomography (CT), and ultrasound

	Sensitivity, %	Specificity, %	Positive likelihood ratio (LR+)	Negative likelihood ratio (LR−)
X-ray	77	50	1.5	0.46
CT	93	100	∞	0.07
Ultrasound	83	100	∞	0.17

Note: 95% confidence intervals not provided in source study.
Source: Data from [7].

performed much better than X-ray and had 100% specificity, allowing for ultrasound to rule in SBO. Furthermore, CT was able to identify the level and cause of the obstruction in 93% and 87% of cases, respectively, compared to ultrasound (70% and 23%) and X-ray (60% and 7%). The causes of bowel obstruction were malignancy (n = 9), inflammation (n = 9), adhesions (n = 3), volvulus (n = 3), strictures (n = 3), intussusception (n = 2), and foreign body (n = 1).

With the advent of bedside ultrasound, emergency physicians have been able to begin the evaluation of patients with suspected bowel obstruction earlier than ever (Figure 40.3). A recent article from Turkey compared the use of bedside ultrasound by emergency medicine and radiology residents in 174 patients, using either surgical findings or 1-month clinical follow-up as a criterion standard.[8] The results (Table 40.2) demonstrate that both emergency medicine and radiology residents were able to effectively rule in bowel obstruction using ultrasound.

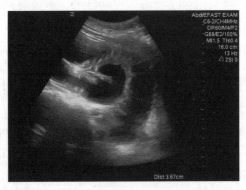

Figure 40.3 Dilated bowel loops indicative of small bowel obstruction seen on ultrasound. (Source: Elke Platz, Heidi Kimberly & Dorothea Hempel, Department of Emergency Medicine, Brigham and Women's Hospital, used with permission).

Table 40.2 Test characteristics of bedside ultrasound for the evaluation of bowel obstruction, performed by both emergency medicine (EM) and radiology residents

	Sensitivity, %	Specificity, %	Positive likelihood ratio (LR+)	Negative likelihood ratio (LR−)
EM residents	97.7	92.7	13.4	0.02
Radiology residents	88.4	100	∞	0.12

Source: Data from [8].

These results were confirmed by a subsequent study by Jang et al who compared X-ray to bedside ultrasound using a criterion standard of CT.[9] They found that emergency physician-performed ultrasound was both more sensitive (91%, CI 75–98%) and more specific (84%, CI 69–93%) than X-ray (sensitivity 46%, CI 20–74%; and specificity 67%, CI 49–81%) for SBO. Notably, the only training given to the emergency physicians prior to the study was a 10-minute training module and five practice ultrasound exams for SBO.

Finally, MRI (which also has no ionizing radiation exposure) is another option for imaging of patients with suspected SBO. In a prospective cross-sectional study of patients with clinical evidence of bowel obstruction, Beall et al reported on 44 patients evaluated with rapid noncontrast MRI, IV contrast CT scanning, or both and found the following test characteristics: MRI sensitivity 95%, specificity 100%, LR+ infinity, and LR− 0.05; and CT sensitivity 71%, specificity 71%, LR+ 2.4, and LR− 0.41. The study used both surgical findings and clinical follow-up as criterion standards, and the total time for MRI, included patient setup and image acquisition, was just under 7 minutes.[10]

Comment

There are few good head-to-head comparative studies in the medical literature of different imaging modalities for the evaluation of patients with suspected SBO, and those that have been performed have been relatively small. Furthermore, studies performed using CT and ultrasound from as recently as 5–10 years ago may not be totally applicable today due to technological advances with each of these modalities (temporal bias, see Chapter 6). Many of the studies, including several of those reviewed in this chapter, suffer from the lack of uniform diagnostic criterion standards, making broad comparisons of several similar studies difficult.

Taking into account these limitations, we believe several take-home points can be learned from the data. With few exceptions, plain abdominal radiography has little role in the evaluation of suspected SBO. The exceptions include expected prolonged delay or absolute unavailability of CT or ultrasound imaging in order to expedite gastric decompression, especially if a more serious time-sensitive etiology (such as a volvulus) is suspected. Plain radiography is still used in other acute abdominal pain situations (foreign body ingestions, penetrating trauma, and suspected pneumoperitoneum), but its use is diminishing.[6] At the opposite end of the spectrum, MRI is not yet ready for widespread use as the diagnostic imaging modality of choice for SBO. Most EDs do not have rapid availability of MRI, and many patients may not tolerate lying supine for the length of time necessary to obtain a MRI without gastric decompression. However, at sites with available MRI and for patients not otherwise appropriate for other types of imaging, the study by Beall et al provides another imaging option for diagnosing SBO.

Computed tomography is clearly the superior imaging modality for SBO when compared to X-ray and ultrasound. The use of abdominal CT imaging has several advantages in that, in addition to making the diagnosis, it can also determine the level and cause of the obstruction. Alternative causes for the patient's abdominal pain – such as an aortic aneurysm, for example – can also be evaluated. Since the principal criticism for the widespread use of CT as the first imaging modality is the concern for radiation exposure, ultrasound should be considered in children, pregnant women, or patients with multiple prior abdominal CTs, as it can effectively rule in the disease without the use of ionizing radiation. As the test characteristics of ultrasound exams are highly operator dependent, they should be used by clinicians who have appropriate training in a setting with appropriate quality assurance and improvement mechanisms in place.

References

1. Abbas S, Bissett IP, Parry BR. Oral water soluble contrast for the management of adhesive small bowel obstruction. Cochrane Database Systematic Reviews. 2005;(1): CD004651.
2. Frager D, Medwid SW, Baer JW, Mollinelli B, Friedman M. CT of small-bowel obstruction: Value in establishing the diagnosis and determining the degree and cause. American Journal of Roentgenology. 1994; 162(1): 37–41.
3. Nagurney JT, Brown DF, Novelline RA, Kim J, Fischer RH. Plain abdominal radiographs and abdominal CT scans for nontraumatic abdominal pain: Added value? American Journal of Emergency Medicine. 1999; 17(7): 668–71.
4. Jackson K, Taylor D, Judkins S. Emergency department abdominal X-rays have a poor diagnostic yield and their usefulness is questionable. Emergency Medicine Journal. 2011; 28(9): 745–9.

5. Ahn SH, Mayo-Smith WW, Murphy BL, Reinert SE, Cronan JJ. Acute nontraumatic abdominal pain in adult patients: Abdominal radiography compared with CT evaluation. Radiology. 2002; 225(1): 159–64.

6. Raja AS, Mortele KJ, Hanson R *et al*. Abdominal imaging utilization in the emergency department: Trends over two decades. International Journal of Emergency Medicine. 2011; 4: 19.

7. Suri S, Gupta S, Sudhakar PJ *et al*. Comparative evaluation of plain films, ultrasound and CT in the diagnosis of intestinal obstruction. Acta Radiologica. 1999; 40(4): 422–8.

8. Unlüer EE, Yava254i O, Eroğlu O, Yilmaz C, Akarca FK. Ultrasonography by emergency medicine and radiology residents for the diagnosis of small bowel obstruction. European Journal of Emergency Medicine. 2010; 17(5): 260–4.

9. Jang TB, Schindler D, Kaji AH. Bedside ultrasonography for the detection of small bowel obstruction in the emergency department. Emergency Medicine Journal. 2011; 28(8): 676–8.

10. Beall DP, Fortman BJ, Lawler BC, Regan F. Imaging bowel obstruction: A comparison between fast magnetic resonance imaging and helical computed tomography. Clinical Radiology. 2002; 57(8): 719–24.

Chapter 41 **Acute Pancreatitis**

Highlights

- Acute pancreatitis accounts for about one in 350 ED visits, is commonly associated with alcohol use and gallstones, and carries an approximate 1–5% mortality rate.
- Serum lipase is useful to rule in and rule out acute pancreatitis. As serum lipase is more sensitive and specific than serum amylase in discriminating acute pancreatitis from other acute abdominal pathology; amylase should not be used to diagnose pancreatitis.
- Clinical and CT-based scoring systems are not useful to rule in or rule out severe pancreatitis or predict mortality in ED patients with acute pancreatitis.

Background

Acute pancreatitis is an acute inflammatory process of the pancreas, which typically presents with severe upper abdominal pain and elevated serum pancreatic enzymes. The majority of adult cases are related to gallstones or alcohol use. Other causes include medications, hyperlipidemia, and hypercalcemia. In children, abdominal trauma is the most common cause of acute pancreatitis. In 2003, about one in 350 (0.3%) emergency department (ED) visits were for acute pancreatitis, and two-thirds of these visits resulted in hospitalization.[1]

Pancreatitis remains a frustrating and humbling condition to treat. While most patients will have a mild, self-limited course, a subset becomes significantly ill. In a review of acute pancreatitis by Banks et al, overall mortality was approximately 5%, increasing to 17% in cases of necrotizing pancreatitis.[2] To date, no interventions, including antibiotics, enzymatic treatments, and surgery, have been definitively shown to improve morbidity and mortality. The mainstay of therapy is excellent supportive care. For this reason,

Evidence-Based Emergency Care: Diagnostic Testing and Clinical Decision Rules, Second Edition.
Jesse M. Pines, Christopher R. Carpenter, Ali S. Raja and Jeremiah D. Schuur.
© 2013 John Wiley & Sons, Ltd. Published 2013 by John Wiley & Sons, Ltd.

the ability to accurately prognosticate is clinically useful and of interest to patients and families. Correspondingly, a number of scoring systems have been developed to predict the severity of acute pancreatitis. In this chapter, we review the diagnostic characteristics of laboratory tests and the accuracy of prognostic systems for acute pancreatitis. As the diagnosis of chronic pancreatitis is largely clinical, we do not address chronic pancreatitis.

Clinical question

What is the role of serum amylase and lipase in the diagnosis of acute pancreatitis?

Serum amylase and lipase are the most frequently used diagnostic tests for pancreatitis in the ED. Lipases are enzymes secreted from pancreatic acinar cells that hydrolyze triglycerides into metabolic substrates. Normally, 99% of lipases are secreted into the pancreatic ductal system, while less than 1% makes its way into the serum, giving the serum lipase level the theoretical advantage of being specific to pancreatic pathology.[3] Amylase is a small enzyme that cleaves starches into smaller carbohydrates. There are two major sources of amylase (the pancreas and salivary glands), but the many physiologic and pathologic causes of amylase elevation give amylase a poor specificity for pancreatitis.[4]

Studies evaluating laboratory tests for pancreatitis have several weaknesses. First, there is no clear criterion standard for acute pancreatitis. Early studies often used the laboratory test in question (usually amylase) as the sole marker or as one of the diagnostic criteria of pancreatitis, inflating the sensitivity of the test. Better constructed studies use a number of factors, including lab tests, CT results, surgical findings, and discharge diagnoses, to define the population with pancreatitis. Second, "normal limits" defined in a sample of healthy young men may differ from the population at risk for pancreatitis. This said, there are several well-conducted studies that can guide the emergency physician's choice of diagnostic tests.

The comparative studies of amylase and lipase in patients with acute pancreatitis all conclude that lipase has equal or greater utility in making the diagnosis. Butler et al conducted an evidence-based review to determine whether lipase was better than amylase in the diagnosis of pancreatitis in patients presenting with abdominal pain.[5] They identified seven studies that compared the tests head-to-head and included almost 2,000 patients. The studies demonstrated that serum amylase (sensitivity 72–95%, specificity 85–99%) had worse test characteristics than serum lipase (sensitivity 86–100%, specificity 95–99%) for pancreatitis.

In one study not included in this systematic review, researchers in New Zealand studied 328 patients admitted to a single hospital over a 3–4-year period in which pancreatitis was a diagnostic consideration.[6] The diagnosis of pancreatitis was based on a combination of factors, none of which included enzymatic determinations (operative or autopsy results, clinical features, and imaging results). Serum enzyme levels were determined on the first day following presentation. A total of 51 patients (16%) were classified as having acute pancreatitis. The authors found that an elevated lipase level (above the diagnostic threshold) was 97% specific, but only 67% sensitive. This was significantly more discriminatory than an elevated amylase level (specificity 97%, sensitivity 45%). The authors used a high cutoff for both tests in order to maximize the specificity of the diagnostic test as a way to avoid excessive false-positive results.

Overall, the comparative studies show serum lipase to be slightly more sensitive and more specific than amylase as a diagnostic marker when used to rule in or rule out pancreatitis. Only two studies looked directly at ED patients with abdominal pain. While other investigators have looked into whether combinations of tests improve diagnostic accuracy, the use of both tests has not improved the test characteristics compared to the use of lipase alone.[4]

Clinical question

Can clinical prediction rules accurately predict the severity of pancreatitis based on features present in the ED?

Acute pancreatitis can be divided into mild (75–85%) and severe or necrotizing pancreatitis (15–25%).[7] Severe pancreatitis is associated with local complications (such as pseudocysts and abscesses), organ failure, respiratory failure, and an approximately 15% mortality.[2] Early identification of high-risk patients is difficult, as clinical features such as pain severity, vital signs, and diagnostic test values (such as serum lipase) do not correlate with severity. Numerous rating scales incorporating clinical features, laboratory test values, and imaging have been developed to prognosticate the severity of acute pancreatitis; however, several well-known scales are not useful to the emergency clinician. Of note, Ranson's score requires values at 48 hours and the CT severity index (CTSI or Balthazar score) requires a contrast-enhanced CT, which is not indicated for all ED patients with acute pancreatitis.[1]

Scoring systems that can be calculated in the ED include: the Acute Physiology and Chronic Health Examination (APACHE) II score,[8] the Systemic Inflammatory Response Syndrome (SIRS) score,[9] and the Bedside Index of Severity in Acute Pancreatitis (BISAP) score.[10] The APACHE II score was originally developed for critically ill patients in intensive care units, and has been the most studied in acute pancreatitis. The APACHE II score includes 12 physiologic measures, age, and chronic disease, making it cumbersome and most easily calculated using a computerized calculator, available in common online textbooks and websites.[11] The SIRS score includes: temperature $>38.5°C$ or $<35.0°C$; heart rate of >90 beats/minute; respiratory rate of >20 breaths/minute or $PaCO_2$ of <32 mm Hg; and white blood cell (WBC) count of $>12,000$ cells/mL, <4000 cells/mL, or $>10\%$ bands. The BISAP score includes: blood urea nitrogen >25 mg/dl, impaired mental status, systemic inflammatory response syndrome (SIRS), age >60 years, and pleural effusions.

Gravante et al conducted a systematic review of studies of prognostic scores for acute pancreatitis and their relationship to mortality.[12] They excluded studies that analyzed factors associated with the severity of disease or the presence of disease-related complications. They identified 195 relevant studies and included 58; however, due to heterogeneous populations and variable test cutoffs, they were unable to calculate pooled diagnostic test characteristics. Among the scores investigated, APACHE II had the greatest positive predictive value (PPV) for mortality (maximum 69%), with sensitivities from 65% to 81% and specificities from 77% to 91%. No scores had high PPV ($>80\%$). While most prognostic variables and scores showed high negative predictive values (NPVs) for mortality ($>90\%$), this was heavily weighted by the relatively low mortality rates. In many studies, clinical assessment for severe pancreatitis (including shock, respiratory distress, or signs of peritonitis) was as accurate as the scoring systems. The authors conclude that despite the number of scoring systems for grading acute pancreatitis, none are ideal for the prediction of mortality.

Two recent prospective studies evaluated multiple prognostic scores. Papachristou et al compared BISAP with the "traditional" multifactorial scoring systems: Ranson's, APACHE-II, and CTSI in predicting severity, pancreatic necrosis, and mortality in a prospective cohort of patients with pancreatitis.[13] They studied 185 consecutive patients over 4 years, of whom 73% underwent contrast-enhanced CT scan. Forty patients (22%) developed organ failure and were classified as having severe acute pancreatitis, 36 (19%) developed pancreatic necrosis, and seven died (3.8%). The sensitivity and specificity of the scoring systems for severe disease ranged from 38% to 86% and from 71% to 92% respectively, and using areas under the curve, no system was better at consistently predicting any of the outcomes.

Bollen et al compared the accuracy of CT and clinical scoring systems for predicting the severity of acute pancreatitis on admission.[14] They studied 346 consecutive patients, of whom 159 received a contrast-enhanced CT scan. Seven CT scoring systems as well as two clinical scoring systems (APACHE-II and BISAP) were evaluated regarding their ability to predict the severity of acute pancreatitis on admission (first 24 hours of hospitalization).

Clinically severe acute pancreatitis (defined as one or more of the following: mortality, persistent organ failure, and/or the presence of local pancreatic complications that require intervention) was diagnosed in 18% of patients, and 6% of patients died. The sensitivity and specificity of the scoring systems ranged from 59% to 87% and from 58% to 85%, respectively, and using areas under the curve, there were no statistically significant differences between the predictive accuracies of CT and clinical scoring systems. Therefore, the authors conclude that a CT on admission solely for severity assessment in acute pancreatitis is not recommended.

Comments

Acute pancreatitis can present as a mild, self-limited illness with no sequelae, or as fulminant multiple-organ failure with circulatory collapse. When evaluating patients in whom there is a clinical suspicion for acute pancreatitis, serum lipase should be used as the routine initial serum test, as it is more sensitive and specific than serum amylase. If lipase is not available, amylase should be used. The outcome for an individual patient diagnosed with acute pancreatitis in the ED is difficult to predict. Most patients with acute pancreatitis will need admission, although a subset who are well appearing and can reliably follow dietary instructions, and whose pain is controlled with oral analgesics, may be appropriate for outpatient management. There is no evidence to support the ED use of any clinical or CT-based scoring system to predict severity of disease, local complication, or death and determine disposition. We recommend that clinicians use their clinical judgment as they would for other potentially critically ill patients to determine the need for ICU placement. This includes vital signs, patient comfort, signs of sepsis, and respiratory status.

References

1. Fagenholz PJ, Fernandez-del Castillo C, Harris NS *et al*. National study of United States emergency department visits for acute pancreatitis, 1993–2003. BMC Emergency Medicine. 2007; 7: 1.
2. Banks PA, Freeman ML, Practice Parameters Committee of the American College of Gastroenterology: Practice guidelines in acute pancreatitis. American Journal of Gastroenterol. 2006; 101: 2379–400.
3. Tietz NW, Shuey DF. Lipase in serum – the elusive enzyme: An overview. Clinical Chemistry. 1993; 39: 746–56.
4. Vissers RJ, Abu-Laban RB, McHugh DF. Amylase and lipase in the emergency department evaluation of acute pancreatitis. Journal of Emergency Medicine. 1999; 17: 1027–37.

5. Butler J, Mackway-Jones K. Towards evidence based emergency medicine: Best BETs from the Manchester Royal Infirmary: Serum amylase or lipase to diagnose pancreatitis in patients presenting with abdominal pain. Emergency Medicine Journal. 2002; 19: 430–1.

6. Treacy J, Williams A, Bais R *et al.* Evaluation of amylase and lipase in the diagnosis of acute pancreatitis. ANZ Journal of Surgery. 2001; 71: 577–82.

7. Bradley EL III. A clinically based classification system for acute pancreatitis: Summary of the international symposium on acute pancreatitis, Atlanta, GA, September 11 through 13, 1992. Archives of Surgery. 1993; 128: 586–90.

8. Ho KM, Dobb GJ, Knuiman M *et al.* A comparison of admission and worst 24-hour acute physiology and chronic health evaluation II scores in predicting hospital mortality: A retrospective cohort study. Critical Care. 2006; 10: R4.

9. Annane D, Bellissant E, Cavaillon JM. Septic shock. Lancet. 2005; 365: 63–78.

10. Wu BU, Johannes RS, Sun X *et al.* The early prediction of mortality in acute pancreatitis: A large population-based study. Gut. 2008; 57: 1698–703.

11. MdCalc website. Available from: http://www.mdcalc.com/apache-ii-score-for-icu-mortality/.

12. Gravante G, Garcea G, Ong SL *et al.* Prediction of mortality in acute pancreatitis: A systematic review of the published evidence. Pancreatology. 2009; 9: 601–14.

13. Papachristou GI, Muddana V, Yadav D *et al.* Comparison of BISAP, Ranson's, APACHE-II, and CTSI scores in predicting organ failure, complications, and mortality in acute pancreatitis. American Journal of Gastroenterology. 2010; 105: 435–41; quiz 442.

14. Bollen TL, Singh VK, Maurer R *et al.* A comparative evaluation of radiologic and clinical scoring systems in the early prediction of severity in acute pancreatitis. American Journal of Gastroenterology. 2011 Apr; 107(4): 612–19.

Chapter 42 **Acute Appendicitis**

Highlights

- The diagnosis of acute appendicitis is clinically challenging as the classic presentation of periumbilical pain followed by nausea and vomiting, with migration of pain to the right lower quadrant, occurs in only about half of patients with appendicitis.
- White blood cell (WBC) count is not useful to rule in or rule out the diagnosis of acute appendicitis.
- The Alvarado Score is not accurate enough to rule in or rule out appendicitis.
- Abdominal CT is more sensitive than abdominal ultrasound in diagnosing appendicitis and is the preferred imaging study in nonpregnant adults. Oral contrast does not improve diagnostic performance of CT.
- Protocols using ultrasound first and CT for equivocal cases show promise in diagnosing appendicitis with less use of CT, but have not been rigorously tested in the United States.
- Increased use of CT has been associated with lower negative appendectomy rates, but clinicians should be aware that false-positive CTs are possible and negative appendectomy rates are still reported to be at least 5%.

Background

Acute appendicitis is frequently in the differential diagnosis of patients presenting to the emergency department (ED) with acute abdominal pain. Approximately one in every 4,000 ED visits (0.03%) is for acute appendicitis,[1] and appendectomy is the most commonly performed emergency surgical procedure. Yet, the diagnosis of appendicitis remains challenging, as the classic presentation of periumbilical pain followed by nausea and vomiting, with migration of pain to the right lower quadrant (RLQ), occurs in only 50–60% of patients with appendicitis.[2] Appendicitis remains a commonly

Evidence-Based Emergency Care: Diagnostic Testing and Clinical Decision Rules, Second Edition.
Jesse M. Pines, Christopher R. Carpenter, Ali S. Raja and Jeremiah D. Schuur.
© 2013 John Wiley & Sons, Ltd. Published 2013 by John Wiley & Sons, Ltd.

missed diagnosis and one of the five most frequent conditions leading to malpractice claims against emergency physicians. The usefulness of specific lab tests and imaging studies in aiding with the diagnosis has been questioned. Traditionally, a surgical consultant was engaged early during the evaluation in patients with any suspicion for having appendicitis. However in the last decade, with the increasing use of computed tomography (CT) to both rule out and rule in appendicitis, many emergency physicians involve a surgeon only after a CT-confirmed diagnosis of appendicitis. Recently, with increasing concern over the effects of ionizing radiation from CT, there is increasing discussion of using ultrasound or clinical suspicion alone to diagnose acute appendicitis.

Clinical question

What is the role of the white blood cell (WBC) count in the diagnosis of acute appendicitis?

Traditional surgical teaching highlights the importance of leukocytosis in the diagnosis of acute abdominal pathology, including appendicitis. Andersson conducted a systematic review and meta-analysis in 2004 of clinical and laboratory values for patients admitted to the hospital with acute appendicitis.[2] The author found 24 articles that met the following inclusion criteria: studies with patients admitted to the hospital for suspected appendicitis, studies including data permitting calculation of likelihood ratios and/or receiver operator characteristic (ROC) curves, and studies including adult patients (pediatric-only studies were excluded). Studies based on unselected patients with abdominal pain, patients taken to surgery for suspected appendicitis, or comparisons of patients with verified appendicitis with healthy controls were excluded. Diagnostic performance was determined using weighted pooled estimates of the area under the ROC curves and likelihood ratios for diagnostic variables of interest. The results for WBC count are in Table 42.1. While increasing WBC count correlates with the diagnosis of acute

Table 42.1 Pooled likelihood ratios of elevated WBC in diagnosing acute appendicitis

White blood cell (WBC) count ($\times 10^9$/l)	Positive likelihood ratio LR+ (CI)	Negative likelihood ratio LR− (CI)
WBC ≥ 10	2.5 (2.1–3.0)	0.3 (0.2–0.4)
WBC ≥ 12	2.8 (2.0–3.8)	0.5 (0.4–0.6)
WBC ≥ 14	3.0 (2.5–3.5)	0.7 (0.6–0.9)
WBC ≥ 15	3.5 (1.6–7.8)	0.8 (0.7–1.0)

Source: Data from [2].

appendicitis, there is a clear trade-off between sensitivity and specificity; no cutoff exists with test characteristics that would change clinical practice.

No other tests, including granulocyte count, proportion of polymorphonuclear cells (PMNs), or C-reactive protein (CRP), were superior to WBC on their own. The author performed numerous permutations of inflammatory marker combinations (WBC, CRP, and proportion of PMNs) and found that only when two or more inflammatory markers were normal, was there sufficient confidence to make appendicitis unlikely. However, this has limited clinical use, as situations in which one test is positive and another is negative are common and have little predictive value (LR between 0.5 and 2.1).

Clinical question

Are clinical prediction rules useful in the diagnosis of acute appendicitis?
Several clinical prediction rules that incorporate elements of the patient's history, physical exam, and lab findings have been developed to aid in the diagnosis of acute appendicitis. Individual values from the history and physical exam are associated with acute appendicitis, but none is individually predictive enough to alter clinical judgment. This is well documented in Andersson's systematic review and meta-analysis described in this chapter, which calculated pooled LRs for history and physical exam findings, and found that none of the findings had LR+ above 3 and that direct tenderness and rebound tenderness had LR− below 0.4.[2]

The clinical prediction rule for acute appendicitis that has been most studied in the ED was developed by Alvarado.[3] He derived the rule retrospectively on a group of 305 hospitalized patients with abdominal pain suggestive of appendicitis, and identified eight factors predictive of acute appendicitis. Based on the weight of their association, each factor was given a score that, when summed, makes up the Alvarado Score (Table 42.2). A systematic review and meta-analysis by Ohle et al evaluated the diagnostic utility of the Alvarado Score for predicting acute appendicitis and included 42 studies.[4] The authors of the meta-analysis assessed the diagnostic accuracy of the score at two thresholds: a cutoff of 5 (1–4 vs. 5–10) and a cutoff of 7 (1–6 vs. 7–10), focusing on three subgroups: men, women, and children. They also analyzed the calibration across low- (1–4), intermediate- (5–6), and high-risk (7–10) strata. They found that the threshold of ≥5 was associated with a pooled sensitivity of 99% (subgroup sensitivities: 96% men, 99% women, and 99% children) and a specificity of 43% (subgroup specificities: 34% men, 35% women, 57% children). At this threshold the pooled LR+ is 1.7 and the LR− is 0.02. At the threshold of ≥7, the score performed poorly with an overall specificity of 81% (subgroup specificities: men 57%, women 73%, and children 76%). They found that the score overpredicts the probability of appendicitis in children in the intermediate- and high-risk

Table 42.2 Alvarado Score for acute appendicitis

Feature	Points
Migration of pain	1
Anorexia	1
Nausea	1
Tenderness in right lower quadrant	2
Rebound pain	1
Elevated temperature (>37.3°C or >99.1°F)	1
Leucocytosis (>10,000)	2
"Left shift" of white blood cell count (e.g., >75% neutrophils)	1

Source: Data from [3].

groups and in women across all risk strata. The authors concluded that the Alvarado Score is useful to rule out acute appendicitis at a cut point of <5 for all patient groups.

The American College of Emergency Physicians (ACEP) Clinical Policy on acute appendicitis, published in 2010, reviewed the literature on the Alvarado Score and came to a different conclusion – that imaging can be warranted even in patients with low Alvarado Scores.[5] They noted that in three studies, a significant proportion (9%, 36%, and 72%) of patients with low-risk Alvarado Scores (<5) ultimately had appendicitis.

Of note, most studies did not answer the critical question – does the Alvarado Score add diagnostic utility beyond the decision making of a typical emergency clinician? It is possible that the Alvarado Score doesn't perform better than clinical gestalt, as most of the components of the score are already used by emergency clinicians when evaluating a patient for possible appendicitis.

Clinical question

Which diagnostic imaging modality is best for diagnosing acute appendicitis?
The two common imaging studies used in the setting of suspected acute appendicitis are abdominal CT and ultrasound. CT is widely available and rapid, but employs both intravenous contrast and ionizing radiation. Ultrasound does not employ ionizing radiation or intravenous contrast, but requires the availability of a technician or radiologist and is operator dependent. Studies have compared the diagnostic performances of these two modalities in algorithms that begin with ultrasound and move on to CT.

A large systematic review of prospective studies examining the accuracy of CT and ultrasound for diagnosing acute appendicitis was published by Doria et al in 2006.[6] Studies from 1986 to 2004 that utilized abdominal

Table 42.3 Summary performance of computed tomography (CT) and ultrasound in diagnosing appendicitis

	Sensitivity (CI)	Specificity (CI)
Children		
Ultrasound	88% (86–90%)	94% (92–95%)
CT	94% (92–97%)	95% (94–97%)
Adults		
Ultrasound	83% (78–87%)	93% (95–96%)
CT	94% (92–95%)	94% (94–96%)

Source: Data from [6].

CT, ultrasound, or both as diagnostic tests for appendicitis in children (26 studies, 9,356 patients) or adults (31 studies, 4,341 patients) with surgical or clinical follow-up were included if they separately reported data to calculate sensitivities and specificities. Overall, CT performed better than ultrasound (Table 42.3). Of note, since many of these studies were performed, the introduction of multidetector CT has improved image resolution and decreased artifact with more rapid scanning times, generally resulting in improved sensitivity and specificity. The authors conclude that while CT has excellent diagnostic accuracy, clinicians must also consider the safety perspective, particularly the radiation associated with CT, especially in children.

Dutch researchers, feeling that prior studies that examined selected patients in academic and university settings using specialized body radiologists were not representative of community practice, conducted a study examining patients with clinical suspicion for acute appendicitis.[7] Of 339 patients with abdominal pain who were eligible for consent, 199 consented and underwent both noncontrast abdominal CT and RLQ ultrasound studies over a 1-hour period. General radiologists (n = 10) and body-specialized radiologists (n = 2) blindly interpreted the studies. Similar to other studies, outcomes were determined by surgical or pathologic reports or by longitudinal follow-up. Surgery was performed in 88% of the enrolled patients, and the prevalence of acute appendicitis was 66%. The diagnostic performances of CT and ultrasound were statistically similar: CT sensitivity was 76% (CI 68–83%), specificity 83% (CI 73–92%), and accuracy 78%; and ultrasound sensitivity was 79% (CI 71–85%), specificity 78% (CI 66–87%), and accuracy 78%.

The main limitation cited by the authors in all of the studies was the use of different criterion standards for patients with positive or negative tests. This is an example of double criterion standard bias (see Chapter 6). Positive CT or US results generally lead to surgery and a pathologic diagnosis, while negative studies were assessed by observation and outpatient follow-up. Surgery is more likely to identify disease, as some patients with mild appendiceal inflammation will spontaneously recover, introducing potential bias when a uniform criterion standard is not utilized. Similarly, most studies included in this assessment reported the severity of disease, which is a form of spectrum bias.

Several studies have evaluated the population effects of widespread use of CT on the diagnosis and outcomes for acute appendicitis. Flum et al performed a population-based analysis of misdiagnosis rates among patients undergoing appendectomies.[8] They examined the hypothesis that with increased imaging among at-risk populations, there would be an expected decrease in the rate of missed appendicitis. Examining population-based data from Washington State, they did not find a statistical change in the misdiagnosis rate over a 12-year period (1987–1998). The rates of ruptured and misdiagnosed appendicitis were stable at approximately 2.6 and 1.6 cases per 10,000 person-years, respectively. Frei et al performed a high-quality chart review of 2,018 patients aged 12–65 years who had an appendectomy between 1998 and 2004.[9] The primary outcomes were delay in treatment, complications (gangrene, perforation, or abscess), negative laparotomy rate, and time to surgery. The proportion of appendectomy patients undergoing CT scan increased from 12% to 84%, and the time to surgery increased over the period of the study. The negative appendectomy rate fell from 16% to 11% in the first year but was relatively constant thereafter. There was a decrease in the complication rate (from 33% to 21%). Wagner et al examined the relationship between the use of preoperative CT and negative appendectomy rates in 1,425 patients undergoing appendectomies from 2000 to 2007.[10] Preoperative CT was performed in 89% of adults and 73% of children. The negative appendectomy rate was 14% in patients not having preoperative CT, and 7% in those having a preoperative CT scan (p = 0.007). The negative appendectomy rate decreased from 11% in 2000 to 5% in 2006, but the decrease was seen only in females, not in males or children. There was not an associated change in perforation rates.

Clinical question

Can ultrasound be used first to reduce the use of CT in the diagnosis of appendicitis?

Several studies have evaluated pathways that first use ultrasound, followed by CT, to diagnose acute appendicitis. The studies have generally found similar diagnostic characteristics for ultrasound and CT as had been described in this chapter. A Dutch study evaluated a diagnostic imaging protocol consisting of initial graded compression ultrasound followed by selective intravenous (IV) contrast-enhanced CT scanning in 151 adults with suspected acute appendicitis.[11] Patients diagnosed with appendicitis on ultrasound went directly to surgery, and those with negative or equivocal ultrasound underwent CT. The criterion standard was the result of surgery or observation for those with negative CTs. Ultrasound was consistent with appendicitis in 79 patients (52%), all of whom had surgery; the negative appendectomy rate was 10%. CT scanning was performed in 60 patients with negative or inconclusive ultrasound, and diagnosed appendicitis in 21 patients, none of whom had a negative appendectomy. None of the 39 patients observed following negative ultrasound and CT required surgical intervention. A second Dutch study prospectively examined a similar pathway at one hospital where 164 of 802 patients with abdominal pain were suspected to have appendicitis.[12] The overall prevalence was 15%, 63% in patients in whom appendicitis was clinically suspected and 2% in whom it was not initially suspected. Imaging was performed in 98% of patients in whom appendicitis was suspected (118 ultrasound studies and 19 CT studies). Ultrasound sensitivity and specificity were 91% and 98%, respectively, and CT sensitivity and specificity were 100% each. Overall, imaging provided an accurate diagnosis in 98% of the patients in whom it was performed, and resulted in a change in management for 20 patients. The negative appendectomy rate was 3%. The overall perforation rate was 24%, but the rate of missed perforated appendicitis was 3%. The authors of these small series concluded that the protocols are safe and avoided CT in about half of patients.

Several studies have evaluated an ultrasound first pathway in children. An Israeli study retrospectively reviewed 2,218 children aged 2–17 with suspected appendicitis from 2002 through 2007.[13] Forty-three percent of children were clinically managed without imaging, ultrasound alone was performed in 43%, both ultrasound and CT scanning were performed in 9%, and 5% had CT alone. Surgery based on clinical findings alone decreased from 55% to 19%, while the use of ultrasound prior to surgery increased from 37% to 64%. The false-positive appendectomy rate among patients undergoing imaging studies decreased from 11% to 2%. The authors advocate initial ultrasound, reserving CT for equivocal cases. Of note, at baseline their practice was to operate without imaging in half of cases, so the protocol increased the use of ultrasound and did not dramatically increase CT use.

Two US studies retrospectively report on similar pathways for children suspected of having appendicitis. Adibe et al at the Children's Hospital of Alabama evaluated 100 children after protocol implementation and compared those to 146 before implementation.[14] They found that the use of CT scanning decreased from 81% to 60% and ultrasound increased from 3% to 21%. Rates of negative appendicitis were 7% before the protocol and 11% after, a nonsignificant increase. Of note, many post-protocol patients with a negative appendectomy had a false-positive CT. Ramarajan et al studied a similar pathway in 680 children evaluated for appendicitis at the Stanford Children's Hospital.[15] Ultrasound was the primary imaging modality, with CT reserved for equivocal cases, but all imaging was at the discretion of managing physicians. The pathway was followed in 60% of the eligible children and yielded a sensitivity of 99% and specificity of 91% for appendicitis. Compared to all children getting a CT scan, the protocol would reduce CT scanning by half.

These studies evaluated ultrasound performed by radiologists or ultrasound technicians with radiology interpretation. There have not been large prospective studies of emergency physicians' ability to perform ultrasound for the diagnosis of appendicitis, and ED-based studies to date have included clinicians with advanced ultrasound training, and are not representative of the average practicing emergency physician.

Clinical question

Is oral or IV contrast useful when performing CT scans for acute appendicitis?
The traditional protocol for abdominal CT for undifferentiated abdominal pain includes the use of oral contrast prior to the study and IV contrast during the study. Alternative protocols for appendicitis have been developed using rectal contrast in lieu of oral contrast. Some centers perform noncontrast CTs for appendicitis, which eliminates several hours of waiting as well as the risks of IV contrast. Anderson et al performed a systematic review of 23 studies and found that the diagnostic performance of CT with and without oral contrast material for the diagnosis of appendicitis in adults was similar (sensitivity, 95% vs. 92%; and specificity, 97% vs. 94%).[16] A second systematic review by Hlibczuk et al evaluated the accuracy of noncontrast multidetector CT in adult ED patients with suspected acute appendicitis.[17] The criterion standard was final diagnosis and surgery or attempted follow-up at a minimum of 2 weeks. They identified seven high-quality studies, including 1,060 patients. Pooled estimates for sensitivity were 93% (90–95%) and specificity 96% (94–98%). The 7% false-negative appendectomy rate was in the same range as that found for CT scanning using contrast (3–17%).

Anderson et al conducted a randomized trial to compare the diagnostic accuracy of IV contrast-enhanced CT with and without the use of oral contrast material in diagnosing appendicitis in patients with abdominal pain.[18] They enrolled a convenience sample of 303 adult patients presenting to an urban academic ED with acute atraumatic abdominal pain and clinical suspicion of appendicitis, diverticulitis, or small bowel obstruction. Patients were randomized to receive IV contrast with or without oral contrast.

Each CT was interpreted by two radiologists, and final diagnosis was based on operative, clinical, and follow-up data. Diagnostic test performance was similar in patients receiving or not receiving oral contrast: sensitivity of 100% (CI 77–100%) and specificity of 97% (CI 93–99%). The authors conclude that for ED patients with abdominal pain and suspected appendicitis, oral contrast does not improve diagnostic accuracy.

Comment

Appendicitis remains a challenging diagnosis in emergency medicine. Clinicians are pulled in several directions when considering diagnostic tests: pressure to not miss the diagnosis, avoiding unnecessary use of CT and its associated radiation, efficiently treating such patients, and pressure from consultants and radiologists about which tests to order. After developing a clinical suspicion of appendicitis, clinicians should not use laboratory tests to alter their suspicion as no laboratory tests, including WBC count, have high likelihood ratios; a clinician is more likely to falsely anchor his or her diagnostic reasoning on a laboratory value than improve the accuracy of diagnosis. Additionally, the Alvarado Score, which combines historical features, physical findings, and WBC count results, is not accurate enough to rule in or rule out appendicitis.

Emergency departments should develop protocols around imaging patients with suspected appendicitis in order to reduce interphysician variability and practice a consistent standard. In children, an ultrasound-first protocol will reduce the number of CTs, but requires the availability of skilled ultrasonographers and surgeons willing to operate based on their findings. In adults, CT remains the diagnostic test of choice in the United States, while in Europe more centers are adopting ultrasound-first pathways. As no large comparative studies have been performed in adults, the safety of such pathways is not yet known.

References

1. Tsze DS, Asnis LM, Merchant RC *et al.* Increasing computed tomography use for patients with appendicitis and discrepancies in pain management between adults and children: An analysis of the NHAMCS. Annals of Emergency Medicine. 2011 May; 59(5): 395–403.
2. Andersson RE. Meta-analysis of the clinical and laboratory diagnosis of appendicitis. British Journal of Surgery. 2004; 91: 28–37.
3. Alvarado A. A practical score for the early diagnosis of acute appendicitis. Annals of Emergency Medicine. 1986; 15: 557–64.
4. Ohle R, O'Reilly F, O'Brien KK *et al.* The Alvarado Score for predicting acute appendicitis: A systematic review. BMC Medicine. 2011; 9: 139.

5. Howell JM, Eddy OL, Lukens TW *et al.* Clinical policy: Critical issues in the evaluation and management of emergency department patients with suspected appendicitis. Annals of Emergency Medicine. 2010; 55: 71–116.
6. Doria AS, Moineddin R, Kellenberger CJ *et al.* US or CT for diagnosis of appendicitis in children and adults? A meta-analysis. Radiology. 2006 Oct; 241: 83–94.
7. Poortman P, Lohle PNM, Schoemaker CMC *et al.* Comparison of CT and sonography in the diagnosis of acute appendicitis: A blinded prospective study. American Journal of Roentgenology. 2003; 181: 1355–9.
8. Flum DR, Morris A, Koepsell T *et al.* Has misdiagnosis of appendicitis decreased over time? A population-based analysis. Journal of the American Medical Association. 2001; 286: 1748–53.
9. Frei SP, Bond WF, Bazuro RK *et al.* Appendicitis outcomes with increasing computed tomographic scanning. American Journal of Emergency Medicine. 2008; 26: 39–44.
10. Wagner PL, Eachempati SR, Soe K *et al.* Defining the current negative appendectomy rate: For whom is preoperative computed tomography making an impact? Surgery. 2008; 144: 276–82.
11. Poortman P, Oostvogel HJ, Bosma E *et al.* Improving diagnosis of acute appendicitis: Results of a diagnostic pathway with standard use of ultrasonography followed by selective use of CT. Journal of the American College of Surgeons. 2009; 208: 434–41.
12. Toorenvliet BR, Wiersma F, Bakker RF *et al.* Routine ultrasound and limited computed tomography for the diagnosis of acute appendicitis. World Journal of Surgery. 2010; 34: 2278–85.
13. Neufeld D, Vainrib M, Buklan G *et al.* Management of acute appendicitis: An imaging strategy in children. Pediatric Surgery International. 2010; 26: 167–71.
14. Adibe OO, Amin SR, Hansen EN *et al.* An evidence-based clinical protocol for diagnosis of acute appendicitis decreased the use of computed tomography in children. Journal of Pediatric Surgery. 2011; 46: 192–6.
15. Ramarajan N, Krishnamoorthi R, Barth R *et al.* An interdisciplinary initiative to reduce radiation exposure: Evaluation of appendicitis in a pediatric emergency department with clinical assessment supported by a staged ultrasound and computed tomography pathway. Academic Emergency Medicine. 2009; 16: 1258–65.
16. Anderson BA, Salem L, Flum DR. A systematic review of whether oral contrast is necessary for the computed tomography diagnosis of appendicitis in adults. American Journal of Surgery. 2005; 190: 474–8.
17. Hlibczuk V, Dattaro JA, Jin Z *et al.* Diagnostic accuracy of noncontrast computed tomography for appendicitis in adults: A systematic review. Annals of Emergency Medicine. 2010; 55: 51–9.e1.
18. Anderson SW, Soto JA, Lucey BC *et al.* Abdominal 64-MDCT for suspected appendicitis: The use of oral and IV contrast material versus IV contrast material only. American Journal of Roentgenology. 2009; 193: 1282–8.

Chapter 43 **Acute Cholecystitis**

Highlights

- History, physical exam findings, and lab values are not sensitive predictors of acute cholecystitis.
- The most appropriate initial imaging technique for patients with suspected cholecystitis is ultrasound, given the test characteristics and availability of US, CT, and HIDA. However, CT can be used if other diagnoses are thought to be likely and HIDA scans can be used in cases in which the diagnosis remains uncertain.
- Emergency physician-performed ultrasound has favorable test characteristics but remains operator dependent.

Background

Acute cholecystitis is a common concern in patients presenting for the evaluation of abdominal pain, accounting for approximately 5–9% of admissions from the emergency department (ED). Patients typically present with pain localized to the right upper quadrant, and the disease involves inflammation of the gallbladder, most commonly due to cystic duct obstruction by a gallstone. Gallstones themselves are relatively common, with a prevalence between 9% and 29% in US patients, depending on ethnicity and gender.[1] Risk factors for gallstones include age (>40 years), gender (women are more than twice as likely as men to have the disease), obesity (>120% of ideal body weight), pregnancy, and the use of oral contraceptives or estrogen replacement therapy.

Once present, gallstones can obstruct the cystic duct leading to the gallbladder inflammation that defines cholecystitis. It is typically diagnosed using ultrasound (with findings of a thickened gallbladder wall, pericholecystic fluid, and a sonographic Murphy sign; Figure 43.1), radionucleotide

Evidence-Based Emergency Care: Diagnostic Testing and Clinical Decision Rules, Second Edition.
Jesse M. Pines, Christopher R. Carpenter, Ali S. Raja and Jeremiah D. Schuur.
© 2013 John Wiley & Sons, Ltd. Published 2013 by John Wiley & Sons, Ltd.

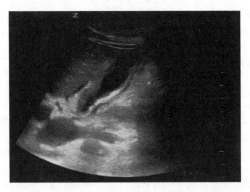

Figure 43.1 Acute cholecystitis with a thickened gallbladder wall and pericholecystic fluid seen on ultrasound. (Source: Elke Platz, Heidi Kimberly & Dorothea Hempel, Department of Emergency Medicine, Brigham and Women's Hospital, used with permission).

cholescintigraphy (the hepatobiliary scintigraphy (HIDA) scan, with a lack of isotope accumulation in the gallbladder, indicating cystic duct obstruction), or computed tomography (CT) (with gallbladder wall thickening, pericholecystic fluid, and inflammation in the pericholecystic fat). Secondary infection due to bile stasis commonly occurs, making empiric antibiotic therapy a mainstay of treatment. Definitive treatment requires removal of the cause of the inflammation, and typically involves immediate cholecystectomy in most patients and either percutaneous cholecystostomy or endoscopic gallbladder drainage (typically via endoscopic retrograde cholangiopancreatography) in patients thought to be too high risk for surgery. Of note, acalculous cholecystitis, which occurs in up to 10% of cases of cholecystitis, can occur due to a number of infectious causes and has a higher morbidity and mortality.

Clinical question

What is the accuracy of the history, physical examination, and laboratory testing for the diagnosis of acute cholecystitis?

Trowbridge et al performed a comprehensive review of studies examining the physical exam, medical history, and lab tests in diagnosing acute cholecystitis.[2] They included 17 studies that evaluated a total of 12 findings in the history and physical examination as well as five laboratory tests, with between 351 and 1,338 patients per finding or test. They found that none of the tested findings, which included fever, the Murphy sign, rebound tenderness, total bilirubin, liver function tests, and leukocytosis, had sufficient

LR+ or LR− to rule in or rule out the disease. Even right upper quadrant tenderness, which had a summary LR− of 0.4, had a CI of 0.2−1.1.

Clinical question

What is the accuracy of CT, ultrasound, or nuclear medicine scans for the diagnosis of acute cholecystitis?

Radiologists at the University of Pennsylvania compared abdominal CT with oral and intravenous (IV) contrast with ultrasonography for the diagnosis of acute biliary disease in a retrospective cohort of patients undergoing both imaging studies.[3] Patients were included if they had right upper quadrant (RUQ) pain and had both RUQ ultrasound and abdominal CT imaging studies performed within 48 hours of each other. Patients with prior cholecystectomy were excluded. CT and ultrasound studies were blindly interpreted by separate radiologists. A final diagnosis of acute cholecystitis was determined by surgical reports, pathology reports, and autopsy findings. The objective in the study was to determine whether CT or ultrasound was the most appropriate first study for these patients. While the focus of this chapter is the diagnosis of acute cholecystitis, this study provides the opportunity to examine the performances of the two imaging studies for the diagnosis of both cholecystitis and other acute biliary diseases that would be included in the differential diagnosis of patients undergoing imaging for suspected acute cholecystitis (including gallstone pancreatitis and choledocholithiasis). The study identified 123 patients, of whom 117 were suspected of having acute biliary disease. A final diagnosis of acute biliary disease was made in 18 patients (incidence 15%) in this study group, and Table 43.1 shows the performance of the two imaging modalities. Only seven of these patients were given a final diagnosis of cholecystitis, and the authors do not include sufficient information to calculate test characteristics for CT and ultrasound for this specific diagnosis.

The authors concluded that RUQ ultrasound was the preferred first study when considering the diagnosis of acute biliary disease, with a significantly better sensitivity and marginally higher specificity than abdominal CT. However, if other abdominal disease processes are considered likely in the differential diagnosis, then CT should still be considered.

HIDA has long been considered the criterion standard for diagnosing acute cholecystitis. In a single-center retrospective analysis of patients suspected of having acute cholecystitis (who had both ultrasound and HIDA scan tests ordered simultaneously) the performance characteristics of the two tests were compared.[4] It was standard practice at the study hospital for both studies to be ordered together when the diagnosis was considered. Consecutive patients were included, and patients were excluded if a test was ordered after the first

Table 43.1 Computed tomography (CT) and ultrasound test characteristics for the diagnosis of acute biliary disease

	Acute biliary Dz (+)	Acute biliary Dz (−)	Totals
CT (+)	7	7	14
CT indeterminate or (−)	11	92	103
Totals	18	99	117
Ultrasound (+)	15	5	20
Ultrasound indeterminate or (−)	3	94	97
Totals	18	99	117

Note: CT: positive likelihood ratio (LR+) 5.6, negative likelihood ratio (LR−) 0.66, sensitivity 39% (CI 17–64%), and specificity 93% (CI 86–97%). Ultrasound: LR+ 16.6, LR− 0.18, sensitivity 83% (CI 59–96%), and specificity 95% (CI 89–98%).
Source: Data from [3].

Table 43.2 Test characteristics of Hepatobiliary scintigraphy (HIDA) scan and ultrasound for cholecystitis

	Acute Biliary Dz (+)	Acute Biliary Dz (−)	Totals
HIDA (+)	28	5	33
HIDA (−)	4	70	74
Totals	32	75	107
Ultrasound (+)	16	9	25
Ultrasound indeterminate or (−)	16	66	82
Totals	32	75	107

Note: HIDA: positive likelihood ratio (LR+) 12.6, negative likelihood ratio (LR−) 0.13, sensitivity 88% (CI 71–97%), and specificity 93% (CI 85–98%). Ultrasound: LR+ 4.2, LR− 0.57, sensitivity 50% (CI 32–68%), and specificity 88% (CI 78–94%).
Source: Data from [3].

test had been completed in an effort to minimize bias based on the initial tests' results. The final diagnosis was determined using surgical, pathology, and autopsy reports or a clinical diagnosis for those who did not die or undergo surgery. A total of 107 patients were examined, 32 (30%) of whom had a final diagnosis of acute cholecystitis. Using data provided in their study, the performance characteristics of the two tests are shown in Table 43.2.

The authors concluded that HIDA was superior to ultrasound in diagnosing acute cholecystitis. They suggest that, since the costs of each of these studies at the time in their institution were similar, the decision should be based on availability and diagnostic performance.

Given the lack of HIDA availability in most EDs as well as the rapid proliferation of bedside ultrasound, a number of recent studies have evaluated the test characteristics of emergency physician-performed point-of-care ultrasound for the diagnosis of acute cholecystitis. A 2011 systematic review by Ross et al reviewed the available literature and found eight articles that described prospective studies with appropriate reference standards (typically radiologist-performed ultrasound or surgical and pathology reports).[5] This pooled dataset contained 710 patients and found an overall sensitivity of 90% (CI 86–93%) and a specificity of 88% (CI 84–91%). The resultant pooled LR+ was 7.5 and the pooled LR− was 0.11, and the individual studies are described in Table 43.3.

While a number of these studies were based on convenience samples and had relatively small sample sizes, the pooled analysis demonstrates favorable test characteristics and relatively narrow confidence intervals. The systematic review's authors' concluded that emergency physician–performed bedside ultrasound can be useful in both making the diagnosis of acute cholecystitis and, if negative, justifying broadening a patient's evaluation to include other possibility etiologies for his or her acute symptomatology.

It should be noted that all of the aforementioned bedside ultrasonography studies were performed on adults; while Tsung et al recently described the feasibility of point-of-care ED ultrasound in a pediatric population, their case series cannot yet support the routine reliance on bedside ultrasound in children with suspected cholecystitis.[14]

Table 43.3 Individual and pooled test characteristics of emergency physician-performed ultrasound to diagnose acute cholecystitis

Study	n	Sensitivity (CI)	Specificity (CI)
Alexander, 2008[6]	50	0.86 (0.67–0.96)	0.95 (0.77–1.00)
Davis, 2005[7]	105	0.81 (0.69–0.90)	0.86 (0.72–0.95)
Ha, 2002[8]	59	0.94 (0.71–1.00)	0.95 (0.84–0.99)
Kendall, 2001[9]	109	0.96 (0.87–1.00)	0.88 (0.77–0.95)
Miller, 2006[10]	127	0.94 (0.88–0.97)	0.96 (0.80–1.00)
Rosen, 2001[11]	110	0.92 (0.83–0.97)	0.78 (0.63–0.89)
Rowland, 2001[12]	35	0.75 (0.48–0.93)	0.84 (0.60–0.97)
Summers, 2010[13]	115	0.89 (0.79–0.95)	0.86 (0.73–0.95)
Pooled	*710*	*0.90 (0.86–0.93)*	*0.88 (0.84–0.91)*

Source: Data from [6–13] as indicated under "Study" column.

Lastly, in their 2008 update to their original 2003 meta-analysis, Trowbridge et al also reviewed bedside ultrasound's test characteristics and found that the combination of bedside ultrasonographic evidence of gallstones and a positive sonographic Murphy sign had good test characteristics, with a LR+ 2.7 (CI 1.7–4.1) and LR− 0.13 (CI 0.04–0.39).[15]

Comments

Given the fact that there are no aspects of the history, physical examination, or laboratory test results that can accurately diagnose or rule out acute cholecystitis, patients in whom the diagnosis is suspected should have ultrasound performed (unless HIDA is available).

While emergency physician–performed bedside ultrasound is well supported by the literature and taught in most US emergency medicine residencies, its ability to detect acute cholecystitis is operator dependent, a limitation acknowledged both by the individual studies cited in this chapter and also by the authors of the systematic review. Brook et al recently reviewed cases of missed cholecystitis at their institution and determined that most of them were due to lack of recognition of the radiological findings of gallbladder wall edema and gallbladder wall thickening, whether on CT and ultrasound.[16] With improved training and quality assurance mechanisms for emergency physician–performed ultrasound, we should continue to see improvements in test characteristics and reliability. Until then, its use should be site and user dependent and based on a well-orchestrated ultrasound quality assurance program involving education, image review, and routine feedback and evaluation.

References

1. Everhart JE, Khare M, Hill M, Maurer KR. Prevalence and ethnic differences in gallbladder disease in the United States. Gastroenterology. 1999; 117(3): 632–9.
2. Trowbridge RL, Rutkowski NK, Shojania KG. Does this patient have acute cholecystitis? Journal of the American Medical Association. 2003; 289(1): 80–6.
3. Harvey RT, Miller WT Jr. Acute biliary disease: Initial CT and follow-up US versus initial US and follow-up CT. Radiology. 1999; 213(3): 831–6.
4. Chatziioannou SN, Moore WH, Ford PV, Dhekne RD. Hepatobiliary scintigraphy is superior to abdominal ultrasonography in suspected acute cholecystitis. Surgery. 2000; 127(6): 609–13.
5. Ross M, Brown M, McLaughlin K et al. Emergency physician–performed ultrasound to diagnose cholelithiasis: A systematic review. Academic Emergency Medicine. 2011; 18(3): 227–35.
6. Alexander DN, Ragg M, Stella J. Emergency department ultrasound for the investigation of right upper quadrant abdominal pain. Emergency Medicine Australasia. 2008; 20(Suppl 1): A21.

7. Davis DP, Campbell CJ, Poste JC, Ma G. The association between operator confidence and accuracy of ultrasonography performed by novice emergency physicians. Journal of Emergency Medicine. 2005; 29(3): 259–64.

8. Ha YR, Kim H, Yoo S et al. Accuracy of emergency ultrasonography for biliary parameters by physicians with limited training. Journal of the Korean Society of Emergency Medicine. 13(4): 407–10.

9. Kendall JL, Shimp RJ. Performance and interpretation of focused right upper quadrant ultrasound by emergency physicians. Journal of Emergency Medicine. 2001; 21(1): 7–13.

10. Miller AH, Pepe PE, Brockman CR, Delaney KA. ED ultrasound in hepatobiliary disease. Journal of Emergency Medicine. 2006; 30(1): 69–74.

11. Rosen CL, Brown DF, Chang Y et al. Ultrasonography by emergency physicians in patients with suspected cholecystitis. American Journal of Emergency Medicine. 2001; 19(1): 32–6.

12. Rowland JL, Kuhn M, Bonnin RL, Davey MJ, Langlois SL. Accuracy of emergency department bedside ultrasonography. Emergency Medicine (Fremantle). 2001; 13(3): 305–13.

13. Summers SM, Scruggs W, Menchine MD et al. A prospective evaluation of emergency department bedside ultrasonography for the detection of acute cholecystitis. Annals of Emergency Medicine. 2010; 56(2): 114–22.

14. Tsung JW, Raio CC, Ramirez-Schrempp D, Blaivas M. Point-of-care ultrasound diagnosis of pediatric cholecystitis in the ED. American Journal of Emergency Medicine. 2010; 28(3): 338–42.

15. Trowbridge RL, Shojania KG. Update: Cholecystitis. In: The rational clinical examination: Evidence-based clinical diagnosis. New York: McGraw-Hill; 2008.

16. Brook OR, Kane RA, Tyagi G, Siewert B, Kruskal JB. Lessons learned from quality assurance: Errors in the diagnosis of acute cholecystitis on ultrasound and CT. American Journal of Roentgenology. 2011; 196(3): 597–604.

Chapter 44 **Aortic Emergencies**

Highlights

- Physical examination findings are insufficiently sensitive to rule out either thoracic aortic dissections or abdominal aortic aneurysms (AAA).
- Chest X-ray cannot rule out the presence of aortic dissection.
- A D-dimer value <500 mg/ml shows promise for the identification of patients who are unlikely to need further aortic imaging for dissection, but additional studies are needed.
- Emergency physician–performed bedside ultrasound is accurate for screening for AAA, given appropriate provider training.

Background

Thoracic aortic dissection and abdominal aortic aneurysm (AAA) are the two aortic emergencies most commonly seen in emergency department (ED) patients. Rupture of AAA is typically a concern in patients presenting with acute abdominal or flank pain, as 4–8% of older men (and slightly fewer women) have occult aneurysms. Similarly, thoracic aortic dissection is a differential diagnostic consideration for patients presenting to the ED with chest pain. Given the low frequency (but high morbidity and mortality) of aortic emergencies, ED evaluation should appropriately focus on screening modalities with high accuracy. While computed tomography (CT) angiography has become the current criterion standard for both disease processes (replacing traditional angiography due to its greater availability), it carries with it the risks of contrast-induced nephropathy and radiation-induced malignancy, as well as the time delay involved with its use in a busy ED. As a result, plain chest radiography and D-dimer have been considered as risk-stratification tools for the presence of an aortic dissection, and the use of bedside ultrasound has been advocated to screen for AAA.

Evidence-Based Emergency Care: Diagnostic Testing and Clinical Decision Rules, Second Edition.
Jesse M. Pines, Christopher R. Carpenter, Ali S. Raja and Jeremiah D. Schuur.
© 2013 John Wiley & Sons, Ltd. Published 2013 by John Wiley & Sons, Ltd.

Clinical question

Which physical examination findings increase or decrease the likelihood of a patient with chest pain having an acute aortic dissection? Is chest radiography or D-dimer appropriate for excluding aortic dissection in patients presenting with chest pain?

A meta-analysis by Klompas in 2002 reviewed the test characteristics of physical examination and radiographic findings for aortic dissection.[1] As few studies met criteria for inclusion, the author was only able to develop pooled data for 1,553 patients and analyze one historical factor (history of hypertension), one symptom (sudden chest pain), two signs (pulse deficit and a diastolic murmur), and one radiographic finding (enlarged aorta or wide mediastinum). The results (Table 44.1) demonstrate that, while the presence of a pulse deficit increases the likelihood for aortic dissection, no element in the history or physical exam is sensitive enough to reliably rule out the disease. Similarly, while a chest x-ray finding of a widened mediastinum was 90% sensitive for thoracic aortic dissection, given the significant morbidity of the disease it was not an appropriate screening exam in patients with a high pretest probability of disease. A later study by von Kodolitsch et al in 2004 confirmed the poor sensitivity of chest x-ray for aortic dissection, finding that it had a sensitivity of only 67% for dissections later verified by either CT or surgery.[2]

A 2011 meta-analysis of 298 patients from seven studies evaluated the use of D-dimer for the exclusion of aortic dissection.[3] A cutoff of 500 ng/ml was used because it is commonly used as the cutoff for the exclusion of pulmonary emboli. All of the studies used CT angiography as the criterion standard and were performed from 2003 to 2009. The results of the pooled analysis demonstrated a D-Dimer sensitivity of 97% (CI 94–99%), a negative predictive value (NPV) of 96% (CI 93–98%), and a LR− 0.05. However, given the number of pathologic situations that can result in an elevated D-dimer, specificity (56%, CI 51–60%), positive predictive value (PPV)

Table 44.1 Accuracy of clinical findings for thoracic aortic dissection

Symptom or sign	Positive likelihood ratio (LR+) (CI)	Negative likelihood ratio (LR−) (CI)
History of hypertension	1.6 (1.2–2.0)	0.5 (0.3–0.7)
Sudden chest pain	1.6 (1.0–2.4)	0.3 (0.2–0.4)
Pulse deficit	5.7 (1.4–23.0)	0.7 (0.6–0.9)
Diastolic murmur	1.4 (1.0–2.0)	0.9 (0.8–1.0)
Enlarged aorta or wide mediastinum	2.0 (1.4–3.1)	0.3 (0.2–0.4)

Source: Data from [1].

(60%, CI 55–66%), and LR+ (2.2) were low. Additionally, these studies are at risk of spectrum bias, as D-dimer testing was not performed on all patients with a suspected aortic dissection. Rather the studies evaluated a group of disease positive patients in whom the test had been performed.

Clinical question

Can abdominal ultrasound be reliably used by emergency physicians to evaluate for and rule out abdominal aortic aneurysms?

Two studies have evaluated the specific use of abdominal ultrasound by emergency physicians to evaluate for AAA (Figure 44.1). The first, by Tayal et al in 2003, enrolled 125 patients, all of whom underwent ultrasound by emergency physicians.[4] Each also underwent one of four confirmatory studies: 28 (22%) underwent radiology ultrasound, 95 (76%) underwent CT, one (1%) underwent MRI, and one (1%) underwent laparotomy. Overall, 29 (23%) were diagnosed with an AAA on emergency physician–performed ultrasound, and 27 of these had an AAA on the confirmatory ultrasound, leading to a sensitivity of 100% (CI 90–100%), a specificity of 98% (CI 93–100%), a PPV of 93%, and a NPV of 100%. Senior emergency medicine residents and emergency medicine attending physicians performed the ultrasound examinations, and each had performed at least 50 ultrasound examinations prior to the study.

The second study, published by Constantino et al in 2005, enrolled 238 patients, all of whom had ultrasound performed by final-year emergency medicine residents (each of whom had performed at least 150 ultrasound exams of any type).[5] All hemodynamically stable patients then received a confirmatory study by a radiologist (either ultrasound or CT). Of the 238

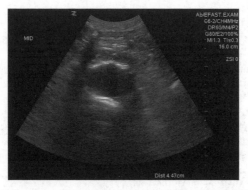

Figure 44.1 Abdominal aortic aneurysm seen on ultrasound. (Source: Elke Platz, Heidi Kimberly & Dorothea Hempel, Department of Emergency Medicine, Brigham and Women's Hospital, used with permission).

patients, 36 were found to have an AAA on the confirmatory study and 34 of these patients were diagnosed with AAA on emergency physician–performed ultrasound, representing a 94% sensitivity. The other two AAA cases were diagnosed as having "abnormal" findings; one ultrasound was correctly read as having an aortic dissection while there was also an incidental 4 cm aneurysm, and the other was read as having a "large intraluminal clot" and had an incorrectly measured aorta due to caliper misplacement.

Comment

Most emergency physicians evaluate patients with possible aortic emergencies every day. For patients with a high pretest probability of aortic disease, it is important to use tests that demonstrate acceptable accuracy. However, reliance on historical characteristics, physical examination findings, or chest radiography is inadequate. While a wide mediastinum on chest x-ray should lead to further consideration of the possibility of aortic dissection, a normal chest x-ray cannot rule out the disease.

The recent meta-analysis of D-dimer use in dissection suggests that this lab test may be useful in the diagnosis of aortic emergencies. However, we do not recommend such a shift in practice until there is more evidence than a meta-analysis of less than 300 patients. Therefore, this finding will need further validation before it becomes the standard of care, particularly to rule out the disease in high-risk situations.

Lastly, the use of bedside ultrasound as a screening modality for AAA should be part of every emergency physician's armamentarium. However, as the study by Constantino aptly demonstrates, the effective use of ultrasound is operator dependent and requires both adequate training and quality assurance.

References

1. Klompas M. Does this patient have an acute thoracic aortic dissection? Journal of the American Medical Association. 2002; 287(17): 2262–72.
2. Von Kodolitsch Y, Nienaber CA, Dieckmann C *et al.* Chest radiography for the diagnosis of acute aortic syndrome. American Journal of Medicine. 2004; 116(2): 73–7.
3. Shimony A, Filion KB, Mottillo S, Dourian T, Eisenberg MJ. Meta-analysis of usefulness of d-dimer to diagnose acute aortic dissection. American Journal of Cardiology. 2011; 107(8): 1227–34.
4. Tayal VS, Graf CD, Gibbs MA. Prospective study of accuracy and outcome of emergency ultrasound for abdominal aortic aneurysm over two years. Academic Emergency Medicine. 2003; 10(8): 867–71.
5. Costantino TG, Bruno EC, Handly N, Dean AJ. Accuracy of emergency medicine ultrasound in the evaluation of abdominal aortic aneurysm. The Journal of Emergency Medicine. 2005; 29(4): 455–460.

Chapter 45 **Ovarian Torsion**

Highlights

- The majority of ovarian torsion cases are missed on initial evaluation.
- Prior diagnostic research on elements of the history and physical exam for ovarian torsion has only assessed disease-positive patients, so specificities and likelihood ratios remain unknown.
- No findings on history or physical exam are sufficiently sensitive to rule out the diagnosis of ovarian torsion.
- The most sensitive ultrasound finding to diagnose ovarian torsion is the absence of ovarian venous flow which is more sensitive than the absence of ovarian arterial flow (67% versus 46%); within 1 day of symptom onset, the sensitivity of absent venous flow is 85%.
- Diagnostic certainty for ovarian torsion can be obtained only via laparoscopic evaluation.

Background

Adnexal torsion, commonly referred to as *ovarian torsion* (OT), occurs when the vascular pedicle is twisted and may involve the Fallopian tubes and ovaries. The majority of patients with OT present for initial evaluation to the emergency department (ED) (75%) rather than the primary care (12%) or gynecology clinics (10%), and usually within 12 hours of the onset of their symptoms.[1] OT is commonly misdiagnosed and is only considered in the differential diagnosis in 47% of cases of the disease.[1] Up to 80% of OT cases are associated with usually benign ovarian tumors or cysts, but only 25% of patients with OT will report a history of a known ovarian cyst or mass.[1] Additional risk factors for OT include both first-trimester pregnancy and chemical

Evidence-Based Emergency Care: Diagnostic Testing and Clinical Decision Rules, Second Edition.
Jesse M. Pines, Christopher R. Carpenter, Ali S. Raja and Jeremiah D. Schuur.
© 2013 John Wiley & Sons, Ltd. Published 2013 by John Wiley & Sons, Ltd.

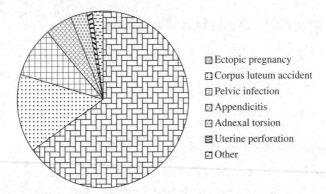

Figure 45.1 Etiology of female abdominal pain requiring emergent surgery.
Source: Data from [3].

induction of ovulation.[1,2] Although OT is the fifth most common reason for emergent surgery in women presenting with abdominal pain (Figure 45.1), the diagnosis is still quite rare, with an annual prevalence of about 3%.[3] Accordingly, diagnostic research is limited to retrospective case series.

The ovaries have a dual blood supply from the uterine and ovarian arteries, so complete arterial obstruction is rare. Attempts at surgical salvage via detorsion are therefore warranted even if the diagnosis is made late in the disease course,[4] with ovarian function having been preserved in 93% of laparoscopically detorsed cases of OT.[5] If detorsion is unsuccessful, one ovary is sufficient to maintain fertility.[6] In pediatric (and probably adult) patients, optimal ovarian salvage rates are obtained in those who are taken to the operating room within 8 hours of diagnosis. In cases where operative detorsion has been delayed for over 24 hours, salvage rates approach zero.[7]

The differential diagnosis of atraumatic abdominal pain in women includes appendicitis, ovarian cysts, ectopic pregnancy, renal colic, urinary tract infection, pelvic inflammatory disease, malignancy, and diverticulitis.[8] In the evaluation of acute female abdominal pain, the choice of which initial imaging modality to obtain should be based upon the most likely etiology after a careful history and physical exam, including a pelvic exam. Ultrasound is generally considered the imaging technique of choice for OT. Computed tomography (CT) is only 34% sensitive for the diagnosis of OT (specificity unknown) and agrees with ultrasound results only 50% of the time.[9,10] Magnetic resonance imaging (MRI) may be considered in pregnant patients, but the diagnostic test characteristics for MRI have not been well described.[11]

Clinical question

What is the diagnostic accuracy of physical exam findings for ovarian torsion in women with abdominal pain?

Right-sided OT is more common (55.8%) than left-sided OT, possibly due to a stabilizing effect of the sigmoid colon on the left.[12] Symptoms of OT include nausea (60–70%) and lower quadrant abdominal pain (90%), which can be characterized as sharp or stabbing in 70% and of moderate to severe intensity in 82% of patients with OT. All other signs, symptoms, and physical exam findings are not sufficiently sensitive to be useful in the ED (Table 45.1). Suspected OT is confirmed operatively in only half of cases.[13]

The specificity of history and physical exam findings, as well as their reproducibility, remains undefined,[1,12] so clinicians have no objective way to quantify the impact of any finding (in isolation or combination) upon a patient's posttest probability for OT. Therefore, emergency physicians must include OT in the differential diagnosis of all women with abdominal pain (who still have their ovaries) in order to maintain a sufficiently safe threshold for further imaging and prompt gynecological consultation to optimize ovarian salvage. Future trials are needed on consecutive patients to fully understand the epidemiology of OT as well as the specificity and likelihood ratios for elements of history and physical exam.

Table 45.1 Sensitivity of history and physical exam findings for ovarian torsion (OT)

Finding	Sensitivity
Any OT risk factors	31%
Any pain	44%
Constant pain	65%
Sudden onset pain	87%
Nausea	59%
Vomiting	54%
Nonmenstrual vaginal bleeding	4%
Palpable abdominal mass	62%
Fever	20%
Leukocytosis (WBC >15,000)	21%

Source: Data from [12].

Clinical question

What is the diagnostic accuracy for adnexal sonography for ovarian torsion in women with abdominal pain?

Two chart reviews have retrospectively evaluated the accuracy of gynecologist-performed ultrasound to evaluate for OT in adult women. Color Doppler evaluation may increase the posttest probability of OT if it is abnormal (however, "abnormal" was not defined by the investigators) with a positive likelihood ratio (LR+) of 5.3, but the absence of an abnormal Doppler signal does not decrease (negative likelihood ratio (LR−) 0.61) the likelihood of ovarian torsion.[13] In adult patients with acute (less than 3 days since symptom onset) lower quadrant abdominal pain, the absence of ovarian venous flow is more sensitive for the diagnosis of OT than is the absence of arterial flow (67% vs. 46%, respectively). Venous flow absence is more sensitive if the time since symptom onset is shorter than 1 day (85%) than if the time is longer (2 days, 75%; ≥3 days, 43%). As judged by ultrasound, all OT patients have enlarged ovaries (mean volume 957 cm^3 in adults with OT versus normal non-OT means 15 cm^3 in reproductive-aged adults) and 56% have an associated cyst or benign mass.[4] Future prospective studies of consecutive patients with and without OT are essential to fully understand the actual diagnostic accuracy (sensitivity, specificity, and likelihood ratios) and reproducibility of history, physical exam, and sonographic findings for the diagnosis of OT.

Comment

All of the OT diagnostic accuracy research evidence is based upon case series. In other words, only disease-positive (confirmed OT) cases were assessed. Therefore, critical readers *can only estimate the sensitivity* for the history, physical exam, laboratory, and sonographic findings that are reported in most of these trials. The remainder of the studies do not report on a cohort of disease negative patients, so we cannot estimate specificity or positive or negative likelihood ratios for findings such as pelvic pain, palpable adnexal mass, and vaginal bleeding. We have no empirical data by which to know whether the presence or absence of these findings increase, decrease, or do not change the posttest probability of OT. Even more disheartening, diagnostic studies that evaluate only disease-positive patients overestimate sensitivity point-estimates.[14]

Another limitation of the OT diagnostic trials is that they focus only upon accuracy. Future trials should use the Standards for the Reporting of Diagnostic Accuracy Studies (STARD) criteria and assess patient-important outcomes in addition to fully describing diagnostic accuracy (sensitivity, specificity, and likelihood ratios) and the reproducibility for each element of history, physical exam, lab testing, and sonography.[15,16] Based upon the available evidence, emergency physicians should include OT in the differential diagnosis of women of all ages with abdominal pain (as long as they still have their ovaries) and maintain a low threshold for further imaging (ultrasound with Doppler, CT, or MRI) and gynecologic consultation while recognizing that these modalities are also imperfect. The most sensitive sonographic finding is the loss of venous blood flow (85% sensitive when ultrasound is performed within 1 day of symptom onset), while loss of arterial blood flow has only a 54% sensitivity within 1 day of symptom onset.

References

1. Houry D, Abbott JT. Ovarian torsion: A fifteen-year review. Annals of Emergency Medicine. 2001; 38(2): 156–9.
2. Hasson J, Tsafrir Z, Azem F, Bar-On S, Almog B, Mashiach R *et al.* Comparison of adnexal torsion between pregnant and nonpregnant women. American Journal of Obstetrics and Gynecology. 2010; 202(6): 536.E1–6.
3. Hibbard LT. Adnexal torsion. American Journal of Obstetrics and Gynecology. 1985; 152(4): 456–61.
4. Shadinger LL, Andreotti RF, Kurian RL. Preoperative sonographic and clinical characteristics as predictors of ovarian torsion. Journal of Ultrasound Medicine. 2008; 27(1): 7–13.
5. Cohen SS, Oelsner G, Seidman DD, Admon D, Mashiach S, Goldenberg M. Laparoscopic detorsion allows sparing of the twisted ischemic adnexa. Journal of American Association of Gynecologic Laparoscopy. 1999; 6(2): 139–43.
6. Lass A. The fertility potential of women with a single ovary. Human Reproduction Update. 1999; 5(5): 546–50.
7. Anders JF, Powell EC. Urgency of evaluation and outcome of acute ovarian torsion in pediatric patients. Archives of Pediatrics and Adolescent Medicine. 2005; 159(6): 532–5.
8. Nichols DH, Julian PJ. Torsion of the adnexa. Clinical Obstetrics and Gynecology. 1985; 28(2): 375–80.
9. Hiller N, Appelbaum L, Simanovsky N, Lev-Sagi A, Aharoni D, Sella T. CT features of adnexal torsion. American Journal of Roentgenology. 2007; 189(1): 124–9.
10. Moore C, Meyers AB, Capotasto J, Bokhari J. Prevalence of abnormal CT findings in patients with proven ovarian torsion and a proposed triage schema. Emergency Radiology. 2009; 16(2): 115–20.
11. Masselli G, Brunelli R, Casciani E, Polettini E, Bertini L, Laghi F *et al.* Acute abdominal and pelvic pain in pregnancy: MR imaging as a valuable adjunct to ultrasound? Abdominal Imaging. 2011 Oct; 36(5): 596–603.

12. White M, Stella J. Ovarian torsion: 10-year perspective. Emergency Medicine Australasia. 2005; 17(3): 231–7.

13. Bar-On S, Maschiach R, Stockheim D, Soriano D, Goldenberg M, Schiff E *et al.* Emergency laparoscopy for suspected ovarian torsion: Are we too hasty to operate? Fertility and Sterility. 2010; 93(6): 2012–5.

14. Newman TB, Kohn MA. Evidence-based diagnosis (practical guide to biostatistics and epidemiology). Cambridge: Cambridge University Press; 2009.

15. Bossuyt PMM, Reitsma JB, Bruns DE, Gatsonis CA, Glasziou PP, Irwig L *et al.* The STARD statement for reporting studies of diagnostic accuracy: Explanation and elaboration. Annals of Internal Medicine. 2003; 138(1): W1–12.

16. Schünemann AHJ, Oxman AD, Brozek J, Glasziou P, Jaeschke R, Vist GE *et al.* Grade: Grading quality of evidence and strength of recommendations for diagnostic tests and strategies. British Medical Journal. 2008; 336(7653).

SECTION 6
Urology

Chapter 46 **Nephrolithiasis**

Highlights

- Nephrolithiasis should be considered in patients presenting with acute flank pain, hematuria, groin pain, and/or vomiting.
- Noncontrast CT imaging is the test of choice for the initial diagnosis of nephrolithiasis.
- Noncontrast CT improves diagnostic accuracy and can provide important information about other unsuspected conditions, some of which may require emergency treatment.
- Repeat CT scanning in patients with a previous documented history results in a change in urgent management in a minority (7%) of cases.

Background

Nephrolithiasis (i.e., kidney stones) affects up to 5% of the population. Patients frequently seek emergency care for the pain associated with nephrolithiasis because it is typically severe and refractory to over-the-counter analgesics. Clinical features of symptomatic nephrolithiasis include acute flank pain radiating to the groin, nausea, vomiting, and microscopic hematuria. The standard imaging modality for the initial diagnosis of nephrolithiasis is noncontrast spiral computed tomography (CT) scan because it provides considerable information, including : (i) whether the symptoms are actually due to nephrolithiasis, (ii) whether the stones are obstructing, and (iii) an estimate of stone burden if the CT is positive for nephrolithiasis. The estimate of stone burden may be helpful for physicians in managing an individual patient's nephrolithiasis after his or her emergency department (ED) visit. Of patients with known nephrolithiasis, almost 50% will develop additional stones within 5–7 years.

Evidence-Based Emergency Care: Diagnostic Testing and Clinical Decision Rules, Second Edition. Jesse M. Pines, Christopher R. Carpenter, Ali S. Raja and Jeremiah D. Schuur. © 2013 John Wiley & Sons, Ltd. Published 2013 by John Wiley & Sons, Ltd.

Clinical question

How does unenhanced CT compare to other diagnostic tests for nephrolithiasis, including intravenous urography and ultrasound?

An early study on the topic in the late 1980s investigated the sensitivity of ultrasound to detect renal calculi in a three-phase study in 100 patients.[1] In the first phase, ultrasound was performed after reviewing abdominal radiography and renal tomograms in 30 patients who had undergone extracorporeal shock wave lithotripsy (ESWL), and the sensitivity for detecting stones was 98%. In the second phase, ultrasound was performed in 30 post-ESWL patients without any prior review of radiographs or tomograms. In the second group, the sensitivity of ultrasound for stone detection was 95%. In the third phase, 40 patients had ultrasound performed in a blinded way in a random mix of post-ESWL patients and patients who had undergone urography for other reasons. In this group, the sensitivity of ultrasound was 91%. In combined data, the authors reported an overall sensitivity of ultrasound of 96%.

A 2003 randomized trial comparing CT to intravenous (IV) urography for patients with suspected nephrolithiasis enrolled 122 patients with acute flank pain.[2] A total of 59 of them were randomized to CT and 63 to intravenous urography. The radiographic studies were independently interpreted by four radiologists. Of patients receiving intravenous urography, mild to moderate adverse reactions from contrast material were seen in three (5%) patients. The mean radiation dose was 3.3 mSv for urography and 6.5 mSv for CT scan. Sensitivity and specificity of CT were 94% and 94%, respectively. For urography, sensitivity and specificity were lower at 85% and 90%, respectively.

Another study investigated the sensitivity of diagnostic ultrasound compared to CT for the detection of kidney stones in 46 patients with acute flank pain, using a combination of tests and clinical follow-up as the criterion standard.[3] CT imaging detected 22 of 23 ureteral calculi (sensitivity: 96%), and ultrasound detected 14 of 23 ureteral calculi (sensitivity: 61%). The specificity for each technique was 100%. When modalities were compared for the detection of any clinically relevant abnormality, the sensitivities of ultrasound and CT were 92% and 100%, respectively.

An additional study was performed in a Spanish hospital and published in 2010.[4] The authors enrolled patients with "persistent renoureteral colic" after standard care. The patients were blindly evaluated by ultrasound and CT and, in the 124 patients studied, nephrolithiasis was present in 60%. The specificity and positive predictive value (PPV) of ultrasound for nephrolithiasis were 100%, but its sensitivity was only 30%.

The most recent study determined the test characteristics of ultrasound for any ureteral stone and for stones $\geq$ 5 mm in size.[5] In 117 patients, the

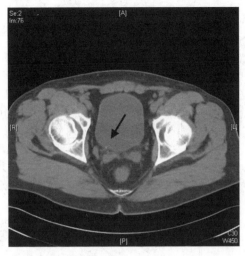

Figure 46.1 Noncontrast computed tomography (CT) scan showing 1–2 mm calculus at the right ureterovesicular junction.

sensitivity for ultrasound was 77% (CI 59–88%) and the specificity was 86% (CI 74–93%) for any stone disease. For stones ≥ 5 mm, the sensitivity was 90% (CI 54–100%) and the specificity was 64% (CI 53–73%).

Clinical question

Is it important to use noncontrast CT to diagnose kidney stones on the first visit for presumed ureteral colic?

A prospective observational study assessed the impact of helical CT in 132 patients with a first episode of suspected nephrolithiasis (see Figures 46.1 and 46.2).[6] Patients with a known history of nephrolithiasis were excluded. Prior to the CT, emergency physicians completed questionnaires detailing their diagnostic certainty of nephrolithiasis as well as the patient's anticipated disposition. The primary study outcome was a comparison of physician diagnostic certainty to CT results. The secondary outcome measure was an alternate diagnosis. Pre-CT diagnostic certainty was divided into four groups (0–49%, 50–74%, 75–90%, and 90–100%), and these groups each had a diagnosis of urinary calculi made in 28.6%, 45.7%, 74.2%, and 80.5% of their patients, respectively. An alternative diagnosis was revealed on CT scan in 40 cases (33%), 19 of whom had another significant pathology. The majority of these other significant diagnoses were previously unrecognized cancers, and some were less significant (such as adrenal adenomas). Prior to CT scanning,

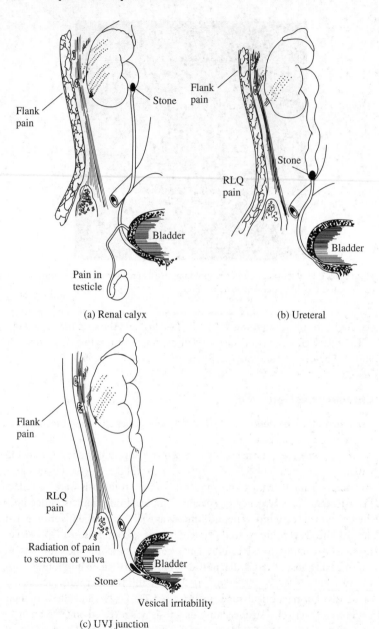

(a) Renal calyx

(b) Ureteral

(c) UVJ junction

Figure 46.2 Radiation of pain with various types of ureteral stone. (Redrawn from Tanagho and McAninch, Smith's General Urology, 16th Edition © 2004 with permission of the McGraw-Hill companies).
Note: RLQ = right lower quadrant.

physicians planned to discharge 115 patients and admit six patients. The authors concluded that patients presenting with a first episode of clinically suspected nephrolithiasis should undergo a CT scan because it enhances diagnostic accuracy and identifies clinically significant alternative diagnoses.

Another more recent study examined the incidence and clinical relevance of alternate diagnoses in a large series of 1,500 patients with acute flank pain and suspected urinary calculi who received a CT scan.[7] In this study, patients with a history of urinary tract calculi were not excluded. Alternate findings on CT were classified as to whether they required immediate or delayed treatment, or were of little or no clinical importance. They found that 69% of their patients had urinary tract calculi, including 30% with nephrolithiasis, 36% with ureterolithiasis, and 34% with both conditions. Of all patients, 1,064 (71%) had other or additional CT findings, 207 (14%) had non-nephrolithaisis-related CT findings requiring immediate or deferred treatment, 464 (31%) had pathological conditions of little clinical importance, and 393 (26%) had pathological conditions of no clinical relevance. The authors concluded that CT in patients with acute flank pain allows for the accurate diagnosis of urinary stone disease and can provide further important information leading to emergency treatment in a substantial number of patients.

Clinical question

Is it helpful to repeat CT imaging in patients with known urinary calculi when they re-present with acute flank pain, similar to previous episodes of nephrolithaisis?

A recent study sought to determine the incidence of "alternative diagnoses" in patients with a history of prior documented nephrolithiasis who underwent repeat CT imaging when they returned to the ED in a single tertiary care hospital.[8] In 231 patients who had been rescanned for similar symptoms of renal colic, 181 (82%) had no change in their diagnosis as a result of the repeat CT scan, 27 (12%) had an alternative diagnosis that did not require an additional intervention, and 15 (7%) were diagnosed with a condition that required an urgent intervention. In the 27 patients with an alternative diagnosis, the most common diagnosis was musculoskeletal pain (18 patients). In the 15 patients who required urgent intervention, the most common diagnosis was acute pyelonephritis (seven patients), followed by diverticulitis (two), appendicitis (two), small bowel obstruction (one), pneumonia (one), pelvic inflammatory disease (one), and cholecystitis (one).

Comment

It appears that noncontrast CT scan is the diagnostic test of choice in patients with suspected nephrolithiasis. CT is considerably more accurate than other testing such as intravenous urography and diagnostic ultrasound. For patients with a first episode of suspected nephrolithiasis, CT scan should be used as it can confirm the presence of kidney stones and has the potential to find other clinically significant pathology in a considerable number of cases. Repeat CT scanning is unlikely to change clinical management in most cases; however, in a minority of cases, the diagnosis can change considerably. Ultrasound demonstrates variable sensitivity for the detection of nephrolithiasis and may be a viable alternative strategy for repeat episodes of suspected nephrolithiasis in patients with documented disease, because the sensitivity is considerably higher in larger, potentially obstructing stones ($\geq$ 5 mm in size).

References

1. Middleton WD, Dodds WJ, Lawson TL, Foley WD Renal calculi: Sensitivity for detection with US. Radiology. 1988; 167: 239–44.
2. Pfister SA, Deckart A, Laschke S et al. Unenhanced helical computed tomography vs intravenous urography in patients with acute flank pain: Accuracy and economic impact in a randomized prospective trial. European Radiology. 2003; 13: 2513–20.
3. Sheafor DH, Hertzberg BS, Freed KS et al. Nonenhanced helical CT and US in the emergency evaluation of patients with renal colic: Prospective comparison. Radiology 2000; 217: 792–7.
4. Rengifo Abbad D, Rodríguez Caravaca G, Barreales Tolosa L et al. Diagnostic validity of helical CT compared to ultrasonography in renal-ureteral colic. Archivos Españoles de Urologia. 2010; 63: 139–44.
5. Moak JH, Lyons MS, Lindsell CJ. Bedside renal ultrasound in the evaluation of suspected ureterolithiasis. American Journal of Emergency Medicine. 2012; 30: 218–21.
6. Ha M, MacDonald RD. Impact of CT scan in patients with first episode of suspected nephrolithasis. Journal of Emergency Medicine 2004; 27: 225–31.
7. Hoppe H, Studer R, Kessler TM et al. Alternate or additional findings to stone disease on unenhanced computerized tomography for acute flank pain can impact management. Journal of Urology 2006; 175: 1725–30.
8. Goldstone A, Bushnell A. Does diagnosis change as a result of repeat renal colic computed tomography scan in patients with a history of kidney stones? American Journal of Emergency Medicine. 2010; 28: 291–5.

Chapter 47 **Testicular Torsion**

Highlights

- Acute testicular torsion is a urological emergency and should be considered in males presenting with testicular or scrotal pain.
- The combination of nausea or vomiting, ipsilateral scrotal skin changes, and the absence of the ipsilateral cremasteric reflex is highly concerning for torsion, especially in the pediatric population.
- Testicular ultrasound is widely available and highly accurate, but does not definitively rule out torsion in patients with classic symptomatology.

Background

The patient with testicular pain presents a diagnostic challenge for emergency physicians. While there are multiple causes for testicular pain, including infectious and inflammatory reasons, neoplasms, hernias, and trauma, torsion is one of the most concerning due to the possibility of organ loss which may be prevented by emergent intervention.[1,2] Torsion should be considered in the differential diagnosis for every male presenting with testicular, scrotal or lower abdominal pain, but it is predominately a condition of the young and very young, occurring in approximately one in 4,000 males under the age of 25. Notably, while adult testicular torsion is rare, adult patients may be more likely to have delayed presentations and diagnoses, and thus lower testicular salvage rates.[3]

Testicular torsion is a urological emergency, as twisting of the spermatic cord compromises first venous, and then arterial blood flow causing acute pain and testicular ischemia. Ruling out testicular torsion is important and time-sensitive because delays in diagnosis and therapy can result in problems with fertility, organ loss, and a poor cosmetic outcome. Viability and salvageability of the torsed testicle decrease as time from onset of symptoms (e.g., pain) increases, with approximately 90% salvageability with detorsion

Evidence-Based Emergency Care: Diagnostic Testing and Clinical Decision Rules, Second Edition. Jesse M. Pines, Christopher R. Carpenter, Ali S. Raja and Jeremiah D. Schuur.
© 2013 John Wiley & Sons, Ltd. Published 2013 by John Wiley & Sons, Ltd.

in <6 hours, nearly 50% viability after 12 hours, and close to 10% after 24 hours. A recent 20-year review of cases by Yang et al included 118 cases with a median duration of symptoms of 64 hours, only 39% of whom had viable testes at surgery.[2] The median duration of symptoms for those with viable testes was 12 hours, while those in whom testes could not be salvaged had a median duration of 90 hours. Due to the importance that time plays in the treatment of testicular torsion, patients with historical and physical exam findings suggestive of the disease should have emergent urologic evaluation. In unclear cases, imaging may be helpful and, in the emergency department (ED), ultrasound has replaced scintigraphy as the standard imaging modality for diagnosing testicular torsion due to its widespread availability and the limited availability of nuclear imaging.

Clinical question

Which historical and physical exam findings can help diagnose or exclude testicular torsion?

Two recent pediatric studies have focused on the diagnostic utility of the history and physical exam findings for testicular torsion. Beni-Israel et al conducted a retrospective review of 523 patients with scrotal pain presenting to their pediatric ED, using ultrasound and surgical findings as their criterion standard.[4] In a population with a mean age of 10 years and 9 months, the authors found an incidence of testicular torsion of 3.3% and, on univariate analysis, determined that five clinical variables were associated with testicular torsion: duration of symptoms <24 hours (OR 6.7, CI 1.6–33), nausea and/or vomiting (OR 8.9, CI 2.6–30), abdominal pain (OR 3.2, CI 1.2–8.9), high position of the testes (OR 58.8, CI 19–167), and abnormal cremasteric reflex (OR 27.8, CI 7.5–100). However, it should be noted that patients who were discharged without ultrasound were not followed up and may have presented elsewhere with missed testicular torsion. This lack of an acceptable criterion standard or meaningful estimates of diagnostic accuracy such as LR+ or LR−, as well as the retrospective nature of this study, preclude any possibility of using these associated symptoms to rule out or rule in torsion.

Srinivasan et al performed a prospective study on 79 consecutive pediatric patients with a mean age of 11 years who were evaluated in the ED by urology residents.[5] There is an inherent selection bias (see Chapter 6) in that not all patients presenting to the ED with scrotal pain were included (urologic consultation had to be obtained), but they were able to follow up all patients enrolled and used either this clinical follow-up or surgical findings as their criterion standards. Using multivariate regression with 11 historical and 12 physical examination parameters, they found three that were predictive of testicular torsion: absence of the ipsilateral cremasteric reflex

Table 47.1 Test characteristics of combinations of: absence of the ipsilateral cremasteric reflex, presence of nausea or vomiting, and scrotal skin changes

	Sensitivity	Specificity	Positive predictive value (PPV)	Negative predictive value (NPV)
0 positive	100%	76%	32%	100%
1 positive	44%	80%	20%	93%
2 positive	25%	97%	50%	92%
3 positive	25%	100%	100%	92%

Source: Data from [5].

(p < 0.001) presence of nausea or vomiting (p < 0.05), and scrotal skin changes (p < 0.001) (Table 47.1).[5] They then developed a decision rule using these three parameters, finding that the absence of all three resulted in a negative predictive value (NPV) of 100% while the presence of all three resulted in a positive predictive value (PPV) of 100%. While this retrospectively derived rule needs validation before it can be used with confidence (see Chapter 4), it may someday form the basis for a decision rule for testicular torsion.

While the two studies noted in this chapter evaluated all patients with suspected torsion, Eaton et al focused primarily on pediatric patients with diagnosed intermittent testicular torsion (ITT) in order to determine whether there were historical or physical examination findings suggestive of the disease.[6] After reviewing the charts of 50 patients with a mean age of 12 years and who had a mean number of 4.3 painful episodes prior to surgery, they found that the only finding suggestive of ITT on exam was a testes with a horizontal lie (p < 0.05). While this finding cannot rule in or rule out torsion, ITT should be considered in patients with rapid onset and resolution of testicular pain.

It should be noted, however, that none of these three recent studies commented on the reliability of the physical examination findings that were tested and their presence may very well be practitioner dependent. In addition, there are no studies of similar quality in the adult population and so these findings should be extrapolated with caution in nonpediatric patients.

Clinical question

What is the diagnostic accuracy of testicular scintigraphy compared to testicular ultrasound for the diagnosis of testicular torsion?
Several studies have compared testicular scintigraphy with testicular ultrasound. Scintigraphy is typically considered positive if a photopenic central area is present and ultrasound is considered positive when arterial

Table 47.2 Performance of color Doppler ultrasound and scintigraphy for diagnosing testicular torsion when the indeterminate studies were considered positive for torsion

	Torsion (+)	Torsion (−)	Totals
Color Doppler ultrasound (+)/ scintigraphy (+)	11/11	7/1	18/12
Color Doppler ultrasound (−)/ scintigraphy (−)	0/0	23/29	23/29
Totals	11	30	41
Sensitivity (CI)	Ultrasound 100% (72–100%), scintigraphy 100% (72–100%)		
Specificity (CI)	Ultrasound 77% (58–90%), scintigraphy 97% (83–100%)		

Source: From reference [7].

flow is either absent or markedly decreased. Unlike ovarian torsion (see Chapter 45), there have been no studies specifically evaluating the utility of absent venous flow on ultrasound in the diagnosis of testicular torsion. A retrospective pediatric study of 41 boys with acute scrotal pain and equivocal physical exams from 1990 to 1996 compared the performance of color Doppler ultrasound with testicular scintigraphy for the diagnosis of testicular torsion.[7] Patients were followed through surgery or clinically until symptom resolution. A total of 11 cases of torsion (27%) were diagnosed, and several studies were interpreted as nondiagnostic. The authors presented two sets of performance tables, one that treated indeterminate studies as positive for torsion (Table 47.2) and another that treated indeterminate cases as negative for torsion (Table 47.3). The data

Table 47.3 Performance of color Doppler ultrasound and scintigraphy for diagnosing testicular torsion when the indeterminate studies were considered negative for torsion

	Torsion (+)	Torsion (−)	Totals
Doppler ultrasound (+)/ scintigraphy (+)	9/10	1/0	10
Doppler ultrasound (−)/ scintigraphy (−)	2/1	29/30	31
Totals	11	30	41
Sensitivity (CI)	Ultrasound 82% (48–98%), scintigraphy 91% (59–100%)		
Specificity (CI)	Ultrasound 97% (83–100%), scintigraphy 100% (88–100%)		

Source: From reference [7].

presented in this way comprise a sensitivity analysis of sorts, showing the effect that indeterminate cases have on the diagnostic performance of the tests.

The weaknesses of the retrospective design of this study prompted a prospective study of children comparing the same diagnostic studies.[8] Forty-six children with acute scrotal pain received both testicular scintigraphy by pediatric nuclear medicine radiologists and ultrasound performed by pediatric sonographers. Final diagnoses were determined surgically in 16 cases and by assessing for clinical resolution in 30 cases. A total of 14 cases of torsion were diagnosed in this study (incidence 34%). Twelve had testicular torsion proven at surgery, one case was detected based on an antecedent torsion and testicular atrophy, and one case of late testicular torsion was detected at follow-up.

The correct diagnosis of torsion was made by ultrasound in 11 of 14 cases (sensitivity 79%, CI 49–95%), and the correct diagnosis of nonsurgical conditions was made in 31 of 32 cases (specificity 97%, CI 84–100%). The PPV and NPV using ultrasound were 92% (CI 62–100%) and 91% (CI 76–98%), respectively. Using ultrasound yielded a diagnostic accuracy of 91%. The correct diagnosis of torsion was made by scintigraphy in 11 of 14 cases (sensitivity 79%, CI 49–96%), and the correct diagnosis of nonsurgical conditions was made in 29 of 32 cases (specificity 91%, CI 75–98%). The PPV and NPV using scintigraphy were 79% (CI 49–95%) and 91% (CI 75–98%), respectively. Scintigraphy resulted in a diagnostic accuracy of 87%.

The lack of a true criterion standard imaging test is demonstrated by the false negatives seen in this study. The authors noted that one of the difficulties in diagnosing normal arterial flow, not to mention detection of abnormal or absent flow, was the small size of the prepubescent testicles.

From 1999 to 2005, European researchers studying the diagnosis of testicular torsion examined 61 infants and children ranging in age from 1 day to 17 years presenting with acute scrotal pain, swelling, and redness.[9] Fifteen cases of torsion were detected (prevalence 25%; 14 by the absence of both arterial and venous flow, and one by the absence of venous flow coupled with decreased arterial pulsation) and all were surgically confirmed with no missed cases at 2-year follow-up. Forty-six nontorsion cases were also diagnosed correctly. Table 47.4 shows the performance using Doppler ultrasound for diagnosing testicular torsion. Within the same manuscript, these authors also performed a retrospective analysis of 75 acute scrotum cases from 1985 to 1994, prior to the start of the study described here. All cases of suspected testicular torsion were explored surgically. Only 25 of the 75 cases (33%) were confirmed as torsion. These data were used as supporting evidence to demonstrate that using testicular ultrasound decreased unnecessary surgical explorations.

Table 47.4 Performance Doppler ultrasound for diagnosing acute testicular torsion in pediatric patients

	Torsion (+)	Torsion (−)	Totals
Color Doppler ultrasound (+)	15	0	15
Color Doppler ultrasound (−)	0	46	46
Totals	15	46	61
Sensitivity (CI)	100% (78–100%)		
Specificity (CI)	100% (92–100%)		
Positive predictive value (PPV) (CI)	100% (78–100%)		
Negative predictive value (NPV) (CI)	100% (92–100%)		

Source: Data from [9].

A more recent large retrospective database study reviewed 1,228 cases of patients presenting with scrotal pain to one children's hospital over 18 years.[2] There were 103 diagnosed cases of testicular torsion, of which ultrasound correctly identified decreased arterial flow in 96 (93.2%). The seven cases missed by ultrasound were explored operatively due to character and duration of the symptoms, highlighting that patients with classic symptomatology should be explored regardless of initial ultrasound results. As the study was retrospective with no follow-up or criterion standard, it is unknown whether other patients with negative ultrasound were subsequently found to have torsion.

While most studies evaluating the use of ultrasound to diagnose suspected testicular torsion have used color Doppler ultrasound to visualize the absence of testicular arterial flow, a recent Irish study by Shaikh et al used a handheld Doppler (HHD, typically used to detect fetal heartbeats and monitor peripheral arterial and venous flow).[10] They evaluated 25 patients (median age 15 years, interquartile range 9–23 years) with acute scrotal pain who presented to a general ED. The HHD evaluation was performed by the surgical resident, and torsion was suspected with either weak or absent audible signals. The results of the HHD were not used in clinical decision making, and patients received color Doppler ultrasound, surgical exploration, or conservative management based on clinical suspicion of torsion.

Of the 25 patients evaluated, nine were diagnosed with torsion, 13 with epididymitis, and three with other disease processes. All patients were followed up at both 6 weeks and 3 months. Sensitivity and specificity of HHD were both 100%, with no signal present in seven of the nine cases of torsion and only weak signals present in the other two cases, providing support for the notion that HHD may be an appropriate evaluative tool for patients with suspected torsion, especially if color Doppler ultrasound is unavailable.

The most recent modality to be tested for the diagnosis of testicular torsion is high-resolution ultrasonography (HRUS). This technique images the spermatic cord to directly visualize and detect twisting of the cord. In a European multicenter study, children with acute scrotal pain were studied with both color Doppler ultrasound as well as HRUS.[11] The study enrolled 919 patients from 1992 to 2005 (age range 1 day to 18 years). Spermatic cord torsion was diagnosed in 208 patients (prevalence 23%). The use of color Doppler ultrasound detected 158 of the 208 cases (sensitivity 76%, CI 70–82%), whereas HRUS demonstrated 199 of the 208 cases (sensitivity 96%, CI 92–98%). Data were not presented to permit calculation of the specificity for color Doppler ultrasound, however the specificity for HRUS was 99% (CI 98–100%), with 705 of 711 cases revealing a linear (normal) spermatic cord. The PPV and NPV for HRUS were 97% (CI 94–99%) and 99% (CI 98–99%), respectively.

Comment

The current practice environment for evaluation of acute scrotal pain requires either prompt surgical evaluation or a diagnostic imaging study to evaluate for testicular torsion. Patients presenting with "classic" findings of acute onset of pain, absence of the ipsilateral cremasteric reflex, presence of nausea or vomiting, and scrotal skin changes should be explored surgically, as a normal ultrasound demonstrating the presence of arterial flow does not rule out the disease given an imperfect sensitivity and a high pretest clinical probability. It is those cases in which the history, the physical findings, or both are equivocal that should prompt the use of a diagnostic imaging study. While no studies have specifically evaluated adult patients with torsion, it seems reasonable to extrapolate pediatric findings to the adult population with the caveat that adults typically present later and have a greater time between presentation and operative intervention.[3]

The array of studies presented demonstrates several key findings. First, regardless of the type of imaging study, none have been shown in any large studies to be perfectly sensitive or specific. Technological advances and newer uses of the existing diagnostic equipment continue to advance the diagnostic thresholds, and these have to be considered when conducting a review of the literature. Cases for which the clinical suspicion is great enough to warrant ordering a study and cases in which the study results are indeterminate or poor quality warrant a urological consultation. Secondly, while none of the studies described specifically addressed this issue, clinicians should consider the experience of the radiologist interpreting the study. Finally, while this discussion has focused on using the imaging studies to rule out testicular torsion, ultrasound has the added advantage of identifying other related diagnoses, such as epididymitis, orchitis, and torsion of the testicular appendages.

The availability of ultrasound is greater than that of nuclear scintigraphy, making ultrasound the study of choice. As there have not yet been studies performed evaluating emergency physician–performed scrotal ultrasound, clinicians without appropriate imaging available should arrange to transfer the patient to a medical facility capable of performing both the diagnostic study and the surgical procedure that a positive study would necessitate. Notably, the recent 25-patient study by Shaikh et al demonstrates that handheld Doppler sonography may be an appropriate screening tool in low-resource settings, but its results warrant corroboration prior to generalization.

References

1. Molokwu CN, Somani BK, Goodman CM. Outcomes of scrotal exploration for acute scrotal pain suspicious of testicular torsion: A consecutive case series of 173 patients. BJU International. 2011; 107(6): 990–3.
2. Yang C, Song B, Tan J, Liu X, Wei G. Testicular torsion in children: A 20-year retrospective study in a single institution. Scientific World Journal. 2011; 11: 362–8.
3. Cummings JM, Boullier JA, Sekhon D, Bose K. Adult testicular torsion. Journal of Urology. 2002; 167(5): 2109–10.
4. Beni-Israel T, Goldman M, Bar Chaim S, et al. Clinical predictors for testicular torsion as seen in the pediatric ED. Am J Emerg Med. 2010; 28(7): 786–789.
5. Srinivasan A, Cinman N, Feber KM, Gitlin J, Palmer LS. History and physical examination findings predictive of testicular torsion: An attempt to promote clinical diagnosis by house staff. Journal of Pediatric Urology. 2011; 7(4): 470–4.
6. Eaton SH, Cendron MA, Estrada CR et al. Intermittent testicular torsion: Diagnostic features and management outcomes. Journal of Urology. 2005; 174(4Pt 2): 1532–5; discussion 1535.
7. Paltiel HJ, Connolly LP, Atala A et al. Acute scrotal symptoms in boys with an indeterminate clinical presentation: Comparison of color Doppler sonography and scintigraphy. Radiology. 1998; 207(1): 223–31.
8. Nussbaum Blask AR, Bulas D, Shalaby-Rana E et al. Color Doppler sonography and scintigraphy of the testis: A prospective, comparative analysis in children with acute scrotal pain. Pediatric Emergency Care. 2002; 18(2): 67–71.
9. Gunther P, Schenk JP, Wunsch R et al. Acute testicular torsion in children: The role of sonography in the diagnostic workup. European Radiology. 2006; 16(11): 2527–32.
10. Shaikh FM, Giri SK, Flood HD, Drumm J, Naqvi SA. Diagnostic accuracy of hand-held Doppler in the management of acute scrotal pain. Irish Journal of Medical Science. 2008; 177(3): 279–82.
11. Kalfa N, Veyrac C, Lopez M et al. Multicenter assessment of ultrasound of the spermatic cord in children with acute scrotum. Journal of Urology. 2007; 177(1): 297–301; discussion 301.

SECTION 7
Neurology

Chapter 48 **Nontraumatic Subarachnoid Hemorrhage**

Highlights

- No clinical decision rules or prediction rules regarding who should undergo testing for subarachnoid hemorrhage or what constitutes a positive lumbar puncture have been shown to be accurate.
- Lumbar puncture should be considered in patients with negative head CTs who are still suspected of having the condition, particularly when there is a high pretest probability based on clinical judgment.

Background

There are about 5 million emergency department (ED) visits per year for headache. Of those, between 1% and 4% have nontraumatic subarachnoid hemorrhage (SAH). The prevalence of acute SAH among ED patients is approximately 0.02%.[1-2] Nontraumatic SAH is frequently caused by a ruptured cerebral aneurysm or an arterio-venous malformation. Extravasation of blood into the subarachnoid space negatively affects local and global brain function. Depending upon the size of the bleed, SAH can be immediately fatal; however, in cases of smaller bleeds, patients can present with severe headaches. SAH is a challenge for emergency providers because it can present in subtle ways and is associated with considerable morbidity and mortality. SAH is typically diagnosed on noncontrast head computed tomography (CT) (Figure 48.1). However, head CT is not 100% sensitive for SAH and is particularly insensitive to diagnose small intracranial bleeds or bleeding that occurred more than 6–24 hours before the ED presentation of headache. Because the greatest risk for re-bleeding occurs in the first month after a sentinel bleed, a timely and accurate diagnosis is vital to managing SAH and minimizing complications. Currently the criterion standard to diagnose SAH is lumbar puncture demonstrating either a high red blood cell count

Evidence-Based Emergency Care: Diagnostic Testing and Clinical Decision Rules, Second Edition.
Jesse M. Pines, Christopher R. Carpenter, Ali S. Raja and Jeremiah D. Schuur.
© 2013 John Wiley & Sons, Ltd. Published 2013 by John Wiley & Sons, Ltd.

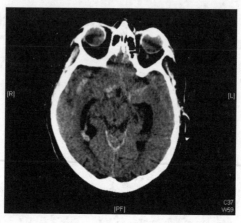

Figure 48.1 Noncontrast head computed tomography (CT) showing an acute subarachnoid hemorrhage.

in the cerebrospinal fluid (CSF) or xanthochromia, a yellowing of the CSF secondary to breakdown products of red blood cells. Lumbar puncture and CSF analysis can also reveal other information that can be useful to clinicians such as elevation in intracranial pressure or the presence of infection.

There is no validated decision rule to predict which patients require testing for SAH in the ED.[3] A decision rule was recently derived for the detection of SAH in ED patients in six centers. Four criteria – (i) arrived by ambulance, (ii) vomited, (iii) diastolic blood pressure ≥100 mm Hg, and (iv) age ≥45 years – were derived in a decision rule that was 100% (CI 97–100%) sensitive and 37% (CI 34–39%) specific for the detection of SAH. Incorporation of this clinical decision rule into practice would have theoretically avoided 34% of the patients from a CT and/or LP without missing any SAH cases. The use of "arrived by ambulance" as a criterion in any decision rule considerably limits the validity and generalizability of the rule, because ambulance use varies regionally and by social factors.

SAH is infrequently found on lumbar puncture (LP) after a negative head CT; however, given that head CT does not completely rule out SAH, physicians often have the difficult decision of whether to perform a LP if the head CT is negative. When patients are at high risk for SAH, lumbar puncture is certainly indicated. Elements that often influence this decision include the pretest probability, the complication rate of LP, patient preferences, and the concern of missing a potentially life-threatening and treatable disease. While LP has been shown to be a safe procedure, it carries a relatively high risk of postdural headaches (up to 20–40% of cases). Furthermore, up to 35% of patients will experience low back pain. Also, in a busy ED, performing an LP can also take considerable time by the emergency physician which increases the ED length of stay for all patients.

Clinical question

What is the sensitivity of noncontrast head CT for subarachnoid hemorrhage?
The sensitivity for noncontrast head CT for SAH has been described in many studies. One of the first diagnostic studies of nontraumatic SAH investigated the need for LP in patients who presented within the first 12 hours of headache onset with normal neurological examinations.[4] They enrolled a consecutive series of 175 patients where SAH was clinically suspected. All patients had a noncontrast head CT followed by a LP (at 12 or more hours from the headache onset) if the head CT was negative. The CT was positive for SAH in 117 patients (prevalence = 67%). Of the 58 patients with negative head CTs, CSF analysis showed SAH in two patients (3%, 95% CI 0.4−12). In both of those cases, there was evidence of a ruptured aneurysm. Therefore, in two out of 119 patients with SAH, the head CT was negative which yields a test sensitivity of 98% (95% CI 92−100).

Another group studied 6 years of data of patients with SAH from 1988 to 1994.[5] They excluded patients who were younger than 2 years or who had a history of head trauma within 24 hours of onset of symptoms. They stratified patients into two groups based on symptom duration (<24 hours and >24 hours). All patients with negative head CTs received a diagnostic LP. In 181 patients, the sensitivity of CT was 93% for patients whose head CT was performed with 24 hours of symptom onset as opposed to 84% for patients whose head CT was performed after 24 hours for an overall sensitivity of 92% indicating that, as time goes by, the sensitivity of CT for the detection of SAH decreases.

In another study, patients received a noncontrast head CT followed by a LP if the CT was negative. Similarly, they stratified patients by time of onset (<12 hours compared with >12 hours).[6] Of 140 patients with SAH, they reported 100% (CI 95−100%) sensitivity in the 80 patients with onset within 12 hours and 82% (CI 70−90%) with symptoms onset >12 hours. They found that 11 out of 140 (8%) patients had a positive CSF for SAH after a negative head CT.

A prospective study examining this issue studied patients who presented with the "worst headache of my life" and received LP if the CT was negative.[7] Of 107 patients with "worst headache," SAH was found on CT scan in 18 patients (prevalence = 17%). Two patients (3%, CI 0−9) had SAH detected on LP after a negative head CT.

In another recent study involving 177 ED patients over a 1-year period who had a CT followed by LP, they found that no patients had a negative head CT and a positive LP.[8]

The most recent study on the topic was a prospective cohort study across 11 tertiary care EDs in Canada from 2000 to 2009.[9] They enrolled neurologically intact adults with a new headache peaking in intensity within 1 hour of onset where the patient had a CT to rule out SAH. In 3,132 patients (of which 82% had their worst headache ever), 240 (8%) had SAH. The sensitivity of CT for SAH was 93% (CI 89–96%) and the specificity was 100% (CI 99–100%). The negative predictive value was 99% (CI 99–100%) and the positive predictive value was 100% (CI 98–100%). In a subgroup analysis of 953 patients who were scanned within 6 hours of symptoms, all 121 patients' with SAH were detected on CT representing a sensitivity of 100% (CI 97–100%) and a specificity of 100% (CI 99–100%).

Comment

The literature addressing ED diagnosis of SAH includes studies with major limitations. Most of the studies presented are retrospective, aside from the most recent study published in *BMJ* in 2011, and did not follow up on patients who were discharged home without any testing or just a negative head CT. This is important because there may have been cases of SAH that were missed, either because no testing was performed or because no LP was performed. Performances of the diagnostic tests would be expected to be different than reported had potentially missed cases been considered.

There were also considerable differences in the prevalence of disease among the populations, ranging from 8% to 67%. As such a high prevalence is not representative of general ED practice, this selection bias (see Chapter 6) may affect the test sensitivity in a number of ways. It may underestimate sensitivity because patients who had a negative head CT but did not subsequently receive the criterion standard test (because either the physician or the patient did not feel the test was indicated) may dramatically increase the denominator of patients for whom SAH was considered in the differential diagnosis. It is also possible that sensitivity could be falsely elevated if some patients with SAH were sent home without any testing. Most of the studies did not follow patients and did not enroll a broad cohort of patients with headache to exclude either of these possibilities.

However, what is clear from these studies is that test sensitivity decreases as time passes from the onset of the acute headache. There were also variable definitions for a positive LP. Because there are no widely accepted, validated criteria for a positive LP, it can be difficult to distinguish a traumatic tap, whereby red blood cells from the mechanical process of performing the procedure get into the CSF, from a true positive tap. In addition, many of these studies had small sample sizes and were performed at only one center, which limits the generalizability of some of these findings.

In the largest study on missed SAH, the most common reason for missing the disease was failure to order a head CT.[9] In patients who present with "worst headache," a new severe headache in patients who do not usually get headaches, or patients with chronic headaches who have a change in their headache symptoms, noncontrast head CT is useful to rule in the diagnosis of SAH. In our practice, the choice to perform LP on patients is highly dependent on the pretest probability for disease. Given the high risk of complications including postdural headache and lower back pain, in centers where multidetector row CT is available, it is reasonable practice to rule out SAH without an LP, after a negative CT if the clinician has a low pretest probability and the headache began within 6 hours. Clinician should be cautious in patients with headaches that began greater than 6 hours prior to arrival, and particularly beyond 24 hours. In such delayed presentations, LP is important to rule out SAH even after a negative CT.

References

1. Edlow JA, Panagos PD, Godwin SA, et al. Clinical policy: critical issues in the evaluation and management of adult patients presenting to the emergency department with acute headache, Ann Emerg Med 2008; 52: 407–436.
2. Vermeulen M, van Gijn K; The diagnosis of subarachnoid haemorrhage, J Neurol Neurosurg Psychiatry 1990; 53: 365–372.
3. Perry JJ, et al. BMJ 2010 Oct 28; 341:c5204.
4. van der Wee N, Rinkel GJ, Hasan D. Detection of subarachnoid haemorrhage on early CT: Is lumbar puncture still needed after a negative scan ? Journal of Neurology, Neurosurgery and Psychiatry. 1995; 58: 357–9.
5. Sames TA, Storrow AB, Finkelstein JA, Magoon MR. Sensitivity of new-generation computed tomography in subarachnoid hemorrhage. Academy of Emergency Medicine. 1996; 3: 16–20.
6. Sidman R, Connolly E, Lemke T. Subarachnoid hemorrhage diagnosis: Lumbar puncture is still needed when the computed tomography scan is normal. Academy of Emergency Medicine. 1996; 3: 827–31.
7. Morgenstern LB, Luna-Gonzales H, Huber JC Jr et al. Worst headache and subarachnoid hemorrhage: Prospective, modern computed tomography and spinal fluid analysis. Annals of Emergency Medicine. 1998; 32: 297–304.

8. Boesiger BM, Shiber Jr. Subarachnoid hemorrhage diagnosis by computed tomography and lumbar puncture: Are fifth generation CT scanners better at identifying subarachnoid hemorrhage? Journal of Emergency Medicine. 2005; 29: 23–7.
9. Perry JJ, Stiell IG, Sivilotti ML *et al*. Sensitivity of computed tomography performed within six hours of onset of headache for diagnosis of subarachnoid haemorrhage: Prospective cohort study. British Medical Journal. 2011; 343: d4277.

Chapter 49 **Acute Stroke**

Highlights

- Rapid evaluation of patients with acute stroke using a noncontrast head CT is critical in differentiating hemorrhagic versus ischemic stroke and identifying patients who may be candidates for intravenous thrombolysis ($\leq$4.5 hours from symptom onset).
- MRI with diffusion-weighted imaging (DWI) is more sensitive ($\sim$97%) than noncontrast head CT for detecting ischemic strokes.
- Noncontrast head CT and MRI can both accurately differentiate ischemic from hemorrhagic stroke, but MRI can provide more information on microhemorrhages.
- Noncontrast CT remains the standard brain-imaging study for the initial ED evaluation of patients with acute stroke symptoms; however, MRI may gain favor as it becomes more widely available.

Background

Stroke is the leading cause of disability and the third-leading cause of death in the United States. Rapid bedside and radiological evaluation of cases of suspected acute stroke within 4.5–6 hours of symptom onset are critical in the assessment of patients potentially eligible for intravenous and intra-arterial thrombolysis with tissue plasminogen activator (tPA). In acute ischemic stroke (Figure 49.1), the central event is an acute vascular occlusion; however, 15% of strokes are hemorrhagic (Figure 49.2). Hemorrhagic strokes treated with tPA do not benefit from thrombolysis, as it can worsen bleeding and increase mortality. Today, intravenous thrombolysis is the treatment of choice for patients with ischemic lesions involving greater than one-third of the middle cerebral artery territory without intracranial

Evidence-Based Emergency Care: Diagnostic Testing and Clinical Decision Rules, Second Edition. Jesse M. Pines, Christopher R. Carpenter, Ali S. Raja and Jeremiah D. Schuur.
© 2013 John Wiley & Sons, Ltd. Published 2013 by John Wiley & Sons, Ltd.

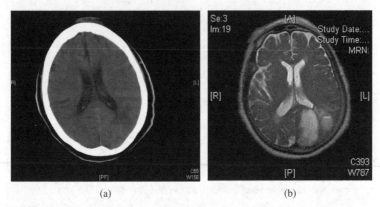

(a)   (b)

Figure 49.1 Noncontrast head CT showing ischemic stroke in the left posterior cerebral artery region (a), confirmed on MRI (b).

hemorrhage who present within 4.5 hours of the onset of symptoms and do not have contraindications for tPA. Traditionally, noncontrast head computed tomography (CT) has been the first imaging modality in acute stroke in the emergency department (ED) (Figure 49.1). By using noncontrast head CT, we are able to differentiate between hemorrhagic and ischemic stroke, and also exclude other potential causes of acute neurological symptoms. A more advanced imaging technique, multimodal magnetic resonance imaging

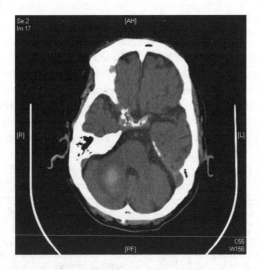

Figure 49.2 Noncontrast head CT showing a right cerebellar hemorrhage.

(MRI) with diffusion weighted imaging (DWI), is frequently performed after CT because it is considered a more accurate diagnostic test for stroke (Figure 49.1). The primary clinical concerns regarding the use of MRI with DWI as a solitary test are (i) reduced ability to detect intracranial hemorrhage in the setting of acute stroke, (ii) less clinical access to potentially unstable patients, (iii) longer testing times, and (iv) poor availability of rapid MRI.

Clinical question

What is the sensitivity of diagnostic modalities (head CT and MRI) in acute stroke, and does MRI miss acute intracranial hemorrhages?
To calculate the sensitivity and specificity of each, a recent article performed a review of the literature comparing non-contrast CT to MRI with DWI when used to diagnose acute stroke.[1] They included articles in which both head CT and MRI were performed within 6–7 hours of the onset of clinical symptoms. A total of eight studies met the authors' inclusion criteria.

The largest study the authors reviewed was a retrospective chart review of 733 patients seen in the ED for signs and symptoms of acute stroke.[2] The inclusion criterion was imaging performed within 6 hours after arrival in the ED. Patients were excluded if they were diagnosed with a transient ischemic attack (i.e., resolved symptoms). Of 691 patients, 509 had a noncontrast head CT and 122 had MRI with DWI within 6 hours of ED arrival. They used a primary discharge diagnosis of stroke as the criterion standard. The study reported a sensitivity of noncontrast head CT of 40% and of MRI with DWI of 97%; the specificity was 92% for both modalities. The PPVs of head CT and MRI with DWI were each 96%. The NPVs were 23% for head CT and 77% for MRI with DWI. This study was limited by its retrospective nature, the presence of incomplete records, and potential selection bias in the cases of patients who received both studies.

The authors went on to review seven other smaller studies (ranging in sample size from 17 to 54), most with considerable methodological issues including variable inclusion criteria, variable criterion standards for stroke, delays between head CT and MRI with DWI, and variable blinding of reviewers.[3–9] They then combined data from all eight studies (despite variable inclusion criteria) to calculate a sensitivity, specificity, positive predictive value (PPV), and negative predictive value (NPV) for each modality. For MRI with DWI, their calculated sensitivity was 97% (CI 94–98%) and their specificity was 100% (CI 88–100%), with a PPV of 100% (CI 98–100%) and a NPV of 91% (CI 75–98%). The sensitivity of head CT was 47 % (CI 43–51%), specificity was 93% (CI 85–97%), the PPV was 97% (CI 94–99%), and the NPV was 23% (CI 19–28%).

Another more recent prospective comparison compared MRI with DWI to noncontrast CT in the ED in a single center in patients with suspected stroke.[10] The scans were interpreted independently by four separate radiologists who were blinded to clinical information. In 356 patients, 217 had a final clinical diagnosis of acute stroke. MRI detected acute stroke (both ischemic and hemorrhagic) and chronic hemorrhage more frequently than CT (p<0.0001, for all comparisons). In the detection of acute intracranial hemorrhage, MRI was similar to CT. MRI detected acute ischemic stroke in 164/356 patients (46%, CI 41–51%) compared with CT in 35/356 patients (10%, CI 7–14%). A subset analysis was performed on patients who were scanned within 3 hours of symptom onset. In those patients, MRI detected acute ischemic stroke in 41/90 (46%, CI 35–56%) and CT detected acute ischemic stroke in 6/90 (7%, CI 3–14%). Using final clinical diagnosis as the criterion standard, they reported a sensitivity of 83% (CI 78–88%) for MRI and 26% (CI 20–32%) for CT. The authors concluded that MRI was better than CT in terms of detecting of acute ischemia. It was also no different in the detection of acute and chronic hemorrhage. They concluded that MRI should be the preferred test for patients with suspected stroke.

Other studies have confirmed that MRI with DWI is as sensitive as CT for the detection of acute intracranial hemorrhage. Fiebach et al performed a multicenter study to test the accuracy of MRI for the detection of acute intracranial hemorrhage in patients with suspected stroke.[11] They compared MRI images from 62 patients with intracranial hemorrhages and 62 without intracranial hemorrhages, all of whom were imaged within 6 hours of symptom onset. They used CT as the criterion standard for the diagnosis of intracranial hemorrhage. Experienced readers of MRI were able to detect intracranial hemorrhage on all cases (100% sensitivity; CI 97–100%).

Kidwell et al also compared the accuracy of MRI and CT in the detection of intracranial hemorrhage in patients within 6 hours of acute focal symptoms of stroke in two centers.[12] In their protocol, patients underwent MRI followed by noncontrast CT. Scans were read by four blinded readers. The authors stopped the study early after only 200 patients were enrolled because an interim analysis found that MRI was detecting cases of hemorrhagic transformation that were not detected by CT. MRI was positive in 71 patients, out of whom CT was positive in only 29 (p<0.001). MRI and CT were equivalent in diagnosing acute hemorrhage, as acute hemorrhage was detected in 25 patients on both MRI and CT. However, in four other patients, acute hemorrhage was detected on MRI but not CT and, in three additional patients, regions that were interpreted as acute hemorrhage on CT were read as chronic hemorrhage on MRI. There was one patient for whom subarachnoid hemorrhage was seen on CT but not on MRI, and chronic hemorrhages (microbleeds) were visualized on MRI in 49 patients that were not seen on CT. The authors concluded that MRI is as accurate as CT in detecting acute hemorrhage in patients with acute focal symptoms of stroke and is more accurate than CT in detecting chronic intracranial hemorrhage.

Comment

In emergency care, the current standard in cases of acute stroke is noncontrast head CT to determine the presence of intracranial hemorrhage, detect large strokes, and potentially exclude other neurological causes for stroke symptoms. Head CT and clinical evaluation are the standards by which the decision to use thrombolysis is typically made. However, head CT has limited sensitivity and, in up to 20% of cases, thrombolytics are used in cases of stroke mimics. In most cases this is followed by MRI with DWI (which is a more sensitive test for acute stroke); however, this modality has limited availability, costs more, takes longer to perform, and requires a higher degree of patient participation. MRI with DWI is also more sensitive than head CT in identifying large-volume strokes that are at increased risk for hemorrhagic transformation and is also more sensitive in detecting chronic intracranial hemorrhage.

A primary historical concern with use of only MRI with DWI in acute stroke is that head CT is more sensitive in detecting acute intracranial hemorrhage. However, recent studies with newer MRI technology have mostly disproved this issue. Soon, increased availability of MRI may make it the best single test for stroke assessment in the ED.

References

1. Davis DP, Robertson T, Imbesi SG. Diffusion-weighted magnetic resonance imaging versus computed tomography in the diagnosis of acute ischemic stroke. Journal of Emergency Medicine. 2006: 31; 269–77.
2. Mullins ME, Schaefer PW, Sorensen AG *et al.* CT and conventional and diffusion-weighted MR imaging in acute stroke: Study in 691 patients at presentation to the emergency department. Radiology. 2002; 224: 353–9.
3. Fiebach J, Jansen O, Schellinger P *et al.* Comparison of CT with diffusion-weighted MRI in patients with hyperacute stroke. Neuroradiology. 2001; 43: 628–32.
4. Fiebach JB, Schellinger PD, Jansen O *et al.* CT and diffusion-weighted MR imaging in randomized order. Stroke. 2002; 33: 2206–10.
5. Urbach H, Flacke S, Keller E *et al.* Detectability and detection rate of acute cerebral hemisphere infarcts on CT and diffusion-weighted MRI. Neuroradiology. 2000; 42: 722–7.
6. Lansberg MG, Albers GW, Beaulieu C, Marks MP. Comparison of diffusion-weighted MRI and CT in acute stroke. Neurology. 2000; 54: 1557–61.

7. Gonzales RG, Schaefer PW, Buonanno FS *et al*. Diffusion-weighted MR imaging: Diagnostic accuracy in patients imaged within 6 hours of stroke symptom onset. Radiology. 1999; 210: 155–62.

8. Barber PA, Darby DG, Desmond PM *et al*. Identification of major ischemic change, diffusion-weighted imaging versus computed tomography. Stroke. 1999; 30: 2059–65.

9. Saur D, Kucinski T, Grzyska U *et al*. Sensitivity and interrater agreement of CT and diffusion-weighted MR imaging in hyperacute stroke. American Journal of Neuroradiology. 2003; 24: 878–85.

10. Chalela JA, Kidwell CS, Nentwich LM *et al*. Magnetic resonance imaging and computed tomography in emergency assessment of patients with suspected acute stroke: A prospective comparison. Lancet. 2007; 369: 293–8.

11. Fiebach JB, Schellinger PD, Gass A *et al*. Stroke magnetic resonance imaging is accurate in hyperacute intracerebral hemorrhage: A multicenter study on the validity of stroke imaging. Stroke. 2004; 35: 502–6.

12. Kidwell CS, Chalela JA, Saver JL *et al*. Comparison of MRI and CT for detection of acute intracerebral hemorrhage. Journal of the American Medical Association. 2004; 292(15): 1823–30.

Chapter 50 **Transient Ischemic Attack**

Highlights

- TIA precedes 23% of strokes; among ED patients, the post-TIA stroke rates are 3% at 2 days and 6% at 7 days.
- Early registry-based validations of the ABCD^2 post-TIA prognostic decision aid were promising, but methodologically rigorous clinical decision rule research has demonstrated that the ABCD^2 is nonspecific at recommended thresholds and that different cutoff values do not improve the ABCD^2 prognostic accuracy.
- No validated, acceptably accurate post-TIA prognostic decision aid currently exists.

Background

Transient ischemic attack (TIA) has been defined as an episode of neurological dysfunction caused by focal brain or retinal ischemia with symptoms resolving in less than 1 hour without evidence of cerebral infarction.[1] TIA precedes 23% of strokes, and the incidence of stroke has been estimated as 200,000–500,000 cases annually.[2,3] The diagnostic and therapeutic management of TIA as a potential medical emergency is a new concept because TIAs were traditionally not linked to strokes. Whereas the post-TIA stroke risk had been historically quantified as 1–2%, Johnston et al reported a 3-month risk of 10.5% with half of those occurring within the first 2 days.[4] Emergency department (ED) patients have higher post-TIA stroke rates than other populations: 3.1% at 2 days and 5.8% at 7 days.[5] Thus post-TIA stroke risk stratification models became a priority amongst neurovascular emergency specialists, and rapid test–treat models were evaluated in a variety of healthcare settings.

The symptoms of TIA are related to the region of the brain suffering ischemia rather than the hemorrhagic, embolic, or atherosclerotic etiology

Evidence-Based Emergency Care: Diagnostic Testing and Clinical Decision Rules, Second Edition.
Jesse M. Pines, Christopher R. Carpenter, Ali S. Raja and Jeremiah D. Schuur.
© 2013 John Wiley & Sons, Ltd. Published 2013 by John Wiley & Sons, Ltd.

of the low flow state, so causative inferences are not possible at the bedside. Potential etiologies of cerebral ischemia include cardiac emboli from valvular disease or atrial fibrillation (10–15%), large vessel extracranial arterial disease (20–25%), and small vessel intracranial atherosclerosis (10–15%).[6] The first two etiologies can be identified by echocardiography, telemetry, and carotid Dopplers. In 50% of cases, the cause of TIA remains undetermined.[7] Observational studies and randomized trials have suggested that stroke specialist care, rapid administration of antiplatelet and lipid-lowering agents, and ED-initiated diagnostic testing within 24 hours can reduce post-TIA stroke rates for up to 1 year.[5,8–12] One potential benefit of admitting TIA patients is that in-hospital thrombolysis using NINDS or ECASS-III protocols is more likely in the inpatient setting.[13–15] However, the cost-effectiveness of hospitalizing TIA patient as opposed to evaluating them in a same-day clinic continues to be debated.[16,17]

Efficacy and cost-effectiveness could be improved if TIA patients at increased risk for short-term stroke could be rapidly and accurately identified in ED settings, but simply diagnosing a TIA is a challenge. TIA mimics complicate clinicians' bedside diagnostic accuracy and include migraine headaches, occult seizures, transient hypoglycemia, and somatization. Consequently, TIAs are frequently misdiagnosed in the ED by neurologists and emergency physicians.[18–20] Features associated with a discordant diagnosis of TIA between neurologists and emergency physicians include headache, involuntary movement, and dizziness, while a high $ABCD^2$ score increases the odds of concordance.[21] Magnetic resonance imaging (MRI) protocols for stroke using axial diffusion-weighted images (DWI) and axial fluid-attenuated inversion recovery imaging can be obtained in 10 minutes, and a normal study can reduce the risk of cerebral ischemia, but this resource is not always readily available. In addition, practice variability and resource constraints limit the uniform application of rapid diagnostic and therapeutic pathways on all TIA patients.[22,23]

Clinical question

Can the ABCD, $ABCD^2$, or any currently available prognostic decision aid accurately risk-stratify TIA patients at increased risk for 7-day stroke risk?
Registry data were used to derive and validate three rules: the California Rule, the ABCD Rule, and the $ABCD^2$ Rule (Table 50.1).[4,24–27] The $ABCD^2$ Rule demonstrated superior prognostic accuracy, so subsequent trials focused on this decision aid. Preliminary validation trials for the $ABCD^2$ were promising.[28–31] However, the only trial that has followed the established methodological rigor for validating a decision instrument prospectively, in

Table 50.1 Transient ischemic attack (TIA) risk stratification instruments

California Rule	
Age >60 years	1 point
Diabetes mellitus	1 point
Symptoms >10 minutes	1 point
Weakness	1 point
Speech deficit	1 point
ABCD Rule	
Age >60 years	1 point
Blood pressure >140/90	1 point
Unilateral weakness	2 points
Language disturbance without weakness	1 point
Duration	
>60 minutes	2 points
10–59 minutes	1 point
ABCD² Rule	
Age >60 years	
Blood pressure >140/90	1 point
Diabetes	2 points
Unilateral weakness	2 points
Language disturbance without weakness	1 point
Duration	
>60 minutes	2 points
10–59 minutes	1 point

Source: Data from [24].

real time using actual clinicians on patients with diagnoses and outcomes unknown at the time the instrument is employed, has yielded disappointing results (Table 50.2).[32,33] Using the cutoff ABCD² score of more than 2 as recommended by American Heart Association Guidelines, the ABCD² was highly sensitive (94.7%) but nonspecific (12.5%) for 7-day stroke risk.[1] Based upon these data, which represent the highest quality validation trial to date, 87.6% of patients would require urgent investigations or hospital admission. Attempts to modify the ABCD² to improve post-TIA risk stratification have not improved its overall accuracy.[34] Therefore, the ABCD² should not be used to stratify TIA patients for short-term stroke risk.

Comment

The development of these TIA decision aids has raised awareness for the natural history of stroke with TIA as a form of "cerebral unstable angina" portending an increased short-term risk of stroke for a subset of patients.

Table 50.2 ABCD^2 likelihood ratio diagnostic accuracy for stroke at 7 and 90 days

ABCD^2 score	Stroke at 7 days	Stroke at 90 days
0	0	0
1	0	0
2	0.61 (0.12–2.38)	0.36 (0.09–1.42)
3	0.13 (0.02–0.91)	0.23 (0.08–0.70)
4	1.07 (0.63–1.84)	1.22 (0.83–1.79)
5	1.53 (0.97–2.39)	1.47 (1.03–2.11)
6	1.19 (0.64–2.22)	1.06 (0.63–1.77)
7	3.89 (1.48–10.19)	4.22 (1.99–8.92)

Source: Data from [32].

The California, ABCD, and ABCD^2 decision aids have consequently improved post-TIA management by refocusing clinicians' contemporary objectives to first correctly diagnosis TIA from amongst the numerous mimics and then to attempt risk stratification to allocate scarce diagnostic tests to those at risk for a disabling stroke. Investigators have recently described the ABCD^{3}I and ABCD^{2}I rules by incorporating brain CT, carotid imaging, and MRI diffusion weighted imaging results into the decision model.[35,36] However, these modified decision aids have not yet been validated using established methods.[33] More importantly, once advanced imaging is required to augment the decision aids, their usefulness and external validity are diminished since access to this technology may be limited in some settings. The ABCD^2 rule relies upon clinical features, neglecting the pathophysiological differences between arteroembolic and cardioembolic stroke or the difficulties in identifying lacunar syndromes using current imaging techniques. Future TIA decision aids will need to incorporate these complexities while maintaining sufficient simplicity to ensure accessibility of the decision aid for heterogeneous emergency settings.

References

1. Easton JD, Saver JL, Albers GW, Alberts MJ, Chaturvedi S, Feldmann E *et al.* Definition and evaluation of transient ischemic attack: A scientific statement for healthcare professionals from the American Heart Association/American Stroke Association Stroke Council; Council on Cardiovascular Surgery and Anesthesia; Council on Cardiovascular Radiology and Intervention; Council on Cardiovascular Nursing; and the Interdisciplinary Council on Peripheral Vascular Disease: The American Academy of Neurology affirms the value of this statement as an educational tool for neurologists. Stroke. 2009; 40(6): 2276–93.

2. Kleindorfer D, Panagos P, Pancioli A, Khoury J, Kissela B, Woo D *et al*. Incidence and short-term prognosis of transient ischemic attack in a population-based study. Stroke. 2005; 36(4): 720–3.

3. Rothwell PM, Warlow CP. Timing of TIAs preceding stroke: Time window for prevention is very short. Neurology. 2005; 64(5): 817–20.

4. Johnston SC, Gress DR, Browner WS, Sidney S. Short-term prognosis after emergency department diagnosis of TIA. Journal of the American Medical Association. 2000; 284(22): 2901–6.

5. Giles MF, Rothwell PM. Risk of stroke after early transient ischaemic attack: a systematic review and meta-analysis. Lancet Neurology. 2007; 6(12): 1063–72.

6. Cucchiara BL, Kasner SE. In the clinic: Transient ischemic attack. Annals of Internal Medicine. 2011; 154(1): Itc11–5.

7. Cucchiara BL, Messe SR, Sansing L, Mackenzie L, Taylor R, Pacelli Journal of *et al*. D-Dimer, magnetic resonance imaging diffusion-weighted imaging, and ABCD2 score for transient ischemic attack risk stratification. Journal of Stroke and Cerebrovascular Disease. 2009; 18(5): 367–73.

8. Cucchiara BL, Messe SR, Taylor RA, Pacelli J, Maus D, Shah Q *et al*. Is the ABCD Score useful for risk stratification of patients with acute transient ischemic attack? Stroke. 2006; 37(7): 1710–4.

9. Calvet D, Lamy C, Touze E, Oppenheim C, Meder JF, Mas JL. Management and outcome of patients with transient ischemic attack admitted to a stroke unit. Cerebrovascular Disease. 2007; 24(1): 80–5.

10. Kennedy J, Hill MD, Ryckborst KJ, Eliasziw M, Demchuk AM, Buchan AM. Fast Assessment of Stroke and Transient Ischaemic Attack to Prevent Early Recurrence (FASTER): A randomised controlled pilot trial. Lancet Neurology. 2007; 6(11): 961–9.

11. Lavallee PC, Meseguer E, Abboud H, Cabrejo L, Olivot JM, Simon O *et al*. A Transient Ischaemic Attack Clinic with Round-the-Clock Access (SOS-TIA): Feasibility and effects. Lancet Neurology. 2007; 6(11): 953–60.

12. Ross MA, Compton S, Medado P, Fitzgerald M, Kilanowski P, O'Neil BJ. An emergency department diagnostic protocol for patients with transient ischemic attack: A randomized controlled trial. Annals of Emergency Medicine. 2007; 50(2): 109–19.

13. The National Institute of Neurological Disorders and Stroke Rt-Pa Stroke Study Group. Tissue plasminogen activator for acute ischemic stroke. New England Journal of Medicine. 1995; 333(24): 1581–7.

14. Hacke W, Kaste M, Bluhmki E, Brozman M, Davalos A, Guidetti D *et al*. Thrombolysis with alteplase 3 to 4.5 hours after acute ischemic stroke. New England Journal of Medicine. 2008; 359(13): 1317–29.

15. Carpenter CR, Keim SM, Milne WK, Meurer WJ, Barsan WG. Thrombolytic therapy for acute ischemic stroke beyond three hours. Journal of Emergency Medicine. 2011; 40(1): 82–92.

16. Nguyen-Huynh MM, Johnston SS. Is hospitalization after TIA cost-effective on the basis of treatment with TPA? Neurology. 2005; 65(11): 1799–801.

17. Joshi JK, Ouyang B, Prabhakaran S. Should TIA patients be hospitalized or referred to a same-day clinic? A decision analysis. Neurology. 2011; 77(24): 2082–8.

18. Kraaijeveld CL, Van Gijn J, Schouten HJ, Staal A. Interobserver agreement for the diagnosis of transient ischemic attacks. Stroke. 1984; 15(4): 723–5.

19. Prabhakaran S, Silver AJ, Warrior L, Mcclenathan B, Lee VH. Misdiagnosis of transient ischemic attacks in the emergency room. Cerebrovascular Disease. 2008; 26(6): 630–5.

20. Castle J, Mlynash M, Lee K, Caulfield AF, Wolford C, Kemp S et al. Agreement regarding diagnosis of transient ischemic attack fairly low among stroke-trained neurologists. Stroke. 2010; 41(7): 1367–70.

21. Schrock JW, Glasenapp M, Victor A, Losey T, Cydulka RK. Variables associated with discordance between emergency physician and neurologist diagnoses of transient ischemic attacks in the emergency department. Annals of Emergency Medicine. 2012; 59(1): 19–26.

22. Giles MF, Rothwell PM. Substantial underestimation of the need for outpatient services for TIA and minor stroke. Age Ageing. 2007; 36(6): 676–80.

23. Johnston SC, Smith WW. Practice variability in management of transient ischemic attacks. European Neurology. 1999; 42(2): 105–8.

24. Carpenter CR, Keim SM, Crossley J, Perry JJ. Post-transient ischemic attack early stroke stratification: The ABCD(2) prognostic aid. Journal of Emergency Medicine. 2009; 36(2): 194–200.

25. Shah KH, Metz HA, Edlow JA. Clinical prediction rules to stratify short-term risk of stroke among patients diagnosed in the emergency department with a transient ischemic attack. Annals of Emergency Medicine. 2009; 53(5): 662–73.

26. Rothwell PM, Giles MF, Flossmann E, Lovelock CE, Redgrave JNE, Warlow CP et al. A Simple score (ABCD) to identify individuals at high early risk of stroke after transient ischaemic attack. Lancet. 2005; 366(9479): 29–36.

27. Johnston SC, Rothwell PM, Nguyen-Huynh MN, Giles MF, Elkins JS, Bernstein AL et al. Validation and refinement of scores to predict very early stroke risk after transient ischaemic attack. Lancet 2007; 369(9558): 283–92.

28. Josephson SA, Sidney S, Pham TN, Bernstein AL, Johnston SS. Higher ABCD2 score predicts patients most likely to have true transient ischemic attack. Stroke. 2008; 39(11): 3096–8.

29. Wasserman J, Perry J, Dowlatshahi D, Stotts G, Stiell IG, Sutherland J et al. Stratified, urgent care for transient ischemic attack results in low stroke rates. Stroke. 2010; 41(11): 2601–5.

30. Cancelli I, Janes F, Gigli GL, Perelli A, Zanchettin B, Canal G et al. Incidence of transient ischemic attack and early stroke risk: Validation of the ABCD2 score in an Italian population-based study. Stroke. 2011; 42(10): 2751–7.

31. Galvin R, Geraghty C, Motterlini N, Dimitrov BD, Fahey T. Prognostic value of the ABCD[2] clinical prediction rule: A systematic review and meta-analysis. Family Practice. 2011; 28(4): 366–76.

32. Perry JJ, Sharma M, Sivilotti MLA, Sutherland J, Symington C, Worster A et al. Prospective validation of the ABCD2 score for patients in the emergency

department with transient ischemic attack. Canadian Medical Association Journal. 2011; 183(10): 1137–45.

33. Stiell IG, Wells GA. Methodologic standards for the development of clinical decision rules in emergency medicine. Annals of Emergency Medicine. 1999; 33(4): 437–47.

34. Raser JM, Cucchiara BL. Modifications of the ABCD(2) score do not improve the risk stratification of transient ischemic attack patients. Journal of Stroke Cerebrovascular Dis. 2012; 21(6): 467–70.

35. Giles MF, Albers GW, Amarenco P, Arsava MM, Asimos A, Ay H *et al*. Addition of brain infarction to the ABCD2 score (ABCD2I): A collaborative analysis of unpublished data on 4574 patients. Stroke. 2010; 41(9): 1907–13.

36. Merwick A, Albers GW, Amarenco P, Arsavo EM, Ay H, Calvet D *et al*. Addition of brain and carotid imaging to the ABCD^2 score to identify patients at early risk of stroke after transient ischaemic attack: A multicentre observational study. Lancet Neurology. 2010; 9(11): 1060–9.

Chapter 51 **Seizure**

Highlights

- The majority of seizures in the ED will not have a clear diagnosis established.
- Withdrawal seizures represent the minority of alcohol-related seizures.
- All reproductive-aged females with a new-onset seizure should have a pregnancy test and careful consideration for eclampsia.
- In adults, assessment of sodium and glucose is often indicated, but routine lab testing in pediatric febrile or afebrile seizures is not recommended.
- Brain CT is indicated in adults after a first unprovoked seizure, but may be deferred to the outpatient setting in some patients.

Background

By the age of 80 years, 3.6% of people in the United States will suffer at least one seizure, excluding febrile seizures which are limited to children aged 6 months to 6 years.[1] Patients with known seizure disorder should be evaluated distinctly from first-episode seizure patients presenting to the emergency department (ED). This chapter will focus on the diagnostic approach to the first-episode seizure patients. One-fifth of first-episode seizure patients are not recognized during their first ED evaluation.[2] Furthermore, migraine headaches and syncope are frequently misdiagnosed as seizure or stroke.[3] After a first seizure, up to 40% of patients will have a recurrence within 2 years.[4] The top three etiologies of seizures in ED patients older than 5 years are toxins (19%), head injury (8%), and epilepsy (7%).[5] Toxins include ethanol, but only 22% of seizures attributed to alcohol abuse can be explained by withdrawal.[6] Therefore, the diagnosis of an alcohol withdrawal seizure should be one of exclusion. Other toxins associated with seizures include cocaine, lidocaine, meperidine, theophylliine, buproprion, carbon monoxide, organophosphates, and nerve agents.[7,8]

Evidence-Based Emergency Care: Diagnostic Testing and Clinical Decision Rules, Second Edition.
Jesse M. Pines, Christopher R. Carpenter, Ali S. Raja and Jeremiah D. Schuur.
© 2013 John Wiley & Sons, Ltd. Published 2013 by John Wiley & Sons, Ltd.

Status epilepticus is defined as seizures persisting for over 30 minutes or multiple seizures without a return to normal consciousness in between. In the ED, status epilepticus represents 7% of seizures.[9] The mortality of status epilepticus is 3% in children and increases to 38% in geriatric adults.[10] One-quarter of status cases are nonconvulsive, which can be a challenging diagnosis, as the patient may present with altered mental status such as lethargy or coma.[11] Additionally, when seizures are not witnessed by bystanders, emergency physicians must differentiate syncope from seizure. Serum creatine kinase measured 4 hours after loss of consciousness can distinguish syncope from tonic-clonic seizure because it is elevated in the latter condition.[12,13]

In children, febrile seizures represent one-third of seizures presenting to the ED.[8] In order to establish the diagnosis of simple febrile seizure, all of the criteria in Table 51.1 must be met.[14] Complex febrile seizures are less well defined and probably represent a heterogeneous mixture. Children with a simple febrile seizure are not at increased risk to develop adult epilepsy compared with those who never had a febrile seizure, but the risk of recurrent febrile seizure is high, ranging from 12% to 50% depending upon whether the seizure occurred in an infant or toddler.

Pregnant women without preexisting epilepsy can develop a gestational seizure disorder called *eclampsia*. Preeclampsia usually precedes the development of seizures with hypertension, proteinuria, and edema beginning after the 20th week of pregnancy. One-quarter of eclampsia seizures occur before labor, one-half during labor, and the rest occur up to 10 days postpartum. Maternal risk factors for preeclampsia include a family history of preeclampsia, multiple gestations, renal disease, diabetes preceding the pregnancy, nulliparity, and extremes of age.[15]

Psychogenic seizures, formerly referred to as *pseudoseizures*, are a diagnosis of exclusion in the ED with a general population prevalence of 0.002–0.33%.[16] About one in three patients receive an anti-epileptic medication for psychogenic seizures, and the mean delay between seizure onset and psychogenic seizure diagnosis is 7 years.[17] Among patients referred to definitive epilepsy diagnostic centers, 30% are ultimately diagnosed with

Table 51.1 Essential criterion to define *simple* febrile seizure

Age 6 months to 5 years
Tonic-clonic seizure
Resolution of convulsions within 15 minutes
Normal mental status after convulsion
Fever <38.0°C
Only one convulsion in 24-hour period
Absence of preceding neurological abnormality

Source: Data from [14].

psychogenic seizures.[18] To further complicate the issue, epilepsy can coexist with psychogenic seizures in 5–40% of cases.[19] Psychogenic seizures may be distinguished from neurogenic seizures by duration (often >90 seconds), presence of corneal reflex, prevention of hand falling on the face, being conversant during the attack, and the absence of a postictal phase or event-related amnesia.[20,21]

Clinical question

What diagnostic tests should be performed in well-appearing adults presenting to the ED following a first-episode *unprovoked seizure?*

The American College of Emergency Physicians has provided evidence-based guidelines upon which to base diagnostic decision making.[22] Some of these recommendations are summarized in Figure 51.1. No Level A evidence-based guidelines were published. The guidelines provide Level B evidence for the following ED diagnostic studies following a first-episode unproved seizure.

• Electroencephalogram (EEG)
• CT or MRI neuroimaging
• Serum glucose
• Serum sodium
• Pregnancy test in reproductive-aged females

The guideline authors found insufficient evidence to support or refute routine toxicology screening or lumbar puncture. Furthermore, when the new-onset seizure patient has returned to a normal baseline, deferred outpatient neuroimaging is sufficient when reliable follow-up is available. The indications for consulting Neurology and/or obtaining an EEG in the ED (versus in outpatient follow-up) are not defined by the guidelines. The sensitivity of EEG decreases with increased time from the event, so arranging urgent outpatient EEG is useful.

Although many electrolyte abnormalities will be suspected on history and physical exam in such patients, unexpected hypoglycemia or hyponatremia will sometimes be identified by laboratory evaluation.[23–25] The same is true for central nervous system (CNS) imaging. In one study of 259 patients with clinically suspected alcohol withdrawal seizures, 16 (6%) had an intracranial lesion on head CT, 10 of which altered subsequent clinical management.[26] A multidisciplinary clinical policy on neuroimaging for such patients recommended that a head CT be obtained in the ED whenever an acute intracranial process is suspected, in the presence of a focal neurological deficit, after acute head trauma, for patients older than 40 years, if focal onset before generalized seizure ensued, or if a history of malignancy, immunocompromising illness, fever, persistent headache, or anticoagulation exists.[27]

Lower quality evidence suggests that serum prolactin levels measured 10–20 minutes after a suspected psychogenic seizure may be useful to distinguish them from tonic-clonic seizures. In tonic-clonic seizures, serum prolactin levels will increase over twice the baseline level (pooled sensitivity 60%, pooled specificity 96%, LR+ 16, and LR− 0.42).[28] This means that an elevated prolactin level supports the diagnosis of generalized tonic-clonic seizure, but a normal prolactin level does not sufficiently diagnose psychogenic seizures. Transient lactic acidosis is also common following a generalized tonic-clonic seizure, but it has never been investigated in the context of psychogenic seizures.[29]

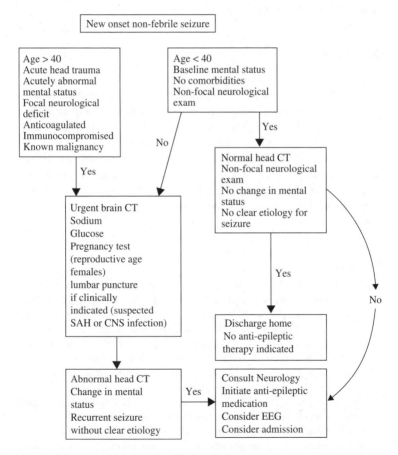

Figure 51.1 Diagnostic evaluation of first-time seizure.

Clinical question

What diagnostic tests should be performed in well-appearing children following a febrile seizure?

Excluding those with prior neurosurgery, significant neurological disorder, or chronic medical illness, in well-appearing children with first complex seizure associated with fever the incidence of significant intracranial pathology is rare (0%, CI 0–4%) and CNS imaging can often be safely deferred.[30-32] Similarly, studies have not demonstrated any role in routinely evaluating electrolytes or glucose in first-episode febrile or afebrile pediatric seizure patients.[14,33-35] However, laboratory testing is indicated in the ill-appearing child with vomiting, diarrhea, dehydration, or failure to return to his or her baseline mental status.

Comment

No trials exist defining the diagnostic accuracy of tests in seizure patients. Additionally, no outcomes-based studies have been published to assess the utility of laboratory or CNS imaging in first-time seizure patients. Figure 51.1 provides an algorithmic approach to the management of seizure patients in the ED that is based upon available guidelines. Future research is needed to explore the subset of patients most likely to benefit from early (versus delayed) CT and EEG, as well as the diagnostic accuracy of history and physical exam to distinguish psychogenic seizures from neurogenic seizures. Clinicians need to approach each seizure patient as a neurogenic seizure until proven otherwise.

References

1. Annegers JF, Hauser WA, Lee JR, Rocca WA. Incidence of acute symptomatic seizures in Rochester, Minnesota, 1935–1984. Epilepsia. 1995; 36(4): 327–33.
2. Leung H, Man CY, Hui ACF, Wong KS, Kwan P. Agreement between initial and final diagnosis of first seizures, epilepsy and non-epileptic events: A prospective study. Journal of Neurology, Neurosurgery and Psychiatry. 2008; 79(10): 1144–7.
3. Moeller JJ, Kurniawan J, Gubitz GJ, Ross A, Bhan V. Diagnostic accuracy of neurological problems in the emergency department. Canadian Journal of Neurological Sciences. 2008; 35(3): 335–41.
4. Berg AT, Shinnar S. The risk of seizure recurrence following a first unprovoked seizure: A quantitative review. Neurology. 1991; 71(7): 965–72.
5. Ong S, Talan DA, Moran GJ, Mower W, Newdow M, Tsang VC *et al.* Neurocysticerocosis in radiographically imaged seizure patients in U.S. emergency departments. Emergency Infectious Disease. 2002; 8(6): 608–13.

6. Krumholz A, Grufferman S, Orr ST, Stern BJ. Seizures and seizure care in an emergency department. Epilepsia. 1989; 30(2): 175–81.

7. Holland RW, Marx JA, Earnest MP, Ranniger S. Grand mal seizures temporally related to cocaine use: Clinical and diagnostic features. Annals of Emergency Medicine. 1992; 21(7): 772–6.

8. Sharma S, Riviello JJ, Harper MB, Baskin MN. The role of emergent neuroimaging in children with new-onset afebrile seizures. Pediatrics. 2003; 111(1): 1–5.

9. Huff JS, Morris DL, Kothari RU, Gibbs MA. Emergency department management of patients with seizures: A multicenter study. Academic Emergency Medicine. 2001; 8(6): 622–8.

10. Delorenzo RJ, Hauser WA, Towne AR, Boggs JG, Pellock JM, Penberthy L et al. A prospective, population-based epidemiologic study of status epilepticus in Richmond, Virginia. Neurology. 1996; 46(4): 1029–35.

11. Drislane FW. Presentation, evaluation, and treatment of nonconvulsive status epilepticus. Epilepsy Behavior. 2000; 1(5): 301–14.

12. Libman MD, Potvin L, Coupal L, Grover SA. Seizure vs. syncope: Measuring serum creatine kinase in the emergency department. Journal of General Internal Medicine. 1991; 6(5): 408–12.

13. Goksu E, Oktay C, Kilicaslan I, Kartal M. Seizure or syncope: The diagnostic value of serum creatine kinase and myoglobin levels. European Journal of Emergency Medicine. 2009; 16(2): 84–6.

14. Hampers LC, Spina LA. Evaluation and management of pediatric febrile seizures in the emergency department. Emergency Medicine Clinics of North America. 2011; 29(1): 83–93.

15. Stead LG. Seizures in pregnancy/eclampsia. Emergency Medicine Clinics of North America. 2011; 29(1): 109–16.

16. Benbadis SR, Allen-Hauser W. An estimate of the prevalence of psychogenic non-epileptic seizures. Seizure. 2000; 9(4): 280–1.

17. Reuber M, Fernandez G, Bauer J, Helmstaedter C, Elger CE. Diagnostic delay in psychogenic nonepileptic seizures. Neurology. 2002; 58(3): 493–5.

18. Friedman JH, Lafrance WC. Psychogenic disorders: The need to speak plainly. Archives of Neurology. 2010; 67(6): 753–5.

19. Bodde NM, Brooks JL, Baker GA, Boon PA, Hendriksen JG, Mulder OG et al. Psychogenic non-epileptic seizures: Definition, etiology, treatment, and prognostic issues: A critical review. Seizure. 2009; 18(8): 543–53.

20. Leis AA, Ross MA, Summers AK. Psychogenic seizures: Ictal characteristics and diagnostic pitfalls. Neurology. 1992; 42(1): 95–9.

21. Jagoda A, Riggio S. Psychogenic convulsive seizures. American Journal of Emergency Medicine. 1993; 11(6): 626–32.

22. ACEP Clinical Policies Subcommittee. Critical issues in the evaluation and management of adult patients presenting to the emergency department with seizures. Annals of Emergency Medicine. 2004; 43(5): 605–25.

23. Turnbull TL, Vanden Hoek TL, Howes DS, Eisner RF. Utility of laboratory studies in the emergency department patient with a new-onset seizure. Annals of Emergency Medicine. 1990; 19(4): 373–7.

24. Tardy B, Lafond P, Convers P, Page Y, Zeni F, Viallon A *et al.* Adult first generalized seizure: etiology, biological tests, EEG, CT scan, in an ED. American Journal of Emergency Medicine. 1995; 13(1): 1–5.

25. Bradford JC, Kyriakedes CG. Evaluation of the patient with seizures: An evidence based approach. Emergency Medicine Clinics of North America. 1999; 17(1): 203–20.

26. Earnest MP, Feldman H, Marx JA, Harris JA, Biletch M, Sullivan LP. Intracranial lesions shown by CT scans in 259 cases of first alcohol-related seizures. Neurology. 1988; 38(10): 1561–5.

27. American College of Emergency Physicians, American Academy of Neurology, American Association of Neurological Surgeons, and American Society of Neuro-radiology. Practice parameter: Neuroimaging in the emergency patient presenting with seizure (summary statement). Annals of Emergency Medicine. 1996; 28(1): 114–8.

28. Chen DK, So YT, Fisher RS. Use of serum prolactin in diagnosing epileptic seizures. Report of the Therapeutics and Technology Assessment Subcommittee of the American Academy of Neurology. Neurology. 2005; 65(5): 668–75.

29. Lipka K, Bülow HH. Lactic acidosis following convulsions. Acta Anaesthesiologica Scandinavica. 2003; 47(5): 616–8.

30. Garvey MA, Gaillard WD, Rusin JA, Ochsenschlager D, Weinstein S, Conry JA *et al.* Emergency brain computed tomography in children with seizures: Who is most likely to benefit? Journal of Pediatrics. 1998; 133(5): 664–9.

31. Maytal J, Krauss JM, Novak G, Nagelberg J, Patel M. The role of brain computed tomography in evaluating children with new onset seizures in the emergency department. Epilepsia. 2000; 41(8): 950–4.

32. Teng D, Dayan P, Tyler S, Hauser WA, Chan S, Leary L *et al.* Risk of intracranial pathologic conditions requring emergency intervention after a first complex febrile seizure episode among children. Pediatrics. 2006; 117(2): 304–8.

33. Gerber MA, Berliner BC. The child with a "simple" febrile seizure: Appropriate diagnostic evaluation. American Journal of Diseases in Children. 1981; 135(5): 431–3.

34. Nypaver MM, Reynolds SL, Tanz RR, Davis AT. Emergency department laboratory evaluation of children with seizures: Dogma or dilemma? Pediatric Emergency Care. 1992; 8(1): 13–6.

35. Sharieff GQ, Hendry PL. Afebrile pediatric seizures. Emergency Medicine Clinics of North America. 2011; 29(1): 95–108.

Miscellaneous: Hematology, Ophthalmology, Pulmonology, Rheumatology, and Geriatrics

Section D
Miscellaneous
Hematology
Ophthalmology
Pulmonology
Rheumatology and
Geriatrics

Chapter 52 **Venous Thromboembolism**

Highlights

- Deep vein thrombosis (DVT) and pulmonary embolism (PE), together known as venous thromboemoblism (VTE), are potentially lethal conditions that can present atypically.
- In evaluating patients with suspected DVT, two-point ultrasound (femoral vein at the groin + popiteal fossa) along with D-dimer are similar to whole-leg ultrasound, which includes the calf.
- Scoring systems like the Wells criteria, the Geneva score, and the PERC rule can guide clinicians about the likelihood of VTE.
- Diagnostic evaluation for VTE involves risk assessment coupled with D-dimer testing for low-risk to very-low-risk patients.
- High-risk patients with suspected PE should receive a chest CTA–CTV to rule out PE.

Background

Diagnosing deep vein thrombosis (DVT) and pulmonary embolism (PE), also together known as venous thromboembolic (VTE) disease, represents a challenge in emergency care because both can present with nonspecific symptoms and can be potentially lethal. Accurate and timely identification of patients with DVT and PE in the ED can minimize complications and morbidity. However, both DVT and PE are relatively rare entities, ones that are often sought but infrequently found. In the United States, approximately 100 persons per 100,000 develop VTE.[1] The challenge in diagnosing DVT and PE in the ED is appropriate selection of patients for diagnostic testing and risk stratification based on clinical findings. While many tests are available for DVT and PE for ED patients, there is a large literature on this topic – mostly directed at the determination of pretest probability using clinical decision rules and the calculation of a diagnostic test's sensitivity and specificity. The following

Evidence-Based Emergency Care: Diagnostic Testing and Clinical Decision Rules, Second Edition. Jesse M. Pines, Christopher R. Carpenter, Ali S. Raja and Jeremiah D. Schuur.
© 2013 John Wiley & Sons, Ltd. Published 2013 by John Wiley & Sons, Ltd.

is not meant to be a comprehensive review of all aspects of the diagnosis of DVT and PE in the ED; rather, it is a compilation of clinically relevant questions and studies providing objective data for specific clinical questions.

There are multiple tests for PE, including D-dimer (enzyme-linked immunosorbent assay (ELISA) or whole-blood assay), chest computed tomography (CT), ventilation–perfusion (V/Q) scan, and pulmonary angiogram. Choosing a test traditionally focuses on assessment of pretest probability of the disease based on objective clinical criteria where lower risk patients can receive D-dimers to rule out PE and higher risk patients traditionally receive more tests that have higher sensitivities, such as chest CT or V/Q scan. Because pulmonary angiogram, long considered the criterion standard test for PE, has a 1.5% incidence of serious complication just from receiving the test, it is rarely used unless absolutely necessary to make a diagnosis and/or guide patient management.

Regarding DVT, venous noncompressibility is the major diagnostic criterion for venous thrombosis using ultrasound. Compression ultrasound, however, is not specific or sensitive for detecting DVT in patients with asymptomatic proximal DVT or in patients with DVT in the calf. It also demonstrates limited accuracy in cases of chronic DVT. The use of ultrasound is further limited in patients who are obese or who have edema. In general, despite its limitations, leg compression ultrasound is used to detect DVT in the ED. Traditionally, only the proximal veins (from the femoral veins down to the calf, where they join the popliteal veins) are studied. While DVTs usually start in the calf, more than 80% of symptomatic DVTs involve the popliteal vein and more proximal leg veins. In patients with calf DVTs that may not be detected on the first ED ultrasound, about 20% will extend more proximally within about a week. As DVTs that do not extend above the calf very rarely cause PE, proximal DVTs are at much higher risk for propagation and for causing PE.

Clinical question

How sensitive is ultrasound in detecting DVT?

A recent review of non-invasive methods for the diagnosis of first and recurrent DVT was performed to answer the question of diagnostic sensitivity of ultrasound in detecting DVT.[2] The authors used contrast venography as the criterion standard for detection of DVT and included only prospective cohort studies and randomized clinical trials. Combined data from individual studies were assessed using a random effects model. The sensitivity of venous ultrasound for a symptomatic proximal DVT in pooled analysis was 97% (CI 96–98%), and for symptomatic calf DVT it was 73% (CI 54–93%). The authors concluded that venous ultrasound is the most accurate non-invasive test for symptomatic DVT.

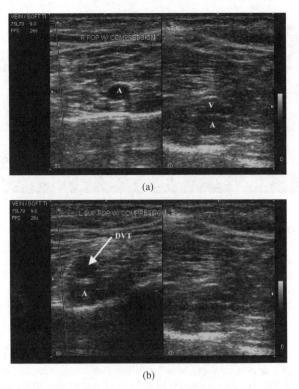

(a)

(b)

Figure 52.1 Compression ultrasound of the right and left popliteal vessels. (a) (top) The screen is split to show the noncompressed normal anatomy on the right-hand side and the compressed anatomy of the left-hand side. (b) (bottom) The left popliteal vein is noncompressible and represents a deep vein thrombosis. (Source: Courtesy of Anthony J. Dean, MD).
Note: A = artery; and V = vein.

Clinical question

What are the sensitivity and specificity of D-dimer testing in the diagnosis of DVT?

The test characteristics of a negative D-dimer to exclude DVT are dependent on the type of assay. Assays are either high sensitivity or moderate sensitivity. As the sensitivity of the assay drops, so too does the ability to use a negative test to rule out DVT. While there are many commercially available D-dimer assays, there are two specific methods that have been studied extensively: ELISA and whole-blood assays. Among the different assays, there is wide variation in the sensitivity, normal reference ranges, and cutoff points. A recently published meta-analysis of different D-dimer assays reported a

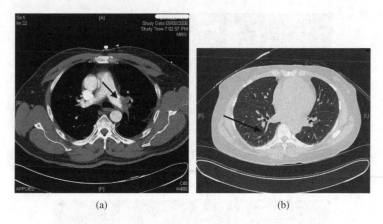

(a)   (b)

Figure 52.2 (a–b) Chest CT images show an acute pulmonary embolism.

sensitivity of ≥95% for ELISA and certain immuno-turbidimetric tests but also reported a low specificity (≥40%) at a cutoff of ≥500 ng/dL to exclude DVT.[3] Other D-dimer assays such as whole-blood and quantitative latex agglutination assays are less sensitive with a reported rate of about 85% but more specific at about 65%.

A recent systematic review examined 14 studies on 8,000 patients examining this question.[4] In the low-, medium-, and high-risk groups using the Wells criteria, the prevalence of DVT was 5%, 17%, and 53%, respectively (Table 52.1). In pooled analysis, the sensitivity and specificity of D-dimer in the low-probability group were 88% (CI 81–92%) and 72% (CI 65–78%), in the medium-probability group were 90% (CI 80–95%) and 58%

Table 52.1 Test characteristics for D-dimer testing in pooled studies to rule out deep vein thrombosis

Specific measure	Pretest probability		
	Low	Moderate	High
Sensitivity	88% (81–92%)	90% (80–95%)	92% (85–96%)
Specificity	72% (65–78%)	58% (49–67%)	45% (37–52%)
Negative predictive value	99% (98–99%)	96% (94–97%)	84% (77–89%)
Positive predictive value	17% (13–20%)	32% (25–41%)	66% (56–75%)

Source: Data from [4].

(CI 49–67%), and in the high-probability group were 92% (CI 85–96%) and 45% (CI 37–52%).

Clinical question

What is the difference in outcomes for patients who received a whole-leg ultrasound (including the calf) compared to a proximal-leg ultrasound with D-dimer to rule out DVT?

A randomized trial was conducted across 14 Italian university or civic hospitals to answer this question surrounding whole-leg ultrasound, which permits the detection of calf vein thrombosis but requires more skilled operators.[5] Patients were included who had their first episode of suspected DVT in the lower extremities, and they were randomized to undergo either two-point ultrasound (where the ultrasound is applied to the common femoral vein at the groin and the popliteal vein at the popliteal fossa) along with a D-dimer test versus whole-leg ultrasound. In the two-point ultrasound group, patients with a normal ultrasound and a positive D-dimer were scheduled for a follow-up ultrasound at 1 week. The major study outcome was the 3-month incidence of symptomatic VTE in patients with an initially normal evaluation. A total of 2,098 patients were randomized (whole-leg ultrasound: 1053; and two-point ultrasound: 1045). Symptomatic VTE was detected in seven out of 801 patients in the two-point ultrasound group versus nine out of 763 patients in the whole-leg ultrasound group. This met the equivalence criterion with an observed difference of 0.3% (CI −1.4% to 0.8%). The authors concluded that the two diagnostic strategies were equivalent in managing patients with suspected DVT.

Clinical question

What are the Wells criteria for pretest probability of DVT and PE?

The initial derivation of the Wells criteria for PE involved the development of a simplified scoring system to calculate pretest probability in patients with suspected PE.[6] The authors used a randomly selected sample of 80% of the patients who had participated in a prospective cohort study of patients with suspected PE who also received D-dimer testing (SimpliRED), and performed logistic regression analysis using 40 clinical variables to create a clinical prediction rule. They created cut points for the new rule and created two separate scoring systems. The first scoring system classified patients as having low, moderate, or high probability of PE and the second system

Table 52.2 The Wells criteria to assess pretest probability for suspected pulmonary embolism

Clinical factor	Point score
Clinical deep vein thrombosis (DVT) (objective leg swelling, tenderness)	3
Heart rate ≥100 beats/minute	1.5
Immobilization >3 days or surgery in previous 4 weeks	1.5
Previous DVT or pulmonary embolus (PE)	1.5
Hemoptysis	1
Malignancy	1
PE as likely as, or more likely than, alternative diagnosis	3

*Interpretation of point total: <2 points: low risk (mean probability = 3.6%); 2–6 points: moderate risk (mean probability = 20.5%); and ≥6 points: high risk (mean probability = 66.7%).
Source: Data from [6].

created two categories, *PE likely* and *PE unlikely*. The goal in the second system was that patients who were PE unlikely and had a negative D-dimer would have a PE prevalence of less than 2%. The authors then applied these probabilities to the remaining 20% of the sample (to validate the scoring system). Seven variables ended up being predictive of PE and were termed the Wells criteria for PE (Table 52.2).

The interpreted point totals did not include D-dimer testing. *PE unlikely* was assigned for patients with a point score of less than or equal to 4 points. Without the use of D-dimer testing, the prevalence of PE in those whose score was >4 was 7.8%. However, when the D-dimer was negative, the rate of PE was only 2.2% (CI 1.0–4.0) in the derivation dataset and 1.7% in the validation dataset. Using a cutoff of <2 points and a negative D-dimer resulted in a PE rate of 1.5% (CI 0.4–3.7%) in the derivation set and 2.7% (CI 0.3–9.0%) in the validation set and occurred in only 29% of patients. The authors concluded that a combination of a score ≤4 and a negative D-dimer may have a negative predictive value where safe discharge is possible in patients with suspected PE.

Wells and colleagues also derived and validated a similar rule for DVT (Table 52.3).[7] In the validation study, all patients had ultrasonography and venography. In 529 patients, the Wells criteria for DVT predicted the prevalence of DVT in high-risk (85%), medium-risk (33%), and low-risk (5%) cases.

Table 52.3 The Wells criteria for deep vein thrombosis (DVT)

Clinical feature	Score
Active cancer (current treatment or within 6 months or palliative)	1
Paralysis, paresis, or recent immobilization	1
Recently bedridden for > than 3 days or major surgery, within 4 weeks	1
Localized calf tenderness	1
Entire leg swollen	1
Calf swelling >3 cm compared with the asymptomatic leg (10 cm below tibial tuberosity)	1
Pitting edema in the symptomatic leg	1
Collateral superficial veins (nonvaricose)	1
Alternative diagnosis as likely as, or greater than, that of DVT	−2

Note: High risk: ≥ 3 points; moderate risk: 1–2 points; and low risk: ≤ 0 points.
Source: Data from [7].

Clinical question

What is the Geneva score for pulmonary embolism, and how does this compare to the Wells score?
The Geneva score is a scoring system that clinicians can use to risk-stratify patients with potential pulmonary embolism. The originally derived scoring system was limited in that it required arterial blood gas analysis, which is painful and is unnecessary in low-risk patients.[8] The revised Geneva score was recently published and does not include arterial blood gas analysis. The scoring system also does not require an assessment by the physician about whether PE is the leading diagnosis, as is required in the Wells score. The revised Geneva score was derived in 965 consecutive patients who were evaluated for PE according to a standardized protocol. A total of 23% in the derivation cohort and 26% in the validation cohort had PE. The area under the receiver operating curve (ROC) was 0.74 (CI 0.70–0.78) in both the derivation and validation datasets. The revised Geneva Score (see Table 52.4) also performed well in an external validation cohort of 756 patients.

Clinical question

Which patients require any testing at all for pulmonary embolism, and can the Pulmonary Embolism Research Consortium (PERC) criteria aid in this decision?
While D-dimer can be helpful in ruling out PE without imaging if applied to low-risk patients, overuse of the D-dimer to screen for possible PE can

Table 52.4 The revised Geneva Score

Risk factors	Points
Age >65 years	1
Previous deep venous thrombosis or pulmonary embolus	3
Surgery or fracture within 1 month	2
Active malignancy	2
Symptoms	
Unilateral lower limb pain	3
Hemoptysis	2
Clinical signs	
Heart rate 75–94 beats/minute	3
Heart rate ≥95 beats/minute	5
Pain on lower limb deep vein palpation and unilateral edema	4

Total score		Prevalence of PE*
0–3	Low risk	7.9%
4–10	Intermediate risk	28%
≥11	High risk	74%

*In the validation cohort.
Source: Data from [8].

have negative consequences because of the low specificity. As patients with elevated D-dimers usually get CT scans to rule out PE and the number of negative CTs for PE is high, selecting which patients need any testing to rule out PE is clinically helpful. A study by Kline et al aimed to derive and test clinical criteria to justify not ordering a D-dimer on ED patients.[9] They constructed a prediction rule, called the *PERC rule*, in 3,148 ED patients to identify patients at such low risk that they would not require any testing at all for PE. The authors sought to find variables that were associated with the absence of PE. In the derivation study, the prevalence of PE was 11%. The final model that was derived consisted of eight criteria (Table 52.5). If all are negative, the patient does not require any testing for PE and PE can be ruled out on clinical grounds.

A validation set included 1,427 low-risk patients, 8% of whom had PE. The rule was negative (did not meet any criteria) in 25% of them. Among those who were PERC rule negative, the proportion with PE was only 1.4% (CI 0.4–3.2%). In these low-risk patients, the authors concluded that they did not need a test for PE. When the same rule was applied retrospectively to a cohort with a 25% prevalence of PE, 6.7% had PE.[10] The PERC criteria has been validated in a prospective study of patients with suspected PE in 13 EDs,

Table 52.5 The Pulmonary Embolism Research Consortium (PERC) criteria for suspected pulmonary embolism

Age <50 years
Pulse <100 beats per minute
Oxygen saturation >94%
Absence of unilateral leg swelling
No hemoptysis
No recent trauma or surgery
No history of deep vein thrombosis or pulmonary embolus
No hormone use

Source: Data from [9].

who had a gestalt pretest probability <15%. The main study outcome was any image-proven VTE or all-cause death within 45 days of presentation.[11] In 8,138 patients, they reported a low suspicion for PE and all PERC criteria being negative in 1,666 patients (20% of the sample). Within 45 days, 561 patients (7%) had been diagnosed with any VTE and 56 had died. For the 1,666 with low suspicion and PERC-negative patients, 15 had VTE and one patient died. Low suspicion and being PERC negative yielded a sensitivity of 97% (CI 96–99%) and a specificity of 22% (CI 21–23%).

Clinical question

Can CT of the chest be used as a diagnostic endpoint in patients at high risk for pulmonary embolism?

First-generation CT scanners initially showed poor sensitivity (70%) for demonstrating pulmonary embolism on chest CT. In the past few years, however, multidetector CT scanning has been tested as a potential replacement to pulmonary angiography. In a prospective study of 756 patients who were referred to the ED with a suspicion of PE (prevalence of 26%), 524 patients with either a high clinical probability or a low or medium clinical probability and a positive D-dimer (ELISA) had both a lower extremity ultrasound and a multidetector row chest CT.[12] A total of three out of 324 (0.9%) had a proximal DVT on ultrasound and a negative chest CT. At 3-month follow-up, the overall risk of DVT and PE was estimated at 1.5% (CI 0.8–3.0%) if the D-dimer assay and CT scanning had been the only tests used to rule out pulmonary embolism. This study suggested that multidetector row CT scanning along with D-dimer for low- or medium-risk patients can be used without employing pulmonary angiogram. These data have been corroborated by another study of 3,306 patients that included mostly outpatients with suspected PE.[13] Patients who were high risk according to the

Wells criteria had a chest CT, and those who were low or medium risk were assessed by the D-dimer. Patients with elevated D-dimers underwent chest CT. The 3-month DVT and PE risk in patients who were not treated on the basis of a negative chest CT was 1.1% (CI 0.6–1.9%). This was independent of the pretest probability for PE.

Comment

Over the past 10 years, the assessment of ED patients for possible DVT and PE has changed considerably. There is considerable information available on test characteristics for laboratory tests and imaging studies, making the application of evidence-based medicine at the bedside a practicable reality. Venous compression ultrasound has replaced contrast venography to evaluate DVT. D-dimer is also useful in evaluating patients at low risk for DVT; however, there is variation and test sensitivity reaches only 88% in the lowest risk group.

There is good evidence that D-dimer can be used safely in patients who are at low or medium risk for PE and that multidetector row chest CT is a safe way to evaluate for higher risk presentations. The recently published results of the PIOPED II study, which was a multicenter trial of CT angiography (CTA) combined with CT venography (CTV), reported that in 824 patients CTA was 83% sensitive and 96% specific for the diagnosis of PE.[14] In about 10% of patients, the results of CTA and CTV together (CTA–CTV) were inconclusive because of poor image quality. Taken together, the sensitivity of CTA–CTV was 90% sensitive and 95% specific for PE. The authors concluded that in patients with suspected PE, the use of multidetector CTA with CTV has a higher sensitivity than CTA alone. They did, however, warn that additional testing should be performed when clinical probability is not consistent with imaging results. These results indicate to us that for higher risk cases of PE, multidetector row CTA with CTV should be the test of choice if it is available. However, when patients are at very high probability of PE based on a clinician's judgment, including use of a clinical scoring system like Wells, a negative CTA–CTV should not be used as a diagnostic endpoint and the criterion standard pulmonary angiogram should be performed.

Deciding which patients to not test for PE is challenging, because a high negative predictive value requires a very low-risk population. Patient selection for any diagnostic testing for PE is highly applicable in the ED because the choice of whether or not to consider a patient at any risk for PE occurs much more frequently than discriminating between medium- and high-risk patients. The PERC rule performed well in the initial derivation and validation study, and it is useful in identifying patients at low risk of

PE who need no further testing. The PERC rule should not be applied to a higher risk group, however, because it does not include all risk factors for VTE and the number of false negatives would be too high for practical use.

Finally, all of the reviewed studies agree that, when the criterion standard test (pulmonary angiogram) is not undertaken, or D-dimer is used for low- and medium-risk patients, there is always a chance that a patient will be sent home with DVT or PE. Where we draw the line – that is, where we set our standard for risk tolerance with our patients – is very physician specific and practice specific. You should make sure to thoroughly explain the risks and benefits of diagnostic strategies to your patients and involve them in the decision-making process for this highly challenging disease.

References

1. White RH. The epidemiology of venous thromboembolism. Circulation. 2003; 107(23 Suppl 1): 14–18.
2. Kearon C, Julian JA, Newman TE *et al*. Noninvasive diagnosis of deep vein thrombosis. Annals of Internal Medicine. 1998; 128: 663–77.
3. Stein PD, Hull RD, Patel KC *et al*. D-dimer for the exclusion of acute venous thrombosis and pulmonary embolism: A systematic review. Annals of Internal Medicine. 2004; 140: 589–602.
4. Wells PS, Owen C, Doucette S *et al*. Does this patient have deep vein thrombosis? Journal of the American Medical Association. 2006; 295: 199–207.
5. Bernardi E, Camporese G, Büller HR *et al*. Serial 2-point ultrasonography plus D-dimer vs whole-leg color-coded Doppler ultrasonography for diagnosing suspected symptomatic deep vein thrombosis: A randomized controlled trial. Journal of the American Medical Association. 2008 Oct 8; 300(14): 1653–9.
6. Wells PS, Anderson DR, Rodger M *et al*. Derivation of a simple clinical model to categorize patients' probability of pulmonary embolism: Increasing the model's utility with the SimpliRED D-dimer. Thrombosis and Haemostasis. 2000; 83: 416–20.
7. Wells PS, Hirsh J, Anderson DR *et al*. Accuracy of clinical assessment of deep-vein thrombosis. Lancet. 1995; 345(8961): 1326–30.
8. Perrier A, Roy PM, Aujesky D *et al*. Diagnosing pulmonary embolism in out-patients with clinical assessment, D-dimer measurement, venous ultrasound, and helical computed tomography: A multicenter management study. American Journal of Medicine. 2004; 116: 291–9.
9. Kline JA, Mitchell AM, Kabrhel C *et al*. Clinical criteria to prevent unnecessary diagnostic testing in emergency department patients with suspected pulmonary embolism. Journal of Thrombosis and Haemostasis. 2004; 2: 1247–55.
10. Righini M, Le Gal G, Perrier A, Bounameaux H. More on: Clinical criteria to prevent unnecessary diagnostic testing in emergency department patients with suspected pulmonary embolism. Journal of Thrombosis and Haemostasis. 2005; 3: 188–9.

11. Kline JA, Courtney DM, Kabrhel C *et al.* Prospective multicenter evaluation of the pulmonary embolism rule-out criteria. Journal of Thrombosis and Haemostasis. 2008; 6: 772–80.

12. Perrier A, Roy PM, Sanchez O *et al.* Multidetector-row computed tomography in suspected pulmonary embolism. New England Journal of Medicine. 2005; 352: 1760–8.

13. van Belle A, Buller HR, Huisman MV *et al.* Effectiveness of managing suspected pulmonary embolism using an algorithm combining clinical probability, D-dimer testing, and computed tomography. Journal of the American Medical Association. 2006; 295: 172–9.

14. Stein PD, Fowler SE, Goodman LR *et al.* Multidetector computed tomography for acute pulmonary embolism. New England Journal of Medicine. 2006; 354: 2317–22.

Chapter 53 **Temporal Arteritis**

Highlights

- Temporal arteritis typically presents as an acute unilateral headache in older adults and can cause permanent visual impairment.
- Definitive diagnosis is achieved with temporal artery biopsies.
- Temporal artery ultrasound is emerging as a non-invasive alternative to diagnosing temporal arteritis.
- Jaw claudication alone (LR+ 4–6) or in combination with scalp tenderness and/or headache (LR+ 15–17) is predictive of temporal arteritis.
- An erythrocyte sedimentation rate (ESR) (LR− 0.2–0.03) is a good screening tool for temporal arteritis.

Background

Temporal arteritis, also known as *giant cell arteritis*, is an inflammatory condition characterized by focal, granulomatous changes of branches of the carotid artery that lead to vessel damage, stenosis, and eventual occlusion. Histopathologic findings from temporal artery biopsies include multinucleated giant cells, necrotic tissue, and lymphocytic infiltration of the inflamed vessel wall. The classic description of the clinical manifestations of temporal arteritis include a new temporal headache that can wax and wane, jaw claudication (and even trismus-like symptoms), and visual symptoms (from floaters to transient monocular vision loss).

Temporal arteritis is a disease process of older adults, and is reported as the most common systemic vasculitis in this age group, estimated to occur in approximately 23 per 100,000 women aged 50 years and older, and approximately one-third as many men. While the mortality associated with temporal arteritis is not different from that for those without the condition, its principle morbidity is the risk for permanent visual impairment, as greater than 20% of patients with temporal arteritis develop permanent

Evidence-Based Emergency Care: Diagnostic Testing and Clinical Decision Rules, Second Edition.
Jesse M. Pines, Christopher R. Carpenter, Ali S. Raja and Jeremiah D. Schuur.
© 2013 John Wiley & Sons, Ltd. Published 2013 by John Wiley & Sons, Ltd.

Table 53.1 American College of Rheumatology (ACR) diagnostic criteria for temporal arteritis

- Age $\geq$ 50 years
- New onset of localized headache
- Temporal artery tenderness or decreased pulse
- Elevated erythrocyte sedimentation rate (ESR) (Westergren) $\geq$ 50 mm/h
- Positive temporal artery biopsy

Data from [2].

visual loss.[1] The American College of Rheumatology diagnostic criteria are listed in Table 53.1.[2] Patients with three of the five criteria are considered to have temporal arteritis; however, it is usually a heightened clinical suspicion that prompts a biopsy that leads to the diagnosis.

While treatments are available that markedly decrease the likelihood of developing permanent visual loss, it is sometimes difficult to determine which patients should receive a biopsy in order to make the diagnosis. Thus, research into the diagnosis of temporal arteritis has focused on the historical features, physical exam findings, and laboratory results that may help determine which patients should be treated and subsequently referred for temporal artery biopsy. Newer research has focused on the use of ultrasound as an additional diagnostic adjunct for the diagnosis of the disease.

Clinical question

Which factors in a patient's history, physical exam, and laboratory values are predictive of having temporal arteritis?

Two large studies have examined signs and symptoms associated with temporal arteritis.[3,4] Both studies included only patients who had undergone biopsies of the temporal artery, and thus both used biopsy as their criterion standard. The prevalence of temporal arteritis in patients sent for temporal artery biopsy in these studies ranged from 33% to 39%, but it should be noted that the prevalence of temporal arteritis in all patients older than 50 years has been estimated to be 1 in 500.[5] Neither study was able to assess the intraobservier reliability of the clinical findings as they were typically taken from retrospective chart reviews. Table 53.2 shows the clinical variables from each study associated with the diagnosis of temporal arteritis.

Jaw claudication, diplopia, and temporal artery beading or prominence had moderate predictive power; however, when combinations of factors were considered that included jaw claudication, LR+s were highly accurate for predicting a positive temporal arteritis biopsy result. Notably, the combination of jaw claudication, a new headache, and scalp tenderness had a LR+

Table 53.2 Clinical findings and laboratory findings in the diagnosis of temporal arteritis

Variable	Positive likelihood ratio (LR+)	Negative likelihood ratio (LR−)
Jaw claudication[3]	4.2 (2.8–6.2)	0.7 (0.6–0.8)
Diplopia[3]	3.4 (1.3–8.6)	0.95 (0.9–0.99)
Beading of temporal artery[3]	4.6 (1.1–18.4)	0.93 (0.88–0.99)
Prominent or enlarged temporal artery[3]	4.3 (2.1–8.9)	0.6 (0.5–0.9)
Elevated erythrocyte sedimentation rate (ESR)* [3]	1.1 (1–1.2)	0.2 (0.08–0.5)
Jaw claudication PM[4]	6.7 (4.9–9.1)	0.6 (0.5–0.7)
Scalp tenderness[4]	3 (2.3–3.9)	0.75 (0.7–0.81)
Jaw claudication + scalp tenderness[4]	17 (8–36)	0.84 (0.8–0.88)
Headache + jaw claudication + scalp tenderness[4]	15 (7–32)	0.86 (0.82–0.9)
Double vision[4]	3.5 (1.4–8.6)	0.97 (0.95–1)
Elevated ESR**[4]	1.16 (1.11–1.21)	0.28 (0.17–0.45)
Elevated ESR***[4]	1.19 (1.15–1.22)	0.03 (0–0.13)

* Among all patients (normal range not defined).
** Among all patients (normal range 0–22 mm/h for men and 0–29 mm/h for women).
*** Among patients not taking steroids (normal range 0–22 mm/h for men and 0–29 mm/h for women).
Source: Data from [3,4] as shown in "Variable" column.

of 15 (CI 7–32). Other symptoms commonly assessed that were positively associated with a diagnosis of temporal arteritis included headache of any type, anorexia, fever, weight loss, fatigue, myalgias, vertigo, or polymyalgia rheumatica; however, none of these symptoms individually had a likelihood ratio that was sufficiency greater than 1.0 to be considered useful.

Erythrocyte sedimentation rate (ESR) values were clinically useful when they were normal (LR− of 0.2–0.28). Among the subset of patients known to not be on steroids at the time of ESR testing, a normal ESR made temporal arteritis very unlikely. Nevertheless, there have been case reports of temporal arteritis despite normal ESR values prior to steroids,[6] so ESR alone should not be used to rule out the disease in patients with otherwise classic symptomatology. Notably, the exact cutoff for an "elevated ESR" was not defined in the meta-analysis by Smenta et al since a number of the studies they pooled did not give exact values, but Younge et al used ESR cutoffs of 22 mm/h for men and 29 mm/h for women.[3,4]

Based on their results given in this section, Younge et al developed a temporal arteritis biopsy formula (Figure 53.1) that estimates the probability

```
Score  =      − 240
              + 48 (if headache present)
              + 108 (if jaw claudication present)
              + 56 (if scalp tenderness present)
              + 70 (if ischemic optic neuropathy present)
              + ESR (mm/h)
              + Age (years)
Risk assessment:
        Score < −110 = Low risk (probability < 10%)
        Score ≥ 70 = High risk (probability > 80%)
```

Figure 53.1 Temporal artery biopsy formula. (Source: Data from [4]).

of a patient referred for temporal artery biopsy having temporal arteritis.[4] They used logistic regression to identify a model that predicted results of the temporal artery biopsy and then developed an equation with coefficients that maximized the receiver operator characteristic (ROC) of their model. While their formula was developed based on a referral population of patients older than 50 years, it is based on the largest series of temporal arteritis patients in the literature and is likely applicable to patients of similar age in the ED.

Clinical question

What are the diagnostic test characteristics of temporal artery ultrasound for the diagnosis of temporal arteritis?

Although considered generally a safe procedure, temporal artery biopsy has a complication rate of around 0.5%, including infection, hematoma formation, and rare injuries to branches of the facial nerve.[7] It is invasive, and patients often undergo bilateral biopsies of arterial sections several centimeters long. Therefore ultrasound has been investigated as a way to avoid the need for biopsy. A 2005 meta-analysis examined a number of temporal artery ultrasound studies.[8] Patients were classified as having temporal arteritis from either biopsy confirmation or meeting the American College of Rheumatology (ACR) criteria (Table 53.1). The study examined 2,036 patients and found that any ultrasound-specific findings including a halo sign, stenosis, or occlusion of the temporal artery were highly predictive of temporal arteritis regardless of whether the ultimate diagnosis was confirmed using biopsy or the ACR criteria.

Two additional systematic reviews, both published in 2010, have also addressed ultrasound of the temporal arteries to diagnose temporal arteritis. The halo sign, when seen during temporal artery ultrasound, is described as a hypoechoic (dark) ring around the temporal artery wall representing edema and inflammation. Arida et al[9] reviewed prospective studies with

Table 53.3 Temporal artery ultrasound findings for temporal arteritis

Variable	Number of patients	Positive likelihood ratio (LR+)	Negative likelihood ratio (LR−)
Any ultrasound abnormality (halo, sign, stenosis, or occlusion) versus biopsy[8]	332	4 (3.1–5.1)	0.15 (0.06–0.39)
Any ultrasound abnormality (halo, sign, stenosis, or occlusion) versus ACR criteria[8]	853	22 (15–31)	0.14 (0.08–0.23)
Halo sign alone versus ACR criteria[9]	525	7.6 (5.3–11)	0.35 (0.28–0.44)
Halo sign alone versus biopsy[10]	357	4.1 (3.2–6)	0.3 (0.22–0.41)

Source: Data from [8].

patients diagnosed with temporal arteritis using the ACR criteria, and examined the diagnostic test characteristics of the halo sign. Ball et al[10] reviewed studies of patients who had undergone temporal arteritis biopsies and reported on the diagnostic test parameters of the halo sign (Table 53.3). Overall, the halo sign had moderate predictive value to be clinically useful, whether compared to biopsy confirmation or the ACR criteria.

Comments

The diagnosis of temporal arteritis can be elusive and should be considered if a patient older than 50 years complains of any number of symptoms including headache, diplopia or visual loss, scalp tenderness, or jaw claudication. Clinicians should maintain a cautious level of concern given the long-term morbidity of permanent visual loss associated with temporal arteritis. Treatment considerations should be modified on the entirety of the clinicians' suspicion based on the timing of the symptoms and any competing alternative diagnoses.

It should be noted that the studies used to generate the associations noted in this chapter were retrospective in nature, and the reported associations represent findings from a highly selective group of patients: those who actually underwent temporal artery biopsy. This form of verification bias, when only those patients in whom there was a sufficiently high suspicion of the disease underwent the criterion standard procedure, needs to be considered when applying and interpreting the findings to unselected patients in an ED setting. Unfortunately the low prevalence of temporal arteritis in the general population would require any prospective study examining predictive factors to enroll a prohibitive number of patients, many of whom would not ultimately undergo temporal artery biopsy.

While not highly specific, an elevated ESR is highly sensitive (especially in patients not taking steroids) and is associated with useful negative likelihood ratios for ruling out the disease. Therefore as an inexpensive, widely available lab test, it is a reasonable test to obtain. Jaw claudication alone is moderately predictive of temporal arteritis but, when combined with a new headache and scalp tenderness, the combination of all three is appropriate for ruling in the disease and initiating treatment in the ED.

Ample prospective evidence indicates that temporal artery ultrasound may be a reasonable noninvasive alternative to artery biopsy for diagnosing temporal arteritis. However, technical competency will likely be limited to centers that perform high volumes of these specialized ultrasound studies, effectively minimizing its widespread usefulness.

References

1. Gonzalez-Gay MA, Martinez-Dubois C, Agudo M *et al*. Giant cell arteritis: Epidemiology, diagnosis, and management. Current Rheumatology Reports. 2010; 12(6): 436–42.

2. Hunder GG, Bloch DA, Michel BA *et al*. The American College of Rheumatology 1990 criteria for the classification of giant cell arteritis. Arthritis and Rheumatism. 1990; 33(8): 1122–8.

3. Smetana GW, Shmerling RH. Does this patient have temporal arteritis? Journal of the American Medical Association. 2002; 287(1): 92–101.

4. Younge BR, Cook BE Jr, Bartley GB, Hodge DO, Hunder GG. Initiation of glucocorticoid therapy: Before or after temporal artery biopsy? Mayo Clinic Proceeding. 2004; 79(4): 483–91.

5. Lawrence RC, Helmick CG, Arnett FC *et al*. Estimates of the prevalence of arthritis and selected musculoskeletal disorders in the United States. Arthritis and Rheumatism. 1998; 41(5): 778–99.

6. Ciccarelli M, Jeanmonod D, Jeanmonod R. Giant cell temporal arteritis with a normal erythrocyte sedimentation rate: Report of a case. American Journal of Emergency Medicine. 2009; 27(2): 255.e1–3.

7. Ikard RW. Clinical efficacy of temporal artery biopsy in Nashville, Tennessee. Southern Medical Journal. 1988; 81(10): 1222–4.

8. Karassa FB, Matsagas MI, Schmidt WA, Ioannidis JPA. Meta-analysis: Test performance of ultrasonography for giant-cell arteritis. Annals of Internal Medicine. 2005; 142(5): 359–69.

9. Arida A, Kyprianou M, Kanakis M, Sfikakis PP. The diagnostic value of ultrasonography-derived edema of the temporal artery wall in giant cell arteritis: A second meta-analysis. BMC Musculoskeletal Disorders. 2010; 11: 44.

10. Ball EL, Walsh SR, Tang TY, Gohil R, Clarke JMF. Role of ultrasonography in the diagnosis of temporal arteritis. British Journal of Surgery. 2010; 97(12): 1765–71.

Chapter 54 **Intraocular Pressure**

Highlights

- Elevated intraocular pressure (IOP) is associated with glaucoma, the leading cause of blindness and visual impairment worldwide.
- The criterion standard for measuring IOP in most studies is Goldmann applanation tonometry; however, it is not typically available in the ED.
- Portable tonometers are good screening tools for the detection of elevated IOP, but they perform with variable accuracy.

Background

Glaucoma is a leading cause of blindness and visual impairment worldwide, and occurs as a result of increased intraocular pressure, which is typically due to either acute narrowing of the anterior chamber angle (angle closure glaucoma) or progressively decreasing aqueous humor outflow and increasing aqueous humor production (open-angle glaucoma). Patients may seek acute care for symptoms related to elevated intraocular pressure (IOP) that include not only eye pain but also visual impairment, nausea, vomiting, and headache. Measuring IOP is an essential component of the evaluation of patients suspected of having glaucoma (of both the acute closed-angle and open-angle types) as well as blunt eye trauma and iritis. Measurements above 20–22 mmHg are abnormal and should prompt evaluation by an ophthalmologist, either in the acute care setting or through urgent referral.

Different methods of measuring IOP are available and are broadly divided into applanation, indentation, noncontact (air puff), rebound, and transpalpebral techniques. The Goldmann applanation tonometer is mounted on a slit lamp and consists of an applanation prism that comes into contact with the patient's fluorescein-stained cornea using a cobalt-blue light filter, creating lighted semicircles. Correct alignment of the semicircles

---

Evidence-Based Emergency Care: Diagnostic Testing and Clinical Decision Rules, Second Edition.
Jesse M. Pines, Christopher R. Carpenter, Ali S. Raja and Jeremiah D. Schuur.
© 2013 John Wiley & Sons, Ltd. Published 2013 by John Wiley & Sons, Ltd.

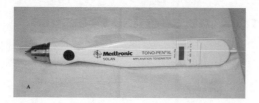

Figure 54.1 The Tono-Pen XL tonometer.

is translated into a pressure reading. The Goldmann applanation method has been accepted as the criterion standard for most studies. The main limitation of the Goldmann tonometer technique is that accurate readings are not possible with cornea irregularities, scarring, or edema. The most common indentation method uses the Tono-Pen (Figure 54.1). This is a handheld device that uses gentle manual indentations of the cornea (Figure 54.2) with the tip of the pen-like instrument to produce electronically averaged readings of IOP. The Tono-Pen is portable and utilizes a disposable rubber tip cover, making it ideal for the acute care setting and rapid sequential uses. The Schiotz tonometer is another common indentation tonometry method that uses a small weighted device to indent the cornea in the supine patient (Figure 54.3). The amount of indentation is measured against a calibrated weight, and the IOP is then determined. Noncontact methods that utilize puffs of air to flatten the cornea, and then measure the IOP by correlating it to the time to corneal flattening, are not typically used in the emergency department (ED). Rebound tonometers, such as the Icare Tonometer (Figure 54.4), bounce a small plastic-tipped metal probe on the cornea and calculate the IOP based on the induction current it creates upon its return through an induction coil. The Icare Tonometer has the advantage

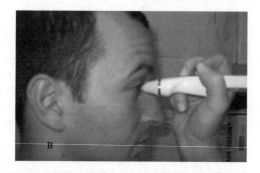

Figure 54.2 Use of the Tono-Pen XL to measure intraocular pressure.

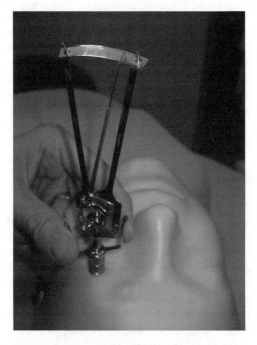

Figure 54.3 Use of the Schiotz tonometer on a supine patient.

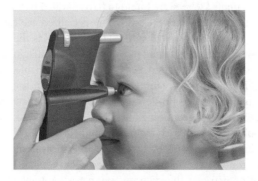

Figure 54.4 Use of the Icare tonometer. (Source: Icare-USA, used with permission).

of not requiring topical anesthetic and has even been trialed as a device that patients can use at home to monitor IOP.[1] Finally, transpalpebral tonometry using the Diaton tonometer allows for IOP measurement through the upper eyelid, eliminating contact with the cornea completely.

While the Goldmann applanation method has been accepted as the criterion standard for most studies, most emergency physicians are not trained in its use. It is bulky, nonportable, expensive, and not widely available in acute care settings. Similarly, noncontact methods using puffs of air are cost prohibitive. These limitations make the search for suitable alternatives to measure IOP in the acute care setting desirable. While indentation devices (including the Schiotz and Tono-Pen) are currently available in most EDs, newer rebound and transpalpebral tonometers are being marketed and are also within the budgetary constraints of most EDs.

Clinical question

Are IOP measurements using the Schiotz tonometer, Tono-Pen, Icare Tonometer, and Diaton Tonometer reliable and accurate compared to IOP measurements using the criterion standard, Goldmann applanation tonometry?

Several small studies have compared IOP measurements using Goldmann tonometry against a Schiotz, the Tono-Pen, or both. Jackson and colleagues in Australia performed and analyzed serial IOP measurements using the Tono-Pen and the Schiotz in 72 patients.[2] Patients were recruited from a general practice, were >50 years old, and had no prior history of glaucoma. IOP was first assessed using a Goldmann tonometer by an ophthalmologist, followed by measurement by the Schiotz and the Tono-Pen. An independent observer recorded the pressure reading, and the physicians were blinded to the results. A total of 19 patients (26%) were found to have elevated IOP ($\geq$21 mmHg), of which 18 followed up after the study for specialized eye care. Only five of these had persistently elevated IOPs. The Schiotz was the most reliable with 64–76% of IOP values falling to within +/− 4 mmHg of the criterion standard measured IOP. The Tono-Pen was extremely variable, with 10–95% of values falling within +/− 4 mmHg of the Goldmann tonometer. Most measurements using the Tono-Pen tended to underestimate the pressure. This study utilized three examining physicians, and there was measurement variation by physician with each method examined.

A small study out of Missouri examined IOP measurements with several portable tonometers, including the Tono-Pen and the Schiotz, with Goldmann tonometry as the criterion standard.[3] A total of 31 patients (58 eyes) from a glaucoma clinic were enrolled and analyzed in the study. Methods of obtaining IOP were standardized, and the orders of examinations were randomized following initial IOP measurements by Goldmann tonometry. Physicians were not blinded to the individual results from each method. Results are shown in Table 54.1. Both Tono-Pen and Schiotz tonometers underestimated IOP by 2–3 mmHg compared to the Goldmann tonometer.

Table 54.1 Results of IOP measurement (n = 58 eyes)

Tonometer	Mean intraocular pressure (mm Hg)	95% CI range (mm Hg)	Standard error	Mean difference from Goldmann (mm Hg)
Goldmann	18.2	Data not shown	0.8	–
Tono-Pen	15.8	7.7	0.6	2.5*
Schiotz	15.3	9.7	0.8	2.9*

*P<0.05.
Source: Data from [3].

In another small Australian study, researchers compared IOP measurements with the Tono-Pen and the Goldmann to determine if measurements were similar (to within 2 mmHg).[4] One hundred and thirty-eight patients were recruited from a glaucoma clinic; 22 more patients were enrolled who had known elevated IOPs. Among the 138 patients, IOPs ranged from 3 to 47. Reproducibility of the results was excellent, as reflected in an intraclass correlation coefficient (ICC) of 0.97 for the Goldmann tonometer and 0.95 with the Tono-Pen. Analysis of paired IOP readings revealed no statistical differences between methods (mean difference Tono-Pen – Goldmann: right eyes = −0.4 mmHg, CI −6 to 5 mmHg; left eyes = −0.3 mmHg, CI −5 to 5 mmHg). Looking at three pressure ranges (0–10, 11–20, and 20–30) revealed divergence of agreement at the high pressures. Results of IOP measurements among the 22 patients with known elevated pressures (range 24–58) revealed a significant difference between methods (mean difference −4.2 mmHg, CI −13.0 to 5.0 mmHg), with the Tono-Pen consistently yielding lower values. These researchers concluded that while Tono-Pen measurements are reproducible, the accuracy at higher IOPs may be underestimated.

British researchers compared IOP measurements using both Goldman tonometry and the Tono-Pen in 105 patients from primary eye and glaucoma clinics with standardized methods across all clinics.[5] Mean IOP with the Tono-Pen was 0.6 mmHg lower than the Goldmann measurements, and these differences did not vary depending on ranges of pressures (Table 54.2).

Table 54.2 Comparisons of IOP measurements using Goldmann and Tono-Pen tonometry

Tonometer (n = 105)	Mean intraocular pressure (mm Hg)	Range (mm Hg)	Standard deviation	Mean difference from Goldmann (mm Hg)
Goldmann	17.2	9–32	4.3	–
Tono-Pen	16.6	7–29	4.4	0.6*

*P = 0.3.
Source: Data from [5].

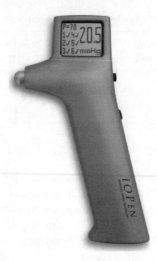

Figure 54.5 The IOPen tonometer. (Source: Medicel AG, used with permission).

Rebound tonometers, such as the Icare and IOPen (Figure 54.5) tonometers, have been garnering more interest given the fact that they can be used without topical anesthetic. In a study comparing the Icare, IOPen, and Goldman tonometers, Jorge et al studied the right eyes of 101 consecutive adult patients with good general and ocular health.[6] The measurements for each device were taken by the same investigator for all patients in order to minimize variation, and the devices were used in random order. The mean (and standard deviation) of the Goldmann applanation tonometer was 15.7 mmHg (4.1), the IOPen was 12.8 mmHg (3.7), and the Icare was 16.0 mmHg (4.6). When compared to the Goldmann IOP measurements, the IOPen measurements were consistently (and significantly) lower, while the Icare measurements were not statistically different (Table 54.3).

Table 54.3 Comparisons of IOP measurements using IOPen and Icare tonometers

Comparison (n = 101)	Mean difference (mm Hg)	Standard deviation	p-value using Wilcoxon signed rank test
IOPen-Goldmann	−2.94	4.65	<0.001
Icare -Goldman	0.27	3.16	0.310

Note: IOP = intraocular pressure.
Source: Data from [6].

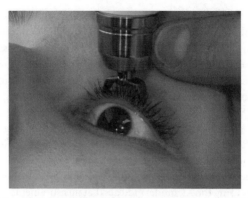

Figure 54.6 The Diaton transpalpebral tonometer. (Source: BiCOM Inc., used with permission).

Similar results were found by Pakrou et al who compared Icare and Goldmann tonometry in 292 eyes of 153 subjects.[7] They found significant agreement between the two methods (intraclass correlation r = 0.95) with mean differences between the two devices of 0.4 mmHg in the right eyes and 0.8 mmHg in the left eyes. Despite the fact that no topical anesthesia was used for the Icare, 74% of patients rated it as more comfortable than the Goldmann applanation tonometer.

Transpalpebral tonometry is the newest non-invasive method for measuring IOP, and the Diaton tonometer is the first commercially available tonometer applying the technique (Figure 54.6). Li et al studied the accuracy of the Diaton tonometer when compared to the Goldmann tonometer in 129 patients.[8] They found that the Diaton results correlated moderately with the Goldmann (criterion standard) results (r = 0.78) and were most closely correlated in patients between the ages of 20 and 50 years (mean difference 0.53 +/− 3.4 mmHg). However, overall, only 76% of patients had less than 3 mmHg difference between the two readings, leading the investigators to conclude that the Diaton is not yet ready for use in routine clinical practice given the significant proportion of patients with wider variation in IOP as measured by both devices.

Comments

The clinical question of concern is whether portable, smaller, and more widely available instruments can be used to reliably and accurately measure IOP. These studies confirm that the reliability of the Tono-Pen is sound. That is, the results are reproducible across different users with acceptable minimal differences in the absolute pressure measurements. While the data are not overwhelmingly convincing with regard to the reliability of the Schiotz and Icare, it is our opinion that they are likely no worse than for the Tono-Pen.

The issue of accuracy is a more technical concern and appears to vary across studies. One study presented measured agreement to within 4 mmHg of the criterion standard, while another study used a 2 mmHg difference as meaningful. Deciding on what constitutes a clinically significant difference from the criterion standard is always a concern. A 2 mmHg difference is seemingly negligible, but a 4 or 5 mmHg difference could significantly affect both the immediate and near-future treatment of a patient. While some early studies of the original Tono-Pen found variable pressure readings, more recent studies using the XL model indicate that measurements are reasonably accurate and do not differ significantly from the Goldmann tonometry measurements. Similar to the discussion of reliability, the accuracy of the Schiotz is not thought to differ greatly from that of the Tono-Pen. While there are fewer studies available for the newer Icare rebound tonometer, it appears to be at least as reliable as the Tono-Pen, while the newest device, the Diaton tonometer, is currently too inaccurate to use in clinical practice.

The Tono-Pen, the Schiotz, or the Icare can serve as screening tools for patients suspected of having abnormal IOPs. Patients should be treated according to the timing, severity, and history of their symptoms in conjunction with the measured IOP values. However, the diagnosis of ocular hypertension or glaucoma should not be excluded solely based on the IOP readings obtained in the ED. An emergent ophthalmology consult should be obtained when there is both sufficient concern by the treating physician and elevated IOP measurements. Borderline or normal IOP measurements should be referred for urgent eye evaluation by a specialist.

References

1. Asrani S, Chatterjee A, Wallace DK, Santiago-Turla C, Stinnett S. Evaluation of the ICare rebound tonometer as a home intraocular pressure monitoring device. Journal of Glaucoma. 2011; 20(2): 74–9.
2. Jackson C, Bullock J, Pitt M et al. Screening for glaucoma in a Brisbane general practice: The role of tonometry. Australian and New Zealand Journal of Ophthalmology. 1995; 23(3): 173–8.
3. Wingert TA, Bassi CJ, McAlister WH, Galanis JC. Clinical evaluation of five portable tonometers. Journal of the American Optometric Association. 1995; 66(11): 670–4.
4. Horowitz GS, Byles J, Lee J, D'Este C. Comparison of the Tono-Pen and Goldmann tonometer for measuring intraocular pressure in patients with glaucoma. Clinical and Experimental Ophthalmology. 2004; 32(6): 584–9.

5. Tonnu P-A, Ho T, Sharma K *et al*. A comparison of four methods of tonometry: Method agreement and interobserver variability. British Journal of Ophthalmology. 2005; 89(7): 847–50.

6. Jorge J, Fernandes P, Queirós A *et al*. Comparison of the IOPen and iCare rebound tonometers with the Goldmann tonometer in a normal population. Ophthalmic and Physiological Optics. 2010; 30(1): 108–12.

7. Pakrou N, Gray T, Mills R, Landers J, Craig J. Clinical comparison of the Icare tonometer and Goldmann applanation tonometry. Journal of Glaucoma. 2008; 17(1): 43–7.

8. Li Y, Shi J, Duan X, Fan F. Transpalpebral measurement of intraocular pressure using the Diaton tonometer versus standard Goldmann applanation tonometry. Graefe's Archive for Clinical and Experimental Ophthalmology. 2010; 248: 1765–70.

Chapter 55 **Asthma**

> **Highlights**
>
> - Asthma is common and is responsible for many ED visits and hospitalizations every year.
> - Hospitalization rates are high for all asthmatics, and relapse following ED visits is frequent among both adults ($\sim$15%) and children ($\sim$10%).
> - Assessment of global function and specific clinical factors is reliable between different providers caring for asthmatics in the ED.
> - Numerous asthma scoring systems have been developed, but few have been rigorously validated and replicated.
> - The Pediatric Assessment Severity Score (PASS) and the Pediatric Respiratory Assessment Measure (PRAM) both distinguish between patients requiring admission and those stable for discharge, but their practical application has not been demonstrated.
> - No uniform set of variables reliably predicts the need for hospitalization or the risk of treatment relapse in adult asthmatics.

Background

Asthma is a chronic disease affecting over 16 million adults and 5 million children in the United States alone, with nearly 20% requiring hospitalization annually. Worldwide estimates place the number of asthmatics at over 300 million.[1] Efforts to improve outpatient care for this disease have been promoted through the development of treatment guidelines, but many patients remain either undertreated or undiagnosed. Visits for asthma exacerbations comprise approximately 1.5% of US emergency department (ED) visits[2] and, while standard ED asthma management is straightforward (including bronchodilators, steroids, and occasionally adjunctive treatments including magnesium), a certain percentage of refractory asthmatics will

Evidence-Based Emergency Care: Diagnostic Testing and Clinical Decision Rules, Second Edition. Jesse M. Pines, Christopher R. Carpenter, Ali S. Raja and Jeremiah D. Schuur. © 2013 John Wiley & Sons, Ltd. Published 2013 by John Wiley & Sons, Ltd.

require hospitalization and monitoring. Since this decision is often the crux of the ED evaluation of a patient with asthma, a number of studies have sought to classify asthma severity and predict which patients will require hospitalization and which, if discharged, will relapse.

Clinical question

Are there scoring systems for ED patients that accurately and reliably predict asthma severity, the need for hospitalization, or relapses after treatment?
Distinct pediatric and adult acute asthma short-term outcome predictors and severity assessment scores exist. Therefore, this section presents pediatric and adult instruments separately.

Reproducibility of the clinical exam

In 2003 Stevens et al examined the interrater reliability of physical exam findings in children with asthma in order to address the concern that findings from clinical trials may not represent actual clinical practice because specially trained staff are usually involved in the research setting.[3] Reproducibility of key physical findings and an overall global gestalt about the severity of a patient's condition by different people across different levels of training is the first step in establishing that any scoring system can be successfully developed and used clinically. The observers in this study included pediatric emergency physicians ($n = 20$), pediatric ED nurses ($n = 50$), and hospital respiratory therapists ($n = 50$). The observers received no prior specialized training on physical exam assessment for the study. Patients aged 1–16 years from a large urban children's hospital presenting with acute asthma were the examination subjects. Observers independently and simultaneously rated the following aspects on a standardized form on a scale of one to three or four: work of breathing, wheezing, decreased air entry, increased expiratory time, breathlessness, mental status, and respiratory rate. A global assessment of "overall" severity (options included asymptomatic, mild, moderate, and severe) was also presented, as was a composite total score.

Weighted kappa statistics for each component of the score (used to determine interrater reliability) for 230 pairs of exams ranged from 0.61 to 0.74, while the overall severity (weighted kappa 0.80) and total scores (weighted kappa 0.82) had excellent agreement. Paired observers who were practitioners of the same profession (physicians, nurses, or respiratory therapists) had slightly better interrater reliability for the elements assessed. The authors felt this supported the use of structured and standardized formats to assess pediatric asthmatic patients. More reassuring was that, among a diverse group of care providers, a high level of agreement was found in the clinical assessment of acute asthmatics.

Severity scores in asthmatic children

Numerous pediatric asthma scores have been developed to assess asthma, including discriminative scores (designed to gauge severity at a single point in time), predictive scores (aimed at predicting particular outcomes), and evaluative scores (allowing documentation of changes over time). Unfortunately, many were developed using small numbers of select subjects, impacting the generalizability of the results. Of the 16 pediatric asthma scores as of 1994, 11 had sample sizes of <100 study subjects, and only one had >300 study subjects.[4] More concerning and critical is that most were not (and have not been) thoroughly evaluated; none have been validated or assessed in terms of their impact on clinical behavior.[5]

In 2004 Gorelick et al published a new pediatric asthma score, the Pediatric Assessment Severity Score (PASS), that was developed and vigorously validated on a large diverse pediatric asthma population, with no exclusions based on severity or disposition (home or admission).[6] The PASS was validated and tested for reliability and responsiveness on a group of 1,221 pediatric asthmatics in two EDs with an enrollment rate of 89% (out of 1,379 eligible patients). Forty-one percent (n = 503) were admitted to an inpatient service. Clinical items examined during the study for inclusion in the final score had been included in prior clinical asthma scores and were acceptable to and pertinent by the clinicians at the study sites. The final three-item score included an assessment of wheezing (none or mild, moderate, or severe or absent due to poor air exchange), work of breathing (none or mild, moderate, or severe), and prolongation of expiration (normal or mildly prolonged, moderately prolonged, or severely prolonged). Items assessed but not included in the final score included air entry, tachypnea, and mental status.

The three-item PASS score discriminated admitted versus discharged patients with a high level of confidence: area under the curve (AUC) for the receiver operator characteristic (ROC) curves for each of the two EDs was 0.83% (CI 0.80–0.86%) and 0.85% (CI 0.81–0.89%). The new score also was responsive to changes (e.g., improvements) on serial assessment; scores improved by 51–79% among those discharged home, whereas in those asthmatics admitted for inpatient care the scores improved only 25–32%. By comparison, the peak expiratory flow rate (PEFR) also improved by 25–32%, but the change was similar between admitted and discharged patients.

In 2008 Ducharme et al assessed whether their previously published Preschool Respiratory Assessment Measure (which had been developed and internally validated in children aged 3–6 years)[7] could be expanded as the *Pediatric* Respiratory Assessment Measure (PRAM).[8] They examined the validity, responsiveness, and reliability of PRAM in children from 2 to 17 years old, and found that it had predictive validity in that higher values of PRAM were associated with higher rates of admission, both at triage and after initial bronchodilation. PRAM was also responsive to change, as demonstrated by a Guyatt responsiveness coefficient of 0.7 (used to detect the ability of an evaluative instrument to detect change over time; 0.5 and 0.8 are considered moderate to large effect sizes, respectively), which was calculated by determining the ratio of the change in PRAM after initial bronchodilation among discharged patients to the standard deviation of the change in PRAM of the patients who were admitted. Last, the overall score was found to have high interrater reliability when assessed by a physician and a nurse ($\kappa = 0.78$) for 254 children aged 2–17 years. PRAM, which contains more components than PASS, measures scalene muscle contraction, suprasternal retractions, wheezing, air entry, and oxygen saturation.

When Gouin et al performed a prospective external validation of both PRAM and PASS on 283 patients in 2010, they found that both scores had good initial discriminative ability.[9] The scores were measured at triage and again after 90 minutes. Their initial performance as predictors of a length of stay of greater than 6 hours and/or admission was equal (PRAM AUC = 0.69 (0.59–0.79) and PASS AUC = 0.70 (0.60–0.80)) but, at 90 minutes, PRAM improved (AUC = 0.82 (0.73–0.90)) while PASS remained steady (AUC = 0.72 (0.62–0.82)). Nevertheless, given that this is the only external comparison of both scores, PASS remains a valid prognostic screening instrument.

Predicting hospitalization in asthmatic children

A large prospective multicenter study by the Multicenter Airway Research Collaboration (MARC) investigators examined risk factors and predictors of hospital admission among children aged 2–17 years seen in 44 EDs from 1997 to 1998.[10] Enrolling sites were from 37 general hospitals and seven children's hospitals across 18 US states and four Canadian provinces. Prospective enrollment occurred 24 hours per day over a median of 2 weeks. Repeat ED visits and patients discharged from the ED against medical advice were excluded.

A total of 1,601 eligible children presenting to EDs with acute asthma were identified, and 1,178 patients were included in the analysis (74%). The admission rate was 23% (CI 21–26%) with an interquartile range of 11–31% across the 44 EDs. Multivariate logistic regression modeling produced patient variables that were independently predictive of hospital admission (Table 55.1). PEFR was not included in the logistic regression model because it could be measured in only 23% of children. However, in those 23% with PEFR measurements, admitted children had lower initial PEFRs compared to non-admitted children (percentage predicted 36% versus 50%, mean difference: 14%). Demographic factors were not predictive of admission.

Table 55.1 Independent predictors of hospital admission in children with asthma from multivariate logistic regression

	Odds ratio	Confidence interval (CI)
Oxygen saturation (per decrease of 5%)	2.2	1.6–3.0
Number of inhaled beta-agonist during ED stay	2.1	1.8–2.4
Prior admission for asthma within past year	1.7	1.1–2.8
Pulmonary Index Score	1.3	1.1–1.4
Not taking corticosteroids at time of emergency department visit	0.3	0.2–0.6
No comorbidities	0.3	0.1–0.7

Source: Data from [10].

The MARC investigators also examined the initial room air oxygen saturation reading to determine if, as a single variable, it could predict hospital admission in asthmatic children.[11] The study differed from prior studies in both the number of enrolled patients and the multicenter study design, strengthening its generalizability. Initial oxygen saturation was documented for 1,040 children with a mean reading of 95%, and the ROC curve predicting hospitalization in the study cohort had an AUC value of 0.76, demonstrating only moderate discriminatory ability, from which we can conclude that initial oxygen saturation is not useful as a single predictor variable for admission.

Treatment relapses in asthmatic children

Another large prospective multicenter study by the MARC investigators examined risk factors and predictors of treatment relapses among children aged 2–17 years seen in 44 EDs.[12] Enrolling sites included 37 general hospitals and seven children's hospitals. Only patients discharged from the ED were included. Again, prospective enrollment and data collection occurred 24 hours per day over a median of 2 weeks. Telephone follow-up was 2 weeks after patient discharge to establish relapses. *Relapse* was defined as any urgent visit to an ED for asthma that was unscheduled in the 2 weeks following initial ED discharge.

A total of 1,184 patients were enrolled with 303 excluded because they were hospitalized or had severe comorbid conditions. A total of 762 of the remaining 881 (86%) patients had complete follow-up and were included in the analysis. Relapse occurred in 10% (CI 8–13%) of children. There was no difference in relapse rates between general and children's hospitals (12% vs. 10%). The four factors independently associated with relapse after multivariate analysis are shown in Table 55.2. The number of ED visits and

Table 55.2 Independent predictors of treatment relapse in children with asthma from multivariate logistic regression

	Odds ratio	Confidence interval (CI)
Asthma medication other than beta-agonists, steroids, cromolyn, or nedocromil	3.7	2.2–6.3
Age (for every 5-year increase)	1.4	1.0–1.8
Asthma-related emergency department visits in past year (per 5 visits)	1.2	1.0–1.5
Cigarette smoke exposure	0.5	0.3–0.9

Source: Data from [12].

cigarette smoke exposure variables were no longer significant in a separate analysis looking only at relapses occurring within 3 days after ED discharge. There were no differences between relapse and no-relapse patients during the initial ED visit with regard to symptom duration, treatment duration, treatment medications, or steroid prescription for home use.

Predicting hospitalization in asthmatics (children and adults)

Australian researchers asked whether a determination of asthma severity after 1 hour of treatment in the ED is a better predictor of need for admission compared to the initial assessment of asthma severity at ED presentation.[13] This observational cohort analyzed 720 patients presenting to 36 Australian EDs during a 2-week period in 2001. Initial, 1-hour, and postdisposition severity assessments were evaluated. Clinical assessments of adult and pediatric patients followed the National Asthma Guidelines endorsed by the Australian National Asthma Campaign. Assessment had ratings of mild, moderate, and severe or life-threatening (with response meanings for each category) and included the following items: altered consciousness, physical exhaustion, talkativeness, pulsus paradoxus, central cyanosis, wheezing intensity, peak expiratory flow (PEF), FEV_1 (percentage predicted), pulse oximetry on presentation, and need for admission.

Adults comprised 44% of the study cohort, and overall 32% of adult patients required hospital admission. Among patients assessed as having mild asthma either at initial presentation or after 1 hour, over 80% were discharged home. Similarly, over 85% classified as severe at either assessment were admitted. A moderate rating at initial presentation was a poor predictor of need for hospitalization. However, a moderate rating at the 1-hour assessment predicted 84% of individuals who needed admission. The authors concluded that response to therapies after 1 hour for patients presenting to

EDs for acute asthma is better than initial severity assessments for predicting hospital admissions.

Predicting hospitalization in asthmatic adults

Investigators used data collected from four prospective cohorts recruited from 64 US and Canadian EDs with 2-week telephone follow-ups in another MARC study that examined patient characteristics associated with hospitalization for acute asthma.[14] The admission rate among the 1,805 patients enrolled with complete data was 20% (CI 18–22%). Table 55.3 lists variables that are independently associated with hospitalization. The multivariate model had an AUC value of 0.91, indicating excellent discrimination; however, no external validation of this model has been performed.

Researchers in 88 EDs across the US and Canada collected data during a median 2 weeks from 1999 to 2002 as part of the MARC research alliance to study acute asthma. In an analysis of older versus younger adults presenting with acute asthma, the investigators sought to examine differences in asthma severity, treatments, and outcomes.[15] Ages were divided into three groups: 18–34, 35–54, and ≥55 years old. Patients reporting a history of chronic obstructive pulmonary disease (chronic bronchitis or emphysema) or who had a smoking history of >10 pack-years were excluded. Patient follow-ups were made by telephone interview 2 weeks after the ED visit.

The study enrolled 2,064 patients (84% of those eligible), of whom 56% were in the youngest age category and 6% were in the oldest age category. Overall 348 patients (17%) required hospital admission. Significantly higher

Table 55.3 Independent predictors of hospitalization in adults with asthma from multivariate logistic regression

	Odds ratio	Confidence interval (CI)
Use of home nebulizers*	2.7	1.6–4.5
Final peak flow (per decrease of 10% predicted)	2.6	2.2–3.1
Female sex	2.1	1.3–3.6
Asthma medications other than beta-agonists or inhaled corticosteroids*	1.9	1.2–3.0
Beta-agonist treatment in the emergency department	1.4	1.3–1.6
Initial peak flow (per increase of 10% predicted)	1.4	1.2–1.7
Initial respiratory rate (per 5 breaths)	1.3	1.1–1.7

*During the past 4 weeks.
Source: Data from [14].

Table 55.4 Independent predictors of hospitalization in adult asthmatics from multivariate logistic regression

	Odds ratio (CI) of need for hospitalization		
	Age 18–35*	Age 35–54	Age ≥ 55
Model** excluding peak expiratory flow (PEF) change	1.0	1.2 (0.8–1.7)	2.0 (1.2–3.4)
Model** including PEF change	1.0	1.2 (0.8–2.0)	0.9 (0.4–2.1)

*Reference category.
**Model included variables shown in Table 55.3.
Source: Data from [15].

admission rates occurred with increasing age categories (13% in the youngest age group, 19% in the middle, and 38% in the oldest). Seriousness of the acute asthma condition at the time of ED presentation based on initial PEF (percentage predicted) was severe for all groups (median 47%). Multivariate modeling revealed that patients aged ≥55 responded the poorest to bronchodilator treatments after controlling for demographic and severity factors. In a logistic regression model that excluded change in PEF, increasing age was an independent predictor of hospital admission. However, age did not predict admission when change in PEF was included in the model (Table 55.4).

Two-week follow-up was available for 64% of all patients. Patients aged ≥55 were hospitalized longer (median stay 2, 3, and 4 days for each progressively older age group) and were more likely to have relapses in the 2 weeks following the initial ED visit (12%, 19%, and 25% for each progressively older age group).

Most recently, Tsai et al used data from the National Emergency Department Safety Study (NEDSS) and MARC to derive and validate a classification tree designed to risk-stratify patients into groups based on likelihood of admission.[16] They used the NEDSS dataset, which included 1,825 patients aged 14–54 years from 63 US EDs for whom eight variables were collected: demographics (age and sex), chronic asthma-related factors (ever hospitalized for asthma), and ED presentation and severity (duration of symptoms, initial oxygen saturation on room air, initial respiratory rate, initial PEF severity, and change in PEF severity). Using recursive partitioning, the authors derived a decision tree based on four clinical variables: change (C) in PEF severity category, any prior hospitalization (H) for asthma, oxygen (O) saturation on room air, and initial PEF (P). This tree was then validated in a validation cohort of 1,335 MARC patients aged 18–54 from 36 EDs across the United States.

The resultant decision tree categorized patients with asthma into seven risk groups based on the four variables noted in this section. Among the seven groups, there was a significant increase in admission risk, from 9% to 48% (p<0.001), between the lowest risk group and the highest risk group, and the tree had satisfactory discriminatory ability, with an AUC of 0.72 in the derivation cohort and 0.65 in the validation cohort. While both these AUCs as well as the fact that no acceptable risk threshold for discharge of asthmatics exists (given the lack of a consensus definition of acceptable risk in this population) currently preclude application of these authors' tree, the methodology used is sound and its application to large datasets of asthmatics is likely to lead to more useful risk stratification tools in the future.

Treatment relapses in asthmatic adults

Using the MARC investigator data collected between 1996 and 1997, Emerman et al examined factors associated with relapses among adult asthmatics following treatment for acute asthma among 641 patients.[17] A total of 17% reported relapse during the 2 weeks following the initial ED visit. Initial, final, and change in PEFR were not different between patients who did and did not relapse. Multivariate logistic regression modeling found that duration of symptoms lasting from 1 to 7 days (OR 2.5, CI 1.2–5.2), use of home nebulizers (OR 2.2, CI 1.5–3.9), multiple urgent care visits for asthma (OR 1.4, CI 1.5–3.9), and multiple ED visits for asthma (OR 1.3, CI 1.5–1.5) were all independent predictors associated with relapse after controlling for age, sex, race, primary care provider status, and number of reported asthma triggers.

Comments

Asthma is a highly-prevalent disease that is responsible for many ED visits and hospitalizations. A number of asthma scoring systems have been developed, primarily for children however, few have been vigorously derived and validated, and none have gained widespread acceptance. While the clinical assessment of acute asthma severity is reproducible, no particular scoring system is more accurate than any other. The PASS and PRAM scores appear to meet the basic criteria for a successful scoring tool: (i) sound derivation and validation on a broad group of unselected study subjects, (ii) using a limited number of clinically relevant items, and (iii) shown to be discriminative and responsive. However, there is not yet a similar tool for use in adult patients, which begs the question: is a separate tool necessary?

Studies have examined sets of predictors of particular outcomes: discharge, hospitalization, and treatment relapse. In children, no set of demographic variables reliably predicts hospital admission. Historical and clinical factors found to be predictive of hospitalization include low initial oxygen saturation, extent of beta-agonist use in the ED (i.e., total number of nebulizer treatments given), prior admissions for asthma in the prior year, and the absence of comorbidities or steroid use at the time of ED visit. Assessment of the need for hospitalization after 1 hour of treatment in the ED appears to be a better predictor of hospitalization compared with the initial assessment because some patients will improve rapidly. For patients treated and discharged, treatment relapse remains high ($\geq$10% in children) and increases with use of asthma medication other than routine medications, as well as annual number of asthma-related ED visits. Among adult asthmatics, several variables appear to predict hospitalization, but none are consistent across studies. Similarly, relapse after treatment in adult asthmatics (>16% in adults) is associated with duration of symptoms, self-treatment at home, and extent of prior urgent care and ED visits related to asthma.

Overall, no uniform set of predictor variables reliably inform the need for hospitalization or risk of treatment relapse. Some variables such as prior admissions, extent of pharmacologic treatment prior to the ED visit, and evaluation after a period of treatment in the ED are intuitive elements that should influence decisions to admit or discharge a patient. The largest and most diverse collection of studies examining acute asthmatics, from the MARC investigators, as well as the promising development of the PASS add breadth and depth to the discussion, yet further studies are certainly warranted. Perhaps sets of factors within subgroups of adult asthmatics can be identified that will be predictive as well as responsive indicators for clinical use, much in the same way that pediatric scores have developed separately from adult predictors. Finally, improvements in therapy will necessitate refinements in any prediction tool. We should continue to base patient disposition on the clinical assessment after a short period of intense treatment in the ED. However, additional elements warrant consideration, including issues surrounding access to care, access to appropriate medications, health literacy, and environmental factors, few of which have been incorporated into the clinical studies performed to date.

References

1. Masoli M, Fabian D, Holt S, Beasley R. The global burden of asthma: Executive summary of the GINA Dissemination Committee report. Allergy. 2004; 59(5): 469–78.
2. Pitts SR, Niska RW, Xu J, Burt CW. National Hospital Ambulatory Medical Care Survey: 2006 emergency department summary. National Health Statistics Reports. 2008; (7): 1–38.
3. Stevens MW, Gorelick MH, Schultz T. Interrater agreement in the clinical evaluation of acute pediatric asthma. Journal of Asthma. 2003; 40(3): 311–15.

4. van der Windt DA, Nagelkerke AF, Bouter LM, Dankert-Roelse JE, Veerman AJ. Clinical scores for acute asthma in pre-school children: A review of the literature. Journal of Clinical Epidemiology. 1994; 47(6): 635–46.

5. McGinn TG, Guyatt GH, Wyer PC *et al*. Users'guides to the medical literature. Journal of the American Medical Association. 2000; 284(1): 79–84.

6. Gorelick MH, Stevens MW, Schultz TR, Scribano PV. Performance of a novel clinical score, the Pediatric Asthma Severity Score (PASS), in the evaluation of acute asthma. Academic Emergency Medicine. 2004; 11(1): 10–18.

7. Chalut DS, Ducharme FM, Davis GM. The Preschool Respiratory Assessment Measure (PRAM): A responsive index of acute asthma severity. Journal of Pediatrics. 2000; 137(6): 762–8.

8. Ducharme FM, Chalut D, Plotnick L *et al*. The Pediatric Respiratory Assessment Measure: A valid clinical score for assessing acute asthma severity from toddlers to teenagers. Journal of Pediatrics. 2008; 152(4): 476–80, 480.e1.

9. Gouin S, Robidas I, Gravel J *et al*. Prospective evaluation of two clinical scores for acute asthma in children 18 months to 7 years of age. Academic Emergency Medicine. 2010; 17(6): 598–603.

10. Pollack CV, Pollack ES, Baren JM *et al*. A prospective multicenter study of patient factors associated with hospital admission from the emergency department among children with acute asthma. Archives of Pediatrics and Adolescent Medicine. 2002; 156(9): 934–40.

11. Keahey L, Bulloch B, Becker AB *et al*. Initial oxygen saturation as a predictor of admission in children presenting to the emergency department with acute asthma. Annals ofEmergency Medicine. 2002; 40(3): 300–7.

12. Emerman CL, Cydulka RK, Crain EF *et al*. Prospective multicenter study of relapse after treatment for acute asthma among children presenting to the emergency department. Journal of Pediatrics. 2001; 138(3): 318–24.

13. Kelly A-M, Kerr D, Powell C. Is severity assessment after one hour of treatment better for predicting the need for admission in acute asthma? Respiratory Medicine. 2004; 98(8): 777–81.

14. Weber EJ, Silverman RA, Callaham ML *et al*. A prospective multicenter study of factors associated with hospital admission among adults with acute asthma. American Journal of Medicine. 2002; 113(5): 371–8.

15. Banerji A, Clark S, Afilalo M *et al*. Prospective multicenter study of acute asthma in younger versus older adults presenting to the emergency department. Journal of American Geriatric Society. 2006; 54(1): 48–55.

16. Tsai C-L, Clark S, Camargo CA Jr. Risk stratification for hospitalization in acute asthma: The CHOP classification tree. American Journal of Emergency Medicine. 2010; 28(7): 803–8.

17. Emerman CL, Woodruff PG, Cydulka RK *et al*. Prospective multicenter study of relapse following treatment for acute asthma among adults presenting to the emergency department. MARC investigators, Multicenter Asthma Research Collaboration. Chest. 1999; 115(4): 919–27.

Chapter 56 **Nontraumatic Back Pain**

Highlights

- Back pain is the leading musculoskeletal complaint in ED patients, but it is usually self-limited.
- The initial diagnostic approach to acute back pain should assess the risk for serious systemic disease to guide subsequent imaging decisions.
- Systemic diseases presenting with back pain include aortic aneurysm, cancer, spinal infections, compression fractures, and ankylosing spondylitis.
- In isolation, most elements of history and physical exam are insufficient to rule in or rule out systemic disease etiologies of back pain.

Background

The lifetime incidence of back pain is 90%, and it accounted for over 2 million emergency department (ED) visits in 2007.[1,2] Fortunately, only 14% of acute back pain episodes last more than 2 weeks. Low back pain may originate from the lumbar spine, vertebral ligaments, annulus fibrosus, vertebral periosteum, facet joints, paravertebral musculature, blood vessels, or spinal nerve roots. In addition, low back pain may be a presenting symptom for many systemic disease processes (Table 56.1). Clinicians should seek to answer three key questions in the evaluation of acute back pain:[3]

1. Is a serious systemic disease causing the pain?
2. Is there neurological compromise that might require surgical evaluation?
3. Do social or psychological situations exist that could amplify or prolong pain?

Systemic diseases can include vascular disease, cancer, spinal infections, compression fractures, and ankylosing spondylitis. A thorough history is superior to extensive ancillary diagnostic testing to identify these disease processes. For example, abdominal aortic aneurysm is typically found in

---

Evidence-Based Emergency Care: Diagnostic Testing and Clinical Decision Rules, Second Edition.
Jesse M. Pines, Christopher R. Carpenter, Ali S. Raja and Jeremiah D. Schuur.
© 2013 John Wiley & Sons, Ltd. Published 2013 by John Wiley & Sons, Ltd.

Table 56.1 Differential diagnoses of acute back pain

Abdominal aortic aneurysm
Ankylosing spondylosis
Compression fracture
Discitis (or spinal osteomyelitis)
Enteropathic
Epidural abscess
Herniated disc
Malignancy
Musculoskeletal
Occult trauma
Pancreatitis
Pyelonephritis
Reactive or psoriatic spondyloarthritis
Spinal stenosis

patients who are older than 60 years, have atherosclerosis, and experience pain at rest.[4] Cauda equina syndrome is often the result of a massive midline herniated disc, most commonly in the L4–5, L5–S1, or L3–4 disc space.[5] The recognition of cauda equina is most often delayed because the diagnosis was not considered.[6,7] Ankylosing spondylitis typically presents with symptom onset before age 40 years with gradual onset, night pain, morning stiffness, and improvement with exercise.[8] Epidural abscesses progress from back pain with fever, to spinal irritation with Lasegue's, Kernig's, and Lhermitte's signs with neck stiffness and sometimes radiation to the arms or legs, to motor-sensory deficits and ultimately paralysis.[9] It is essential that clinicians recognize that the duration of each phase is highly variable and may be extremely short. Risk factors for epidural abscess include intravenous drug abuse, alcohol abuse, obesity, distal bacterial infections, trauma, and invasive procedures.[9–11] ED diagnostic delays in epidural abscesses have occurred in 83.6% of cases, but implementation of a guideline to systematically assess signs and symptoms, erythrocyte sedimentation rate (ESR) and C-reactive protein (CRP), and then MRI reduced delays to 9.7%.[12] The prevalence of these systemic diseases has not been defined in ED populations. By contrast, in primary care patients with back pain, 4% will have a compression fracture, 3% spondylolisthesis, 0.7% spinal malignancy, 0.3% ankylosing spondylitis, and 0.01% spinal infections.[2]

In the current diagnostic evaluation of acute low back pain, 30% have an X-ray and 9.6% have either an MRI or a CT based upon National Hospital Ambulatory Medical Care Survey (NHAMCS) ED data. The use of MRI or CT increased from 3.2% to 9.6% between 2002 and 2006.[13] Others have confirmed these estimates.[14–16] In primary care settings, using MRI as the first-line imaging test for low back pain has failed to improve functional disability, but did result in more surgical interventions and a higher cost of care.[17] Similarly, multiple randomized trials have failed to demonstrate any measurable benefit to immediate imaging in the absence of features suggesting serious problems.[18] Emergency physicians are generally more conservative than primary care physicians in the radiographic evaluation of low back pain.[15,19] Paper-based explicit criteria that emergency physicians review prior to imaging back pain patients have been shown to produce a sustained reduction in inappropriate testing.[20] Electronic decision support systems have also reduced the inappropriate utilization of lumbar MRI.[21]

Following back pain diagnostic guidelines reduces costs and improves outcomes, but clinicians rarely follow these recommendations.[22] Although no emergency medicine guidelines exist for the diagnostic evaluation of acute atraumatic back pain, multiple specialty societies have published guidelines upon which an evidence-based approach can be formulated.[23] In general, the diagnosis being contemplated should guide the initial imaging choice and urgency. "Red flags" generally signal clinicians to expedite advanced imaging considerations, and 22 "red flags" have been identified in various guidelines (Table 56.2).[23] Guidelines for the imaging of

Table 56.2 Red flags and imaging recommendations

Disease	Red flags	Imaging choices
Cauda equina syndrome	Fecal incontinence Gait abnormality Limb weakness Saddle numbness Urinary retention Widespread neuro symptoms	MRI Surgical evaluation
Malignancy	Age > 50 Cancer history Pain at multiple sites Pain at rest Refractory pain Unexplained weight loss Urinary retention	X-ray MRI
Spine fracture	Age ≥50 years Osteoporosis Steroid use Structural deformity	X-ray CT MRI
Spine infection	Fever Immunosuppression Intravenous drug abuse Systemic illness or toxicity	X-ray MRI Blood cultures

Source: Data from [23].

suspected spine fractures sometimes diverge because multidetector CT is the method of choice for bony structures, but MRI is the investigation of choice for the spinal cord and ligaments.[24] The duration of back pain should also be included when deciding whether and when to image patients.[25]

Two key considerations in contemplating test ordering are noteworthy. First, although guidelines are based upon evidence appraisal and expert consensus, they often ignore clinical realities such as malpractice risk and third-party payors' management recommendations.[23] Second, clinicians mistakenly assume that negative or positive diagnostic test results offer reassurance to anxious patients, while the evidence suggests the opposite.[26] In fact, ordering tests that are unlikely to yield diagnoses for which effective therapies exist (such as back pain) can independently increase the duration of symptoms.[27]

Clinical question

What is the diagnostic accuracy of history and physical exam to identify the various etiologies of acute nontraumatic back pain?

Ankylosing spondylitis patients are usually older than 40 years (Table 56.3). Reduced chest expansion (≤ 2.5 cm) has a positive LR of 9. None of the other history-related risk factors have a useful positive or negative LR for ankylosing spondylitis.[28] The only clinically significant positive finding for cancer is a past history of cancer, but the absence of findings does not significantly reduce the probability of malignancy as the etiology of the back pain.[29] Steroid use increases the risk of compression fractures, but again the absence of these risk factors does not significantly reduce the posttest probability.[2] The presence of sciatica significantly increases the risk of a disc herniation and the absence reduces the risk significantly.[30,31] The only physical exam finding that increases the risk of a herniated disc is the single-leg sit-to-stand test in which the patient attempts to rise from a chair using only one leg. This test differentiates an L3–L4 herniation (if unable to perform) from an L5–S1 herniation and has excellent reliability (kappa = 0.85) (Table 56.4).[32] The ipsilateral straight-leg raise may decrease the probability of a lumbar disc herniation, but the negative LR has a wide range across seven studies extending up to 0.54.[33] No other physical exam finding significantly decreases the probability of a disc herniation.[32–35] No high-quality diagnostic research was identified to describe the diagnostic accuracy of physical exam for spinal stenosis, cancer, compression fractures, or ankylosing spondylitis.[2,36]

Table 56.3 Diagnostic accuracy of history for systemic disease etiology of back pain

Disease	Element of history	Positive likelihood ratio (LR+)	Negative likelihood ratio (LR−)
Ankylosing spondylitis	4 of 5 Calin responses positive[1]	1.3	0.94
	Age at onset ≤40	1.1	0
	Pain not relieved when supine	1.6	0.41
	Morning back stiffness	1.6	0.61
	Pain duration >3 months	1.5	0.54
	Reduced chest expansion[2]	9	0.92
Cancer	Age ≥50	2.7	0.32
	Cancer history	15.5	0.70
	Unexplained weight loss	2.5	0.90
	Failure to improve after 1 month of therapy	3.1	0.77
	No relief with bed rest	1.7	0.22
	Duration of pain >1 month	2.6	0.62
	Age ≥50 or history of cancer or unexplained weight loss or failure of conservative therapy	2.5	0
Compression fracture	Age ≥50 years	2.1	0.26
	Age ≥70 years	5.5	0.81
	Corticosteroid use	12	0.94
	Trauma	2	0.82
Herniated disc	Sciatica	7.9	0.06
Spinal stenosis	Age ≥50 years	3	0.14

1. Calin questions were: (i) Onset of back discomfort before age 40 years? (ii) Did the problem begin slowly? (iii) Persistence for at least 3 months? (iv) Morning stiffness? And (v) improved by exercise?
2. Expansion ≤2.5 cm.
Source: Data from [2].

Clinical question

What is the diagnostic accuracy of radiologic imaging for acute nontraumatic back pain?

One systematic review has formally assessed the diagnostic accuracy of common imaging modalities.[37] X-rays are useful in the evaluation of cancer if positive, but lack the accuracy to reduce posttest probability of disease

Table 56.4 Diagnostic accuracy of physical exam for herniation with radiculopathy

Physical exam finding	Positive likelihood ratio (LR+)	Negative likelihood ratio (LR−)
Ankle dorsiflexion weakness	1.2	0.93
Ankle plantar flexion weakness	1.2	0.99
Crossed straight-leg raise	1.6–5.8	0.59–0.90
Great-toe extensor weakness	1.7	0.71
Impaired ankle reflex	1.3	0.83
Ipsilateral straight-leg raise	0.99–2.0	0.04–0.54
Sit-to-stand test	26.0	0.35
Sensory loss	1.0	1.0

Source: Data from [2].

Table 56.5 Diagnostic accuracy of imaging for back pain

Imaging choice	Disease	Positive likelihood ratio (LR+)	Negative likelihood ratio (LR−)
X-ray	Cancer	12–120	0.40–0.42
	Infection	1.9	0.32
	Ankylosing spondylitis	?*	0.55–0.74
Computed tomography	Herniated disc	2.1–6.9	0.11–0.54
	Stenosis	4.5–22	0.10–0.12
Magnetic resonance imaging	Cancer	8.3–31	0.07–0.19
	Infection	12	0.04
	Herniated disc	1.1–33	0–0.93
	Stenosis	3.2	0.10–0.14
Nuclear medicine	Cancer (SPECT)	9.7	0.14
	Infection	4.1	0.13
	Ankylosing spondylitis	?*	0.74

*No value for LR+ has been identified in the existing literature.
Source: Data from [37].

if negative in cancer, infections, or ankylosing spondylitis (Table 56.5). CT is useful in the evaluation of stenosis whether positive or negative, but has a wide range of likelihood ratios for herniated discs. Over half of individuals without back pain will have a herniated disc on MRI, and a wide range of likelihoods have been reported.[38] MRI is quite helpful if positive and particularly if negative in cancer and infection. A negative MRI will significantly reduce the posttest probability of stenosis. Radionuclide scanning (SPECT) can significantly increase or decrease the probability of cancer. Nuclear medicine is less useful than MRI for infections and is not useful for ankylosing spondylitis.

Comment

Back pain is the most common musculoskeletal complaint in ED visits in the United States. Even though back pain has a self-limited natural history in over 90% of patients, clinicians must consider more serious etiologies for each case within the context of the patient's age, comorbid illnesses, psychosocial stressors, potentially occult mechanisms of injury, neurological findings, and symptom duration. Emergency medicine clinical decision aids for the more serious causes of back pain have yet to be developed and validated, so costly imaging procedures that delay ED throughput and are most often inconsequential to patient-centric outcomes must be carefully weighed against initial clinical concern and each test's diagnostic accuracy. Guideline-derived algorithms have been shown to increase the efficiency of back pain test ordering in primary care and emergency settings and currently represent the best approach to reduce variability without compromising patient care.

References

1. Niska R, Bhuiya F, Xu J. National Hospital Ambulatory Medical Care Survey: 2007 emergency department summary. National Health Statistics Reports. 2010(26): 1–31.

2. Deyo RA, Rainville J, Kent DL. What can the medical history and physical examination tell us about low back pain? In: Simel DL, Rennie D, editors. The rational clinical examination:Evidence-based clinical diagnosis. New York: McGraw-Hill; 2009: 75–86.

3. Deyo RA. Early diagnostic evaluation of low back pain. Journal of General Internal Medicine. 1986; 1(5): 328–38.

4. Lederle FA, Simel DL. The rational clinical examination: Does this patient have abdominal aortic aneurysm? Journal of the American Medical Association. 1999; 281(1): 77–82.

5. Shapiro S. Medical realities of cauda equina syndrome secondary to lumbar disc herniation. Spine. 2000; 25(3): 348–51.

6. Small SA, Perron AD, Brady WJ. Orthopedic pitfalls:Cauda equina syndrome. American Journal of Emergency Medicine. 2005; 23(2): 159–63.

7. Jalloh I, Mnihas P. Delays in the treatment of cauda equina syndrome due to its variable clinical features in patients presenting to the emergency department. Emergency Medicine Journal. 2007; 24(1): 33–4.

8. Chou R, Qaseem A, Snow V, Casey D, Cross JT, Shekelle P *et al.* Diagnosis and treatment of low back pain: A joint clinical practice guideline from the American College of Physicians and the American Pain Society. Annals of Internal Medicine. 2007; 147(7): 478–91.

9. Reihsaus E, Waldbaur H, Seeling W. Spinal epidural abscess:A meta-analysis of 915 patients. Neurosurgical Review. 2000; 23(4): 175–204.

10. Angsuwat M, Kavar B, Lowe AJ. Early detection of spinal sepsis. Journal of Clinical Neuroscience. 2009; 17(1): 59–63.

11. Tompkins M, Panuncialman I, Lucas P, Palumbo M. Spinal epidural abscess. Journal of Emergency Medicine. 2010; 39(3): 384–90.

12. Davis DP, Salazar A, Chan TC, Vilke GM. Prospective evaluation of a clinical decision guideline to diagnose spinal epidural abscess in patients who present to the emergency department with spine pain. Journal of Neurosurgery: Spine. 2011; 14(6): 765–70.

13. Friedman BW, Chilstrom M, Bijur PE, Gallagher EJ. Diagnostic testing and treatment of low back pain in United States emergency departments: A national perspective. Spine. 2010; 35(24): E1406–E11.

14. Elam KC, Cherkin DC, Deyo RA. How emergency physicians approach low back pain: Choosing costly options. Journal of Emergency Medicine. 1995; 13(2): 143–50.

15. Weiner AL, MacKenzie RS. Utilization of lumbosacral spine radiographs for the evaluation of low back pain in the emergency department. Journal of Emergency Medicine. 1999; 17(2): 229–33.

16. Isaacs DM, Marinac J, Sun C. Radiograph use in low back pain: A United States emergency department database analysis. Journal of Emergency Medicine. 2004; 26(1): 37–45.

17. Jarvik JG, Hollingworth W, Martin B, Emerson SS, Gray DT, Overman S *et al.* Rapid magnetic resonance imaging vs radiographs for patients with low back pain: A randomized controlled trial. Journal of the American Medical Association. 2003; 289(21): 2810–8.

18. Chou R, Fu R, Carrino JA, Deyo RA. Imaging strategies for low-back pain: Systematic review and meta-analysis. Lancet. 2009; 373(9662): 463–72.

19. Webster BS, Courtney TK, Huang YH, Matz S, Christiani DC. Survey of acute low back pain management by specialty group and practice experience. Journal of Occupational and Environmental Medicine. 2006; 48(7): 723–32.

20. Gallagher EJ, Trotzky SW. Sustained effect of an intervention to limit ordering of emergency department lumbosacral spine films. Journal of Emergency Medicine. 1998; 16(3): 395–401.

21. Blackmore CC, Mecklenburg RS, Kaplan GS. Effectiveness of clinical decision support in controlling inappropriate imaging. Journal of the American College of Radiology. 2011; 8(1): 19–25.

22. Becker A, Leonhardt C, Kochen MM, Keller S, Wegscheider K, Baum E *et al.* Effects of two guideline implementation strategies on patient outcomes in primary care: A cluster randomized controlled trial. Spine. 2008; 33(5): 473–80.

23. Dagenais S, Tricco AC, Haldeman S. Synthesis of recommendations for the assessment and management of low back pain from recent clinical practice guidelines. Spine Journal. 2010; 10(6): 514–29.

24. Roudsari B, Jarvik JG. Lumber spine MRI for low back pain:Indications and yield. American Journal of Roentgenology. 2010; 195(3): 550–9.

25. Negrini S, Giovannoni S, Minozzi S, Barneschi G, Bonaiuti D, Bussotti A *et al.* Diagnostic therapeutic flow-charts for low back pain patients: The Italian clinical guidelines. Europa Medicophysica. 2006; 42(2): 151–70.

26. van Ravesteijn H, van Dijk I, Darmon D, van de Laar F, Lucassen P, olde Harman T *et al.* The reassuring value of diagnostic tests: A systematic review. Patient Education and Counseling. 2012; 86(1): 3–8.

27. Swedish Council on Technology Assessment in Health Care (SBU). Back pain, neck pain: An evidence based review. Stockholm: Swedish Council on Technology Assessment in Health Care; 2000. Report No. 145.

28. Gran JT. An epidemiological survey of the signs and symptoms of ankylosing spondylitis. Clinical Rheumatology. 1985; 4(2): 161–9.

29. Deyo RA, Diehl AK. Cancer as a cause of back pain: Frequency, clinical presentation, and diagnostic strategies. Journal of General Internal Medicine. 1988; 3(3): 230–8.

30. Deyo RA, Tsui-Wu YJ. Descriptive epidemiology of low-back pain and its related medical care in the United States. Spine. 1987; 12(3): 264–8.

31. Spangfort EV. The lumbar disc herniation: A computer-aided analysis of 2,504 operations. Acta Orthopaedica Scandinavica. 1972; 142: 1–95.

32. Rainville J, Jouve C, Finno M, Limke J. Comparison of four tests of quadricepts strength in L3 or L4 radiculopathies. Spine. 2003; 28(21): 2466–71.

33. van den Hoogen HMM, Koes BW, van Eijk JTM, Bouter LM. On the accuracy of history, physical examination, and erythrocyte sedimentation rate in diagnosing low back pain in general practice:A criteria-based review of the literature. Spine. 1995; 20(3): 318–27.

34. Jönsson B, Strömqvist B. Symptoms and signs in degeneration of the lumbar spine: A prospective, consecutive study of 300 operated patients. Journal of Bone and Joint Surgery, British Volume. 1993; 75(3): 381–5.

35. Deville WLJM, van der Windt DAWM, Dzaferagic A, Bezemer PD, Bouter LM. The test of Lasègue:Systematic review of the accuracy in diagnosing herniated discs. Spine. 2000; 25(9): 1140–7.

36. Turner JA, Ersek M, Herron L, Deyo R. Surgery for lumbar spinal stenosis: Attempted meta-analysis of the literature. Spine. 1992; 17(1): 1–8.

37. Jarvik JG, Deyo RA. Diagnostic evaluation of low back pain with emphasis on imaging. Annals of Internal Medicine. 2002; 137(7): 586–97.

38. Jensen MC, Brant-Sawakski MN, Obuchowski N, Modic MT, Malkasian D, Ross JS. Magnetic resonance imaging of the lumbar spine in people without back pain. New England Journal of Medicine. 1994; 331(2): 69–73.

Chapter 57 **Intravascular Volume Status**

Highlights

- Accurately assessing volume status in acutely ill ED patients is an important clinical skill and can impact outcomes.
- No studies have assessed the diagnostic accuracy of history for hypovolemia.
- The only useful finding on physical exam to rule in hypovolemia is an abnormal capillary refill, while the most helpful features to rule out hypovolemia are the absence of a dry mouth or tongue furrows.
- The diagnostic accuracy of laboratory tests has not been evaluated in acutely ill ED patients.
- Bedside tests such as the passive leg raise, ultrasonic cardiac output monitors, and sonographic inferior vena cava diameter are being evaluated as readily available data to predict fluid responsiveness in critically ill patients.

Background

This chapter focuses on the assessment of volume status in adults because the literature on children is vast and not always applicable to older populations.[1] In patients with trauma or other bleeding states, hot weather, congestive heart failure, sepsis, and gastrointestinal loss conditions, volume management decisions are frequently encountered in the emergency department (ED). The optimal fluid management strategy is not always clear and can carry increased morbidity and mortality with either over- or undervolume resuscitation of patients.[2−5] When encountering a hemodynamically unstable patient, it's not always obvious where the patient is on the Starling curve or if the volume issue is one of preload, afterload, cardiac contractility, or none of the above.

Evidence-Based Emergency Care: Diagnostic Testing and Clinical Decision Rules, Second Edition.
Jesse M. Pines, Christopher R. Carpenter, Ali S. Raja and Jeremiah D. Schuur.
© 2013 John Wiley & Sons, Ltd. Published 2013 by John Wiley & Sons, Ltd.

Consequently, only about one-half of hemodynamically unstable, critically ill patients respond to a fluid bolus.[6]

The terminology for volume deficiency conditions can be confusing. Whereas *volume depletion* refers to extracellular space sodium losses, *dehydration* is the loss of intracellular water that increases plasma sodium levels and osmolality.[7] Clinicians and investigators tend to lump these volume state descriptors together as evidenced by the accepted criterion standard of either an elevated serum urea nitrogen-to-creatinine ratio (which measures volume depletion) or an elevated serum sodium or osmolality (which measures dehydration). Hypernatremia occurs predominantly in geriatric adults with intravascular volume depletion and is associated with a 40% mortality rate. Hypernatremia-related deaths are associated with the type and rate of fluid administration as well as the duration of hypotension.[8,9] In this chapter, we will use the term *hypovolemia* to denote the constellation of dehydration and volume depletion.

Physical exam findings for dehydration or volume depletion include assessing postural vital signs (orthostatics), skin turgor, mucous membrane dryness, capillary refill, urine output, and neurological status. One caveat for orthostatic vital signs is that clinicians must wait at least 2 minutes before measuring supine vital signs, and 1 minute after standing before measuring upright vital signs. Sitting vital signs are far less accurate than standing ones. Also, counting the pulse for 30 seconds is more accurate than for 15 seconds.[10] Capillary refill time is assessed by gently pressing the fingernail of the patient's middle finger while it is positioned at the same level as the heart for 5 seconds before releasing and noting the time required for the nailbed's normal color to return (normally 3 seconds for adults and 4 seconds for the elderly). Skin turgor describes the skin's ability to return to its normal position after being pinched between the examiner's fingers and is a function of elastin-related recoil. No studies on normal recoil times have been identified, but skin turgor decreases (i.e., there is a greater time to return to normal skin position) with age as elastin levels are reduced.

Investigators have evaluated the diagnostic accuracy of postural vital signs following acute blood loss in healthy volunteers following experimental phlebotomy, but with the exception of young otherwise healthy patients with hemorrhage, these lab trials are not applicable to the usual course of events, associated illness or injury, or patient populations routinely evaluated in ED settings.[7] In summary, these studies suggest that a postural pulse change from lying to standing of ≥30 or severe postural dizziness has 97% sensitivity and 98% specificity for a large blood loss. whereas postural hypotension (>20 mm Hg systolic decrease) or supine tachycardia or hypotension are insensitive tests.[7]

Clinical question

In adult patients presenting to the ED with vomiting, diarrhea, or decreased oral intake, what is the diagnostic accuracy of physical exam for hypovolemia?

Three ED-based studies have reported the diagnostic test characteristics for physical exam (Table 57.1).[11–13] Schriger et al evaluated 32 ED patients with suspected hypovolemia (and frank hypotension or abnormal orthostatic vital signs, mean age 44 years) and 47 volunteer blood donors to assess capillary refill, excluding those on cardiovascular medications. The criterion standard for hypovolemia in the "suspected hypovolemia" subset is not clearly stated in their manuscript. The likelihood ratios for "abnormal capillary refill time" reported in Table 57.1 are in reference to the age- and sex-specific upper limits of normal for capillary refill.[11] Gross et al evaluated 55 patients older than 60 years presenting to one of two academic EDs with suspected dehydration to assess 38 signs and symptoms. As their criterion standard, they used a nonvalidated Physician Dehydration Rating Scale that relied upon gestalt, vital signs, serum sodium, osmolality, and urea creatinine.[12] Johnson et al assessed 23 pregnant patients in the ED because of hyperemesis gravidarum to assess the diagnostic accuracy of postural vital signs. Their inclusion criteria were a positive β-hCG, $\leq$16-week gestation by dates, and either a urine-specific gravity $\geq$1.025 or a urine ketone $\geq$40 mg/dL. They used percentage dehydration via pre- and posthydration body weight as the criterion standard for hypovolemia.[13] Eaton et al conducted a fourth non-ED-based study of geriatric adults assessing axillary sweating in 100

Table 57.1 Diagnostic accuracy of physical exam in ED patients to identify hypovolemia not due to blood loss

Finding	Positive likelihood ratio (LR+)	Negative likelihood ratio (LR−)
Orthostatic pulse change >30	1.7	0.8
Orthostatic systolic BP change >20 mm Hg	1.5	0.9
Dry axilla	2.8	0.6
Dry mouth	2.0	0.3 (0.1–0.6)
Longitudinal tongue furrows	2.0	0.3 (0.1–0.6)
Sunken eyes	3.4	0.5
Confusion	2.1	0.6
Extremity weakness	2.3	0.7
Speech not clear	3.1	0.5
Abnormal capillary refill time	6.9 (range 3.2–15)	0.7

Source: Data from [11–13].

consecutive patients admitted to the medicine service (mean age 80 years). Axillary sweating was assessed within 24 hours of admission by applying pre-weighed tissue paper to the right axilla for 15 minutes with the arm held adducted. The tissue paper was then re-weighed. The criterion standard for hypovolemia was a serum urea:creatinine ratio over 1:10 and a plasma osmolality above 295 mmol/kg.[14]

Abnormal capillary refill is the only physical exam finding to significantly increase the posttest probability of hypovolemia. The absence of tongue furrows or a dry mouth are the only physical exam findings to significantly decrease the probability of hypovolemia. Combinations of physical exam findings have not been reported. One study of critically ill patients developed and internally validated a simple decision rule to predict circulating blood volume, but the rule did not follow established standards for developing a clinical decision rule (see Chapter 4), has not been validated, and was derived on intensive care unit patients, limiting its applicability in the ED.[15] No high-quality studies have evaluated the accuracy of history in the diagnosis of hypovolemia.

Clinical question

In adult patients presenting to the ED with suspected hypovolemia not caused by blood loss, what is the diagnostic accuracy of lab testing?

Although serum urea nitrogen, sodium, and osmolality have been used as the criterion standard for hypovolemia in the highest quality diagnostic accuracy trials, the accuracy of these labs has not been evaluated in healthy or acutely ill populations. Elevated urine-specific gravity ($\geq$1.020) has also been used as a component of the criterion standard for hypovolemia in several studies. Bartok evaluated the diagnostic accuracy of urine-specific gravity in 25 male collegiate wrestlers using weight-based dehydration as the criterion standard. The laboratory-based urine-specific gravity $\geq$1.020 had 96% sensitivity and 96% specificity, while the dipstick technique had 87% sensitivity and 91% specificity.[16] The diagnostic accuracy of urine-specific gravity has not been assessed in acutely ill ED patients.

Clinical question

In adult patients with hemodynamic instability and uncertain volume status, what is the diagnostic accuracy of emergency physician–performed ultrasound or other bedside tests to predict volume resuscitation responsiveness?

Passive leg raising has been assessed as a rapid fluid-loading mimic that is simple and reversible.[17,18] Biais et al evaluated 34 spontaneously breathing

Table 57.2 Diagnostic accuracy of bedside tests to predict volume responsiveness

Bedside test	Positive likelihood ratio (LR+)	Negative likelihood ratio (LR−)
Passive leg raise echo stroke volume increase ≥ 13%		
Biais (2009)	5.0	0.00
Thiel (2009)	11.6	0.20
Passive leg raise Flotrac stroke volume increase ≥ 16%	8.5	0.17

Source: Data from [17,18].

patients with transthoracic echocardiography stroke volume and Vigileo (FloTrac) stroke volume measurements after passive leg raising in a semi-recumbent position. Increases of echocardiography stroke volume ≥13% or Flotrac stroke volume ≥16% during passive leg raising were sensitive and specific to predict volume expansion.[17] (See Table 57.2.) Thiel et al evaluated the transthoracic ultrasound change in stroke volume following a fluid challenge to assess passive leg raise in intensive care unit patients requiring volume expansion. A change in the passive leg raise stroke volume by ≥15% was predictive of volume responsiveness.[18] Other potential bedside tests for emergency physicians have been described, but their accuracy and reliability have not been systematically assessed. The most promising such tests include ultrasonic cardiac output monitors and the inferior vena cava diameter.[6,19–21]

Comment

Accurate assessment of volume responsiveness in any clinical setting is a challenge, but in the ED this challenge is magnified by incomplete histories and short evaluation times. Understanding the limitations of history and physical exam is key to safe, efficient volume resuscitation. Unfortunately, the diagnostic accuracy of history has not been studied, and very few elements of the physical exam are helpful to increase or decrease the probability of hypovolemia. High-quality diagnostic trials are needed to determine the accuracy and reliability of history and physical exam in isolation and in various combinations for ED patients with suspected hypovolemia. Additionally, these ED-based diagnostic trials should assess subsets of hypovolemia patients including blood loss hypovolemia, gastrointestinal loss hypovolemia, and critical illness–related hypovolemia to ascertain their reliability, diagnostic accuracy, and volume-responsiveness prognostic potential. To do so, researchers will need to establish a valid criterion standard for hypovolemia and assess the accuracy of clinical gestalt. No clinical decision rule for hypovolemia risk currently exists, but such an aid would be particularly useful in ED subsets at increased risk for adverse outcomes if the assessment of volume status results in the wrong therapy (fluids for the volume-overloaded patient or fluid restriction for the hypovolemia patient). The most helpful elements of physical exam to rule in hypovolemia include an abnormal capillary refill time, sunken eyes, and a dry axilla, while the absence of a dry mouth is the most useful finding to exclude hypovolemia.

References

1. Steiner MJ, DeWalt DA, Byerley JS. Is this child dehydrated? Journal of the American Medical Association. 2004; 291(22): 2746–54.
2. Bandstrup B, Tønnesen H, Beier-Holgersen R, Hjortsø E, Ørding H, Lindorff-Larsen K et al. Effects of intravenous fluid restriction on postoperative complications: Comparison of two perioperative fluid regimens: A randomized assessor-blinded multicenter trial. Annals of Surgery. 2003; 238(5): 641–8.
3. Vincent JL, Sakr Y, Sprung CL, Ranieri VM, Reinhart K, Gerlach H et al. Sepsis in European intensive care units: Results of the SOAP study. Critical Care Medicine. 2006; 34(2): 344–53.
4. Wiedemann HP, Wheeler AP, Bernard GR, Thompson BT, Hayden D, deBoisblanc B et al. Comparison of two fluid-management strategies in acute lung injury. New England Journal of Medicine. 2006; 354(24): 2564–75.
5. Wheeler AP, Bernard GR, Thompson BT, Schoenfeld D, Wiedemann HP, deBoisblanc B et al. Pulmonary-artery versus central venous catheter to guide treatment of acute lung injury. New England Journal of Medicine. 2006; 354(21): 2213–24.
6. Michard F, Teboul JL. Predicting fluid responsiveness in ICU patients: A critical analysis of the evidence. Chest. 2002; 121(6): 2000–8.
7. McGee S, Abernethy WB, Simel DL. Is this adult patient hypovolemic? In: Simel DL, Rennie D, editors. The rational clinical examination. New York: McGraw-Hill; 2009: 315–27.
8. Snyder NA, Feigal DW, Arieff AI. Hypernatremia in elderly patients: A heterogeneous, morbid, and iatrogenic entity. Annals of Internal Medicine. 1987; 107(3): 309–19.
9. Mandal AK, Saklayen MG, Hillman NM, Markert RJ. Predictive factors for high mortality in hypernatremic patients. American Journal of Emergency Medicine. 1997; 15(2): 130–2.
10. Hollerbach AD, Sneed NV. Accuracy of radial pulse assessment by length of counting interval. Heart Lung. 1990; 19(3): 258–64.
11. Schriger DL, Baraff LJ. Capillary refill: Is it a useful predictor of hypovolemic states? Annals of Emergency Medicine. 1991; 20(6): 601–5.

12. Gross Cr, Lindquist RD, Woolley AC, Granieri R, Allard K, Webster B. Clinical indicators of dehydration severity in elderly patients. Journal of Emergency Medicine. 1992; 10(3): 267–74.
13. Johnson DR, Douglas D, Hauswald M, Tandberg D. Dehydration and orthostatic vital signs in women with hyperemesis gravidarum. Academic Emergency Medicine. 1995; 2(8): 692–7.
14. Eaton D, Bannister P, Mulley GP, Connolly MJ. Axillary sweating in clinical assessment of dehydration in ill elderly patients. British Medical Journal. 1994; 308(6939): 1271.
15. Stéphan F, Flahault A, Dieudonné N, Hollande J, Paillard F, Bonnet F. Clinical evaluation of circulating blood volume in critically ill patients: Contribution of a clinical scoring system. British Journal of Anaesthesiology. 2001; 86(6): 754–62.
16. Bartok C, Schoeller DA, Sullivan JC, Clark RR, Landry GL. Hydration testing in collegiate wrestlers undergoing hypertonic dehydration. Medicine and Science in Sports and Exercise. 2004; 36(3): 510–7.
17. Biais M, Vidil L, Sarrabay P, Cottenceau V, Revel P, Sztark F. Changes in stroke volume induced by passive leg raising in spontaneously breathing patients: Comparison between echocardiography and Vigileo/FloTrac device. Critical Care. 2009; 13(6): R195.
18. Thiel SW, Kollef MH, Isakow W. Non-invasive stroke volume measurement and passive leg raising predict volume responsiveness in medical ICU patients: An observational cohort study. Critical Care. 2009; 13(4): R111.
19. Barbier C, Loubières Y, Schmit C, Hayon J, Ricôme JL, Jardin F et al. Respiratory changes in inferior vena cava diameter are helpful in predicting fluid responsiveness in ventilated septic patients. Intensive Care Medicine. 2004; 30(9): 1740–6.
20. Dey I, Sprivulis P. Emergency physicians can reliably assess emergency department patient cardiac output using the USCOM continuous wave Doppler cardiac output monitor. Emergency Medicine Australasia. 2005; 17(3): 193–9.
21. Schefold JC, Storm C, Bercker S, Pschowski R, Oppert M, Krüger A et al. Inferior vena cava diameter correlates with invasive hemodynamic measures in mechanically ventilated intensive care unit patients with sepsis. Journal of Emergency Medicine. 2010; 38(5): 623–37.

Chapter 58 **Geriatric Syndromes**

Highlights

- Cognitive dysfunction is present in 30–40% of community-dwelling geriatric patients in the emergency department, but is usually not detected by clinicians without focused screening efforts.
- Few brief screening instruments for dementia or delirium have been evaluated in ED settings.
- The Short Blessed Test or the Brief Alzheimer's Screen can significantly reduce the probability of dementia, but neither can significantly increase the probability of dementia.
- Although the Confusion Assessment Method (CAM) requires validation in ED settings, the physician-administered CAM can accurately rule in or rule out the diagnosis of delirium.
- Falls studies have not reported the diagnostic accuracy of individual or aggregate risk factors in ED populations, but past falls and cognitive dysfunction appear to be strongly associated with future falls among elders in the ED.

Background

Worldwide, the proportion of emergency department (ED) visits by geriatric adults is growing – the symptom of an aging society benefiting from vast improvements in public health and medical science over the last century.[1–3] The current utilization rate is 50 ED visits per year for every 100 persons over the age of 65 years in the United States, and the fastest growing segment of the population is the "oldest old" – those aged 85 years and older. Geriatric patients present to the ED with atypical disease manifestations and often undiagnosed complicating comorbidities like dementia or delirium that can prolong their length of stay, overall ED resource consumption, and admission

Evidence-Based Emergency Care: Diagnostic Testing and Clinical Decision Rules, Second Edition. Jesse M. Pines, Christopher R. Carpenter, Ali S. Raja and Jeremiah D. Schuur.
© 2013 John Wiley & Sons, Ltd. Published 2013 by John Wiley & Sons, Ltd.

rates.[4,5] The prevalent comorbidities that contribute to the aging phenotype have been labeled as *geriatric syndromes*, and include incontinence, falls, delirium, dementia, frailty, functional decline, and polypharmacy.[6] Although ED clinical problem solving has not traditionally incorporated the geriatric care model, as society ages, emergency physicians will be expected to identify and initiate management of prevalent geriatric syndromes.[7,8]

The term *cognitive dysfunction* incorporates mild cognitive impairment, delirium, and dementia into one descriptor, and aligns well with the clinical description that an ED physician may elicit on a brief first-time encounter with a patient. If systematically screened, up to 42% of geriatric ED patients have some degree of cognitive dysfunction.[9–13] ED physicians miss the majority of cognitive dysfunction presenting to the ED.[9,14] The medical cost of these disorders is significant with the worldwide cost of dementia estimated at $422 billion in 2009 and delirium-related expenses costing $152 billion annually.[15,16] In addition, cognitive dysfunction in geriatric ED patients is associated with accelerated functional decline or short-term readmissions,[17–19] falls,[20] impaired driving safety,[21] lower patient satisfaction,[22] and lower caregiver quality of life.[23]

Dementia is a neurodegenerative process, and Alzheimer's disease, which is the most common cause of dementia, will afflict 1 in 85 individuals by the year 2050.[24] Other causes of dementia include strokes, Parkinson's disease, and head injuries.[25] Mild cognitive impairment is characterized by memory or language problems that do not interfere with daily activities but can be detected by certain screening tests.[26] The prevalence and optimal screening instruments for mild cognitive impairment in the ED have not yet been evaluated.

Delirium is a transient disorder of cognitive capabilities that is a symptom of an acute illness or toxic exposure. The *Diagnostic and Statistical Manual of Mental Disorders* (DSM) criteria to establish a diagnosis of delirium require the documentation of a fluctuating disturbance in consciousness and change in cognition developing over time and caused by an acute physiological stressor.[27] This is in direct contradistinction with dementia, which has a gradual onset over months to years with no component of altered consciousness or inattention. Although delirium can be detected in 8–30% of ED patients, up to 87% of the time it is not recognized by emergency clinicians.[14,28,29] The ED identification of delirium is considered a quality indicator with optimal screening and management strategies that are the topic of ongoing multidisciplinary research.[30,31] Delirium accelerates Alzheimer's-related cognitive decline,[32] increases hospital length of stay,[33] and is associated with increased mortality.[34] Delirium also impedes effective patient–physician communication in the ED.[35] Hypoactive delirium predominates in the ED, representing 92% of cases.[29] The Confusion Assessment Method (CAM) is the most frequently evaluated screening instrument for delirium, but like the MMSE the CAM has never been formally validated in ED settings.[36,37]

Falls are the leading cause of trauma-related mortality in older adults, and the rate of injurious falls is outpacing the rapidly expanding geriatric demographic.[38] Currently, about one-third of individuals over the age of 65 fall each year, and up to 15% fall more than once during that timeframe.[20] Screening for geriatric fall risk has been advocated in all clinical settings as a secondary preventative intervention.[39] One multidisciplinary ED-based secondary falls prevention intervention demonstrated a 20% absolute risk reduction in falls at 1 year, but others have not replicated this success.[40,41] Fall risks differ between subgroups of patients including nursing home versus community-dwelling individuals, as well as inpatients versus outpatients. To be effective, all ED-based falls prevention programs require willing and compliant patients, multidisciplinary professional teams with reliable and continual communication streams, and dependable follow-up across socioeconomic strata.[42] However, the first barrier to overcome is identifying individuals at highest risk of falling and most likely to benefit from ED interventions to reduce injurious falls.[31]

Clinical question

In geriatric ED patients at risk for cognitive dysfunction, what are the most accurate brief dementia screening instruments?

For the immediate diagnosis of dementia, the Mini Mental State Examination (MMSE) is the most extensively evaluated tool in research settings, but is too lengthy for routine ED use and has not been formally validated in the ED.[43–45] The MMSE is particularly inaccurate in identifying mild cognitive impairment with a sensitivity as low as 18%.[46] In addition, the MMSE has unacceptably high false-positive rates in poorly educated and lower socioeconomics subgroups.[47,48]

One systematic review noted that 25 screening instruments have been evaluated in 29 studies, but none were ED-based analyses.[44] Four trials have evaluated the diagnostic accuracy of brief (<1 minute) instruments that do not require any special equipment to administer in ED settings, using an MMSE ≤23 as the criterion standard (Table 58.1).[10–12,49] The Six-Item Screener (SIS) was inferior to the Short Blessed Test (SBT; Figure 58.1) and the Brief Alzheimer's Screen (BAS; Figure 58.2) for exclusion of dementia. None of the screening instruments is sufficiently accurate to rule in the

Table 58.1 Diagnostic test characteristics of the Short Blessed
Test (SBT), Brief Alzheimer's Screen (BAS), Six-Item Screener
(SIS), and Caregiver-Completed AD8 (cAD8)

Test	Positive likelihood ratio (LR+)	Negative likelihood ratio (LR−)
SBT	2.7	0.08
BAS	2.0	0.10
SIS	3.3	0.33
cAD8	2.2	0.27
SBT+cAD8*	1.2	0.32
BAS+cAD8**	1.1	0.27
SIS+cAD8***	3.0	0.16

*Abnormal SBT or abnormal cAD8.
**Abnormal BAS or abnormal cAD8.
****Abnormal SIS or abnormal cAD8.
Source: Data from [11].

diagnosis of dementia, but the SBT and BAS can significantly reduce the
probability that an individual patient has dementia. Although the caregiver-
administered AD8 (Figure 58.3) was inferior to the SIS, it had the advantage
that it does not rely upon a conscious or cooperative patient in assessing the
functional impact of cognitive decline from the perspective of a close family
member. The SBT and BAS also identified all cases of delirium.[11]

Clinical question

*In geriatric ED patients at risk for cognitive dysfunction, what are the diagnostic
test characteristics of bedside delirium screening instruments?*
One systematic review evaluated 25 studies that included over 3,000
subjects with delirium prevalence ranging from 9% to 63% while evaluating 11 bedside delirium instruments.[37] Among these 11 instruments,
only four instruments demonstrated useful positive and negative likelihood ratios (LR+ and LR−, respectively) *and* could be administered
in less than 5 minutes: the CAM, Delirium Observation Screening Scale
(DOSS), Global Attentiveness Rating (GAR), and Nursing Delirium Screening Scale (Nu-DESC; see Table 58.2). None of the instruments had been
explicitly evaluated in ED settings. Although the geriatrician-administered
GAR demonstrated superb accuracy in a single trial, the CAM had several
advantages over the other instruments including simplicity (Figure 58.4),
enhanced external validity (most often studied in a variety of settings),
and excellent diagnostic accuracy. The CAM had a summary LR+ of
7.3 (CI 1.9–27) and a summary LR− of 0.08 (CI 0.01–0.38) when

Instructions to the patient: Now I would like to ask you some questions to check your memory and concentration. Some of them may be easy and some of them may be hard.

	Correct	**Incorrect**
1) What year is it now?	0	1
2) What month is this?	0	1

Please repeat this name and address after me:
      John Brown, 42 Market Street, Chicago
      John Brown, 42 Market Street, Chicago
      John Brown, 42 Market Street, Chicago
      (Underline words repeated correctly in each trial.)
      Trials to learn _____ (if unable to do in 3 trials = C)

3) Without looking at your watch or clock, tell me what time it is. (If response is vague, prompt for specific response within 1 hour.)

	Correct	**Incorrect**
	0	1

4) Count aloud backward from 20 to 1. (Mark correctly sequenced numerals – if subject starts counting forward or forgets the task, repeat instructions and score one error.)

                                               0 1 2 Errors

20 19 18 17 16 15 14 13 12 11 10 9 8 7 6 5 4 3 2 1

5) Say the months of the year in reverse order. If the tester needs to prompt with the last name of the month of the year, one error should be scored – mark correctly sequenced months.

D N O S A JL JN MY AP MR F J   **0 1 2 Errors**

6) Repeat the name and address you were asked to remember.

(John Brown, 42 Market Street, Chicago)   **0 1 2 3 4 5 Errors**
_____, _____, ____, _____, _____

Item	Errors	Weighting Factor	Final Item Score
1		× 4	
2		× 3	
3		× 3	
4		× 2	
5		× 2	
6		× 2	

Sum total (range 0–28) =
0–4 = Normal cognition
5–9 = Questionable impairment
≥ 10 = Impairment consistent with dementia

Figure 58.1 Short Blessed Test.

Instructions to the patient: I would like to ask you some questions that ask you to use your memory. I am going to name three objects. Please wait until I say all three words, then repeat them. Remember what they are because I am going to ask you to name them again in a few minutes. Please repeat these words for me: APPLE – TABLE – PENNY. (May repeat names three times if necessary; repetition not scored.)

Did the patient correctly repeat all three words?   **YES**   **NO**

1) What is the date? (D)   **Correct   Incorrect**

2) Name as many animals as you can in 30 seconds. (A) _____ (number)

3) Spell "world" backwards. (S)   Number correct
                                                   0   1   2   3   4   5

4) Three-item recall (R)   Number correct
                                                   0   1   2   3

Brief Alzheimer's Screen = $(3.03 \times R) + (0.67 \times A) = (4.75 \times D) + (2.01 \times S)$

BAS ≤ 26 is consistent with dementia.

Figure 58.2 Brief Alzheimer's Screen.

If the patient has an accompanying reliable informant, the informant is asked the following questions: Has this patient displayed any of the following issues? Remember that a "Yes" response indicates that you think there has been **a change in the last several years** caused by thinking and memory (cognitive) problems.

1) Problems with judgment (for example, falls for scams, bad financial decisions, or buys gifts inappropriate for recipients)?

2) Reduced interest in hobbies or activities?

3) Repeats questions, stories, or statements?

4) Trouble learning how to use a tool, appliance, or gadget (VCR, computer, microwave, or remote control)?

5) Forgets correct month or year?

6) Difficulty handling complicated financial affairs (for example, balancing checkbook, income taxes, or paying bills)?

7) Difficulty remembering appointments?

8) Consistent problems with thinking and/or memory?

Each affirmative response is one point. A score of ≥ 2 is considered high risk for cognitive impairment.

Figure 58.3 AD8.

Table 58.2 Summary diagnostic test characteristics of brief delirium screening instruments

Test	Number of trials	Positive likelihood ratio (LR+)	Negative likelihood ratio (LR−)
Confusion Assessment Method (CAM)	12	9.6	0.16
Delirium Observation Screening Scale (DOSS)	2	5.2	0.10
Global Attentiveness Rating (GAR) <7	1	65	0.06
Mini Mental Status Exam (MMSE) <24	1	1.6	0.12
Nursing Delirium Screening Scale (Nu-DESC) >0	1	3.1	0.06

Source: Data from [37].

performed by nurses. Alternatively, when the CAM is administered by physicians the summary LR+ is 65 (CI 9.3–458) and the summary LR− is 0.06 (CI 0.01–0.38).

Clinical question

In geriatric ED patients who have suffered a standing-level fall, which features of the history and physical exam most accurately predict future falls?

Two studies have evaluated fall risk factors in ED patients.[50,51] Close et al identified the following independent risk factors for 1-year falls following ED evaluation for a fall: previous falls (OR 1.5), indoor falls (OR 2.4), inability to

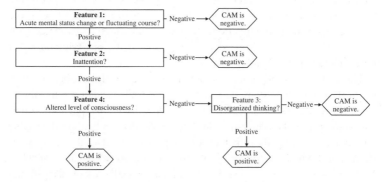

Figure 58.4 The Confusion Assessment Method.

Table 58.3 One-year risk factors for ≥1 falls

Risk factor	Positive likelihood ratio (LR+)	Negative likelihood ratio (LR−)
Dementia	17	0.99
Fall last 1 month	3.8	0.84
Fall last 1 year	2.8	0.86
≥5 errors on Short Portable Mental Status Questionnaire (SPMSQ)*	4.2	0.88
≥4 days in bed last 1 month	3.7	0.94
Medications*	27	0.88
Parkinson's	5.0	0.98
Residual stroke findings**	15	0.91
Unable to rise from chair***	4.3	0.77

*Benzodiazepine, phenothiazine, or antidepressant.
**In women.
***In men, without using arms.
Source: Data from [20].

rise after a fall (OR 5.5), moderate alcohol consumption (OR 0.6), abnormal mental status (OR 0.7), and hospital admission for the index fall (OR 0.3).[50] Carpenter et al enrolled geriatric ED patients who had not suffered a fall with 6-month follow-up identifying the following fall risk factors: nonhealing foot sore (HR 3.7), past falls (HR 2.6), inability to cut own toenails (HR 2.0), and self-reported depression (HR 1.7). The incidence of falls at 6 months was 39%, ranging from 4% of individuals with no risk factor to 42% of those with all four risk factors.[51] Of note, neither ED study demonstrated the ability for functional tests such as the Get Up and Go test to predict future falls. These prospective studies evaluated a variety of functional tests at the bedside, but none of the functional tests were subsequently associated with fall risk. Neither study reported sensitivity, specificity, or likelihood ratios for individual or aggregate risk factors.

The accuracy of individual risk factors has been well described in other medical settings. A systematic review of nine trials yielded the likelihood ratios noted in Table 58.3.[20] Medications (benzodiazepines, phenothiazines, and antidepressants), dementia, and old stroke deficits that are detectable on physical exam significantly increase the probability of a fall within 1 year. Dementia also increases the probability of two or more falls over 1 year (LR+ 13, CI 2.3–79). No risk factors significantly decrease the risk of falls with the lowest LR− (0.8).

Comment

Brief screening instruments for dementia have been validated in ED settings to significantly reduce the probability of dementia, but they cannot accurately rule in the diagnosis. Monette et al has been referenced as an ED validation of the CAM, but this trial did not have an emergency nurse or physician CAM validated by an independent specialist diagnosis using DSM criteria, so it was not included in this review and might not be considered a true validation trial.[52] Similarly, the Confusion Assessment Method for the Intensive Care Unit (CAM–ICU) has been used as a criterion standard for delirium in prior ED research, but has not yet been validated in this setting.[29,34,35,53] One approach to incorporate this compilation of cognitive dysfunction screening instruments in case finding for dementia and delirium is proposed in Figure 58.5. The optimal systems design defining who should conduct

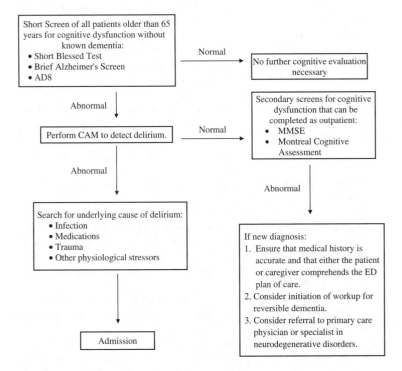

Figure 58.5 Diagnostic algorithm to detect occult cognitive dysfunction.

this screening in busy ED settings, when during the course of ED care the screening should occur, and how abnormal screening results should influence emergency clinician management and decision making remains largely undefined.

Accurately assessing fall risk in geriatric ED patients remains a challenge. Certain medications, dementia, Parkinson's disease, and past falls are associated with increased fall risk in geriatric outpatients. Medications that increase the risk of falls include benzodiazepines and phenothiazines.

References

1. Chu K, Brown A, Pillay R. Older patients' utilisation of emergency department resources: A cross-sectional study. Australian Health Review. 2001; 24(3): 44–52.

2. Downing A, Wilson R. Older people's use of accident and emergency services. Age and Ageing. 2005; 34(1): 24–30.

3. Roberts DC, Mckay MP, Shaffer A. Increasing rates of emergency department visits for elderly patients in the United States, 1993 to 2003. Annals of Emergency Medicine. 2008 51(6): 769–74.

4. Singal B, Hedges J, Rousseau E, Sanders A, Berstein E, Mcnamara R *et al.* Geriatric patient emergency visits. Part I: Comparison of visits by geriatric and younger patients. Annals of Emergency Medicine. 1992; 21(7): 802–7.

5. Aminzadeh F, Dalziel W. Older adults in the emergency department: A systematic review of patterns of use, adverse outcomes, and effectiveness of interventions. Annals of Emergency Medicine. 2002; 39(3): 238–47.

6. Inouye SK, Studenski S, Tinetti ME, Kuchel GA. Geriatric syndromes: Clinical, research, and policy implications of a core geriatric concept. Journal of the American Geriatric Society. 2007; 55(5): 780–91.

7. Hwang U, Morrison RS. The geriatric emergency department. Journal of the American Geriatric Society. 2007; 55(11): 1873–6.

8. Hogan T, Losman E, Carpenter C, Sauvigne K, Irmiter C, Emanuel L *et al.* Development of geriatric competencies for emergency medicine residents using an expert consensus process. Academic Emergency Medicine. 2010; 17(3): 316–24.

9. Hustey FM, Meldon SW. The prevalence and documentation of impaired mental status in elderly emergency department patients. Annals of Emergency Medicine. 2002; 39(3): 248–53.

10. Wilber ST, Carpenter CR, Hustey FM. The Six-Item Screener to detect cognitive impairment in older emergency department patients. Academic Emergency Medicine. 2008; 15(7): 613–6.

11. Carpenter CR, Bassett ER, Fischer GM, Shirshekan J, Galvin JE, Morris JC. Four sensitive screening tools to detect cognitive impairment in geriatric emergency department patients: Brief Alzheimer's screen, Short Blessed Test, Ottawa3DY, and the Caregiver Administered AD8. Academic Emergency Medicine. 2011 18(4): 374–84.

12. Carpenter CR, Despain B, Keeling TK, Shah M, Rothenberger M. The Six-Item Screener and AD8 for the detection of cognitive impairment in geriatric emergency department patients. Annals of Emergency Medicine. 2011; 57(6): 653–61.

13. Hirschman KB, Paik HH, Pines JM, Mccusker CM, Naylor MD, Hollander JE. Cognitive impairment among older adults in the emergency department. Western Journal of Emergency Medicine. 2011; 12(1): 56–62.

14. Elie M, Rousseau F, Cole M, Primeau F, Mccusker J, Bellavance F. Prevalence and detection of delirium in elderly emergency department patients. Canadian Medical Association Journal. 2000; 163(8): 977–81.

15. Wimo A, Winblad B, Jonsson L. The worldwide societal costs of dementia: Estimates for 2009. Alzheimers& Dementia. 2010; 6(2): 98–103.

16. Leslie DL, Marcantonio ER, Zhang Y, Leo-Summers L, Inouye SK. One-year health care costs associated with delirium in the elderly population. Archives of Internal Medicine. 2008; 168(1): 27–32.

17. Mccusker J, Bellavance F, Cardin S, Trepanier S, Verdon J, Ardman O. Detection of older people at increased risk of adverse health outcomes after an emergency visit: The ISAR screening tool. Journal of the American Geriatric Society. 1999; 47(10): 1229–37.

18. Runciman P, Currie CT, Nicol M, Green L, Mckay V. Discharge of elderly people from an accident and emergency department: Evaluation of health visitor follow-up. Journal of Advanced Nursing. 1996; 24(4): 711–8.

19. Meldon S, Mion L, Palmer R, Drew B, Connor J, Lewicki L et al. A brief risk-stratification tool to predict repeat emergency department visits and hospitalizations in older patients discharged from the emergency department. Academic Emergency Medicine. 2003; 10: 224–32.

20. Ganz DA, Bao Y, Shekelle PG, Rubenstein LZ. Will my patient fall? Journal of the American Medical Association. 2007; 297(1): 77–86.

21. Carr DB. Commentary: The role of the emergency physician in older driver safety. Annals of Emergency Medicine. 2004; 43(6): 747–8.

22. Nerney MP, Chin MH, Jin L, Karrison TG, Walter J, Mulliken R et al. Factors associated with older patients' satisfaction with care in an inner-city emergency department. Annals of Emergency Medicine. 2001; 32(2): 140–5.

23. Banerjee S, Samsi K, Petrie CD, Alvir J, Treglia M, Schwam EM et al. What do we know about quality of life in dementia? A review of the emerging evidence on the predictive and explanatory value of disease specific measures of health related quality of life in people with dementia. International Journal of Geriatric Psychiatry. 2009; 24(1): 15–24.

24. Brookmeyer R, Johnson E, Ziegler-Graham K, Arrighi HM. Forecasting the global burden of Alzheimer's disease. Alzheimer &Dementia. 2007; 3(3): 186–91.

25. Kawas C. Early Alzheimer's disease. New England Journal of Medicine. 2003; 349(11): 1056–63.

26. Morris JC. Mild cognitive impairment is early-stage Alzheimer disease: Time to revise diagnostic criteria. Archives of Neurology. 2006; 63(1): 15–6.

27. American Psychiatric Association. Diagnostic and statistical manual of mental disorders. 4th ed., text revision. Washington (DC): American Psychiatric Association; 2000.

28. Lewis L, Miller D, Morley J, Nork M, Lasater L. Unrecognized delirium in ED geriatric patients. American Journal of Emergency Medicine. 1995; 13(2): 142–5.

29. Han J, Zimmerman E, Cutler N, Schnelle J, Morandi A, Dittus R *et al.* Delirium in older emergency department patients: Recognition, risk factors, and psychomotor subtypes. Academic Emergency Medicine. 2009; 16(3): 193–200.

30. Terrell K, Hustey F, Hwang U, Gerson L, Wenger N. Quality indicators for geriatric emergency care. Academic Emergency Medicine. 2009 16(5): 441–9.

31. Carpenter C, Shah M, Hustey F, Heard K, Miller D. High yield research opportunities in geriatric emergency medicine research: Prehospital care, delirium, adverse drug events, and falls. Journal of Gerontology: Medical Sciences. 2011; 66(7): 775–83.

32. Fong TG, Jones RN, Shi P, Marcantonio ER, Yap L, Rudolph JL *et al.* Delirium accelerates cognitive decline in Alzheimer disease. Neurology. 2009; 72(18): 1570–5.

33. Saravay SM, Kaplowitz M, Kurek J, Zemen D, Pollack S, Novik S *et al.* How do delirium and dementia increase length of stay of elderly general medical inpatients? Psychosomatics. 2004; 45(3): 235–42.

34. Han JH, Shintani A, Eden S, Morandi A, Solberg LM, Schnelle J *et al.* Delirium in the emergency department: An independent predictor of death within 6 months. Annals of Emergency Medicine. 2010; 56(3): 244–52.

35. Han JH, Bryce SN, Ely EW, Kripalani S, Morandi A, Shintani A *et al.* The effect of cognitive impairment on the accuracy of the presenting complaint and discharge instruction comprehension in older emergency department patients. Annals of Emergency Medicine. 2011; 57(6): 662–71.

36. Inouye SK, Van Dyck CH, Alessi CA, Balkin S, Siegal AP, Horwitz RI. Clarifying confusion: The confusion assessment method: A new method for detection of delirium. Annals of Internal Medicine. 1990; 113(12): 941–8.

37. Wong CL, J. H-L Simel DL, Straus SE. Does this patient have delirium? Value of bedside instruments. Journal of the American Medical Association. 2010; 304(7): 779–86.

38. Kannus P, Parkkari J, Koskinen S. Fall-induced injuries and deaths among older adults. Journal of the American Medical Association. 1999; 281: 1895–9.

39. Panel on Prevention of Falls in Older Persons. Summary of the updated American Geriatrics Society/British Geriatrics Society clinical practice guideline for prevention of falls in older persons. Journal of the American Geriatric Society. 2011; 59(1): 148–57.

40. Close J, Ellis M, Hooper R, Glucksman E, Jackson S, Swift C. Prevention of falls in the elderly trial (PROFET): A randomised controlled trial. Lancet. 1999; 353(9147): 93–7.

41. Gates S, Lamb SE, Fisher JD, Cooke MW, Carter YH. Multifactorial assessment and targeted intervention for preventing falls and injuries among older people in

community and emergency care settings: A systematic review and meta-analysis. British Medical Journal. 2008; 336: 130–3.

42. Ganz DA, Alkema GE, Wu S. It takes a village to prevent falls: Reconceptualizing fall prevention and management for older adults. Injury Prevention. 2008; 14: 266–71.

43. Folstein MF, Folstein SE, Mchugh PR. Mini-Mental State: A practical method for grading the cognitive state of patients for the clinician. Journal of Psychiatric Research. 1975; 12(3): 189–98.

44. Holsinger T, Deveau J, Boustani M, Williams JW. Does this patient have dementia? Journal of the American Medical Association. 2007; 297(21): 2391–404.

45. Carpenter CR. Does this patient have dementia? Annals of Emergency Medicine. 2008; 52(5): 554–6.

46. Nasreddine ZS, Phillips NA, Bédirian V, Charbonneau S, Whitehead V, Collin I et al. The Montreal Cognitive Assessment, Moca: A brief screening tool for mild cognitive impairment. Journal of the American Geriatric Society. 2005; 53(4): 695–9.

47. Ihl R, Frolich L, Dierks T, Martin EM, Maurer K. Differential validity of psychometric tests in dementia of the Alzheimer type. Psychiatry Research. 1992; 44(4): 93–106.

48. Scazufca M, Almeida OP, Vallada HP, Tasse WA, Menezes PR. Limitations of the Mini-Mental State Examination for screening dementia in a community with low socioeconomic status: Results from the Sao Paulo Ageing & Health Study. European Archives of Psychiatry and Clinical Neuroscience. 2009; 259(1): 8–15.

49. Wilber S, Lofgren S, Mager T, Blanda M, Gerson L. An evaluation of two screening tools for cognitive impairment in older emergency department patients. Academic Emergency Medicine. 2005; 12: 612–6.

50. Close J, Hooper R, Glucksman E, Jackson S, Swift C. Predictors of falls in a high risk population: Results from the Prevention of Falls in the Elderly Trial (Profet). Emergency Medicine Journal. 2003; 20(5): 421–5.

51. Carpenter CR, Scheatzle MD, D'Antonio JA, Ricci PT, Coben JH. Identification of fall risk factors in older adult emergency department patients. Academic Emergency Medicine. 2009; 16(3): 211–9.

52. Monette J, Galbaud Du Fort G, Fung SH, Massoud F, Moride Y, Arsenault L et al. Evaluation of the Confusion Assessment Method (CAM) as a screening tool for delirium in the emergency room. General Hospital Psychiatry. 2001; 23(1): 20–5.

53. Ely EW, Inouye SK, Bernard GR, Gordon S, Francis J, May L et al. Delirium in mechanically ventilated patients: Validity and reliability of the Confusion Assessment Method for the Intensive Care Unit (CAM-ICU). Journal of the American Medical Association. 2001; 286(21): 2703–10.

Index

Page numbers in *italics* refer to Figures; those in **bold** to Tables.

Evidence-Based Emergency Care: Diagnostic Testing and Clinical Decision Rules, Second Edition.
Jesse M. Pines, Christopher R. Carpenter, Ali S. Raja and Jeremiah D. Schuur.
© 2013 John Wiley & Sons, Ltd. Published 2013 by John Wiley & Sons, Ltd.